Bifurcation Stenting

Bifurcation Stenting

EDITED BY

Ron Waksman, MD, FACC

Washington Hospital Center, Washington, DC, USA and
Georgetown University School of Medicine, Washington,
DC, USA

And

John A. Ormiston, MBChB FRACP, FRANZCR, FRCP, FACC, ONZM

Mercy Angiography, Mercy Hospital, Auckland, New Zealand

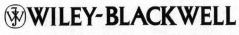

A John Wiley & Sons, Ltd., Publication

Library of Congress Cataloging-in-Publication Data

Bifurcation stenting / edited by Ron Waksman and John A. Ormiston.
     p. ; cm.
  Includes bibliographical references and index.
  ISBN 978-1-4443-3462-3 (cloth)
 1. Stents (Surgery) 2. Coronary heart disease–Surgery. I. Waksman, Ron. II. Ormiston, John A.
  [DNLM: 1. Coronary Disease–surgery. 2. Stents. 3. Cardiac Surgical Procedures. 4. Coronary Angiography. WG 300]
  RD598.35.S73B54 2012
  617.4'12–dc23

                                   2011018729

A catalogue record for this book is available from the British Library.

Set in 9.5/12pt Minion by Thomson Digital, Noida, India.
Printed and bound in Malaysia by Vivar Printing Sdn Bhd

1 2012

Contents

Contributors

Alexandre Abizaid, MD, PhD
Chief of Coronary Interventions
Instituto Dante Pazzanese de Cardiologia
Chairman, Cardiovascular Research Center
São Paulo, SP, Brazil
Visiting Professor of Medicine
Columbia University Medical Center
New York, NY, USA

Pierfrancesco Agostoni, MD, PhD
University Medical Center Utrecht
Department of Interventional Cardiology
Utrecht, The Netherlands

Remo Albiero, MD
Director Cardiac Cath Lab
Emodinamica, Istituto Clinico San Rocco
Ome (Brescia), Italy

Giombattista Barrano, MD
Postgraduate School of Cardiology
University of Catania
Catania, Italy

Anouar Belkacemi, MD
University Medical Center Utrecht
Department of Interventional Cardiology
Utrecht, The Netherlands

Hiram G. Bezerra, MD, PhD
Assistant Professor
Medical Director Cardiovascular Imaging Core Laboratories
Case Western Reserve University
University Hospitals Case Medical Center
Cleveland, OH, USA

Gary Binyamin, PhD
Director of Science and Technology
TriReme Medical, Inc.
Pleasanton, CA, USA

Katrin Boeke-Purkis, BSc, CCIR
Abbott Vascular
Santa Clara, USA

Marco A. Costa, MD, PhD, FACC, FSCAI
Professor of Medicine
Director, Interventional Cardiovascular Center
Director, Center for Research and Innovation
Harrington-McLaughlin Heart and Vascular Institute
University Hospitals, Case Western Reserve University
Cleveland, OH, USA

Ricardo A. Costa, MD
Department of Interventional Cardiology
Instituto Dante Pazzanese de Cardiologia
Director, Angiographic Core Laboratory
Cardiovascular Research Center
São Paulo, SP, Brazil

Luca Costanzo, MD
Postgraduate School of Cardiology
University of Catania
Catania, Italy

Frederic de Vroey, MD
Cardiac Investigation Unit
Auckland City Hospital
Auckland, New Zealand

Alfredo R. Galassi, MD, FACC, FESC, FSCAI
Associate Professor of Cardiology
Postgraduate School of Cardiology
Head of the Catheterization Laboratory and Cardiovascular
Interventional Unit
Clinical Division of Cardiology
Ferrarotto Hospital
University of Catania
Catania, Italy

Eberhard Grube, MD
Professor of Cardiology
University of Bonn
Departement of Medicine II
Bonn, Germany

Juan Luis Gutiérrez-Chico, MD, PhD, FESC
Erasmus Medisch Centrum, Thoraxcentrum
Interventional Cardiology Department
Rotterdam, The Netherlands

Niels R. Holm, MD
Research Fellow
Department of Cardiology
Aarhus University Hospital, Skejby
Aarhus, Denmark

Gary M. Idelchik, MD
Division of Interventional Cardiology
Scottsdale Healthcare Hospitals
Scottsdale, AZ, USA

Soo-Jin Kang, MD, PhD
Assistant Professor of Medicine
Asan Medical Center
Seoul, Korea

Young-Hak Kim, MD, PhD
Associate Professor of Internal Medicine
University of Ulsan College of Medicine
Asan Medical Center
Seoul, Korea

Pieter H. Kitslaar, MSc
Department of Cardiology
Leiden University Medical Center
Leiden, The Netherlands

Eitan Konstantino, PhD
Chief Executive Officer
TriReme Medical, Inc.
Pleasanton, CA, USA

Alexandra J. Lansky, MD
Associate Professor, Cardiovascular Medicine
Director, Yale Cardiovascular Research Group
Co-Director, Valve Program
Yale University School of Medicine
New Haven, CT, USA

Jens Flensted Lassen, MD, PhD, FESC
Associate Professor of Cardiology
Consultant, Invasive Cardiology
Department of Cardiology B
Aarhus University Hospital, Skejby
Aarhus, Denmark

Thierry Lefèvre, MD, FESC, FSCAI
Director of the Cardiac Catheterization
Department at Institut Cardiovasculaire Paris Sud
Hôpital Privé Jacques Cartier, Massy
France

Victor Legrand, MD, PhD, FESC, FACC
Professor of Clinical Medicine
University of Liège, Liège, Belgium

Director of Centre Intégré d'Interventions
Transluminales
CHU de Liège, Liège, Belgium

Jurgen Ligthart, BSc
Department of Cardiology
Erasmus Medisch Centrum, Thoraxcentrum
Rotterdam, The Netherlands

Li Hui-Ling, MD, PhD
Department of Cardiology
Erasmus Medisch Centrum, Thoraxcentrum
Rotterdam, The Netherlands

Yves Louvard, MD, FSCAI
Institut Cardiovasculaire Paris Sud,
Massy, France

Michael Maeng, MD, PhD
Department of Cardiology
Aarhus University Hospital, Skejby
Aarhus, Denmark

Michael Mahmoudi, MD, PhD
Division of Cardiology
Washington Hospital Center
Washington, DC, USA

Vivian G. Ng, MD
Columbia University Medical Center
New York, NY, USA

John A. Ormiston, MBChB
Mercy Angiography
Auckland, New Zealand

Seung-Jung Park, MD, PhD
Professor of Internal Medicine
University of Ulsan College of Medicine
Asan Medical Center
Seoul, Korea

Evelyn Regar, MD, PhD, FESC
Associate Professor
Interventional Cardiology Department
Erasmus Medisch Centrum, Thoraxcentrum
Rotterdam, The Netherlands

Johan H.C. Reiber, PhD
Department of Cardiology
Leiden University Medical Center
Leiden, The Netherlands

David G. Rizik, MD, FACC, FSCAI
Director of the Division of Heart & Vascular Medicine
Scottsdale Healthcare Hospitals
Scottsdale, AZ, USA

Patrick W. Serruys, MD, PhD, FESC, FACC
Erasmus Medisch Centrum, Thoraxcentrum
Interventional Cardiology Department
Rotterdam, The Netherlands

Samin K. Sharma, MD, FACC
Professor of Medicine Cardiology
Catheterization Laboratory of the Cardiovascular Institute
Mount Sinai Hospital
New York, USA

John E. Shulze, BSEE, MBA
Chief Technical Officer
Biosensors International
Morges, Switzerland

Oana Sorop, PhD
Department of Cardiology
Erasmus Medisch Centrum, Thoraxcentrum
Rotterdam, The Netherlands

Pieter R. Stella, MD, PhD
Professor of Cardiology
Medical University Ho Chi Minh (VN)
Associate Professor of Cardiology, UMCU
Director Heart Catheterization Laboratories, UMCU
Director Clinical Cardiovascular Research, UMCU
University Medical Centre Utrecht
The Netherlands

Joseph M. Sweeny, MD
Assistant Professor of Medicine Cardiology
Catheterization Laboratory of the Cardiovascular Institute
Mount Sinai Hospital
New York, USA

Satoko Tahara, MD, PhD
Research fellow
Cardiovascular Imaging Core Laboratories
University Hospitals Case Medical Center
Harrington-McLaughlin Heart & Vascular Institute
Cleveland, OH, USA

Leif Thuesen, MD, DMSci
Director PCI Research Unit
Department of Cardiology
Aarhus University Hospital, Skejby
Denmark

Salvatore Davide Tomasello, MD, PhD
Department of Cardiology
Morriggia-Pelascini Hospital, Italia Hospital Gravedona,
Como, Italy

Brett Trauthen, MS
Chief Scientific Officer
Devax Inc.
Irvine, CA, USA

Heleen M.M. van Beusekom, PhD
Department of Cardiology
Erasmus Medisch Centrum, Thoraxcentrum
Rotterdam, The Netherlands

Willem J. van der Giessen, MD, PhD
Professor of Cardiology
Erasmus Medisch Centrum, Thoraxcentrum
Rotterdam
Interuniversity Cardiology Institute of the Netherlands
ICIN-KNAW
The Netherlands

Robert Jan M. van Geuns, MD, PhD, FESC
Associate Professor of Cardiology
Erasmus Medisch Centrum, Thoraxcentrum
Interventional Cardiology Department
Rotterdam, The Netherlands

Stefan Verheye, MD, PhD
Interventional Cardiology
Antwerp Cardiovascular Center
ZNA Middelheim
Antwerp, Belgium

Michiel Voskuil, MD, PhD
University Medical Center Utrecht,
Department of Interventional Cardiology
Utrecht, The Netherlands

Ron Waksman, MD
Division of Cardiology
Washington Hospital Center
Washington, DC, USA

Bruce Webber, MHSc
Mercy Angiography
Auckland, New Zealand

Mark Webster, MBChB
Mercy Angiography
Auckland, New Zealand

Foreword

Marie-Claude Morice, MD

Institut Cardiovasculiare Paris Sud, Hôpital Privé Jacques Cartier, Massy, France

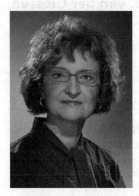

The coronary arteries can be compared to tree trunks in that they produce branches: it would, therefore, be preposterous to treat a trunk without taking into account its branches.

The coronary network is a succession of bifurcations branching off into gradually narrower segments in an uneven pattern.

For a long time, the percutaneous treatment of diseased coronary bifurcations was voluntarily left aside because most interventional cardiologists were daunted by the anticipated inherent complexity of the procedures. Indeed, the tubular configuration and constant diameters of balloon-catheters and stents seemed to preclude any successful attempt at tackling and efficiently navigating the coronary bifurcation anatomy.

However, in view of the significant incidence of coronary bifurcation disease documented in 15–20% of patients undergoing PCI and with the support of increasingly enhanced technology, several teams gradually decided to overcome this obstacle and work towards a better understanding of the flow pattern, anatomical variations and physical principles governing coronary bifurcations. They endeavored to put into perspective the intricacies of bifurcation anatomy and the pattern of atheroma build-up in branching coronary segments.

Their efforts resulted in classifications of bifurcation types and potential customized treatments.

Increasingly subtle, refined and complex techniques were devised in order to adapt our tubular stents to diseased vessel segments with a proximal diameter larger than their distal extremity, and to access branches from the middle of tubular stents.

Of the multiple strategies suggested by diligent and very imaginative minds, experience showed that the implantation of a single stent was associated with a better outcome in lesions amenable to this strategy. This is why provisional stenting has become the standard treatment.

Several dedicated stents were designed by creative engineers but very few of these devices made their way from bench to bedside. The ones that did are presented here.

All specificities and technical strategies implemented in the treatment of the most important of all coronary bifurcations, the left main, are thoroughly addressed in this book.

Each chapter is written by the most prominent expert in the subject involved.

This impressive collaborative work provides an exhaustive account of all potential issues and concerns that may be raised by the treatment of coronary bifurcations.

There is no doubt that the reader will find here an invaluable source of information, which is based on the experience of seasoned specialists who share their findings with the interventional cardiology community in order to provide state-of-the-art therapeutic approaches and optimal care to our patients.

Acknowledgements

Chapter 2

The authors thank Catherine Dupic for assistance in manuscript preparation.

Chapter 3

Participating centres (Nordic-Baltic Bifurcation Studies I-III):

Finland: Oulu University Hospital, Tampere University Hospital, Turku University Hospital, Kajaani Central Hospital, Rovaniemi Central Hospital, Kemi Central Hospital, Kuopio University Hospital, Helsinki University, Hospital, Satakunta Central Hospital, Pori
Denmark: Aarhus University Hospital, Skejby, Odense University Hospital, Aalborg University Hospital, Gentofte University Hospital, Rigshospitalet, Copenhagen
Sweden: Örebro Central Hospital, Falun Hospital, Uppsala University Hospital
Norway: The Feiring Clinic, Feiring, University Hospital of Tromsoe, Oslo University Hospital, Rikshospitalet, Ullevaal University Hospital, Oslo, St. Olav Hospital, Trondheim, Haukeland University Hospital, Bergen
Latvia: Paul Stradins Clinical Hospital, Riga

Chapter 14

The work for this chapter was supported by a grant from Abbott Vascular Inc.

Chapter 17

The author would like to thank Mark Paquin for his time and contribution in preparing this chapter.

CHAPTER 1

Classification of coronary artery bifurcation lesions

Victor Legrand, MD, PhD, FACC, FESC

Centre Intégré d'Interventions Transluminales, CHU de Liège, Liège, Belgium

Bifurcation lesions constitute 12–15% of the lesions treated with percutaneous coronary intervention (PCI) [1–3]. They represent a distinct lesion subset associated with an increased risk of procedure-related complications and were recognized early in the development of PCI [3,4]. Consequently, this stenosis morphology was considered to represent a moderately increased risk (type B) if side branches were protectable by a guidewire and high risk (type C) if they could not be protected, in the AHA/ACC Task Force classification [5].

Technical improvements, including development of dedicated stents and the use of drug-eluting stents, together with better medical management and treatment strategy have considerably reduced the risk of acute complications, restenosis and late stent thrombosis [6]. These advances were gained mostly from clinical experience, which showed that the likelihood of side branch occlusion depends on the relative position of the plaque to the bifurcation and whether the side branch originates from the primary lesion in the main vessel, as well as its degree of angulations [7]. These observations underlined the need for a comprehensive classification scheme to guide the treatment strategy. Classification of coronary artery bifurcation lesions is also of paramount importance to permit accurate comparisons of techniques, results and outcomes in homogeneous lesion groups.

A fundamental challenge in assessing bifurcation is to consider simultaneously lesion length and

severity of the main vessel and the side branch, knowing that both vessels are not in the same plane and that angulations must be viewed in a three-dimensional space. Additionally, some morphologic considerations may be added, including the extent of calcification, the presence of coronary ectasia and irregularities, plaque ulceration and thrombus [8,9]. Therefore, it is not surprising that many classifications have been proposed to describe this complex anatomical subset. Moreover, these inherent lesion complexity and imaging challenges also represent pitfalls and limitations for conventional quantitative angiographic analysis.

In order to guide interventional cardiologists, we reviewed the coronary artery bifurcation classifications that have been proposed and the challenges for a representative design of a coronary bifurcation. To achieve consistency in the reporting of bifurcation analyses we propose a simple comprehensive and universal approach that could help to better select a particular technique and define the risks of PCI.

Coronary bifurcation classifications

According to American College of Cardiology/American Heart Association (ACC/AHA) task force classification [5] a bifurcation lesion is "a lesion located in a bifurcation point with a side branch >2 mm in diameter". The lesion

Bifurcation Stenting, First Edition. Edited by Ron Waksman and John A. Ormiston.
© 2012 Blackwell Publishing Ltd. Published 2012 by Blackwell Publishing Ltd.

being defined as >50% diameter stenosis in the proximal and/or distal parent vessel and/or a >50% diameter stenosis in the ostium of the contiguous side branch. A less restrictive definition could be "any lesion located in a bifurcation point". Conversely, a more clinically oriented definition could be a "lesion located in a bifurcation point with a side branch that you don't want to lose". The position of a contiguous stenosis, relative to the bifurcation point is important. Should it be within the 2 mm of the bifurcation point or is a bifurcation lesion any side branch covered by an inflated balloon or covered by a stent? Differences in interpretation of these basic definitions may have important implications in treatment strategy and results as well as in comparisons between different studies and registries.

In order to clarify the definition of a coronary artery bifurcation lesion, the European Bifurcation Club proposed that a bifurcation lesion is "a coronary artery narrowing occurring adjacent to, and/or involving, the origin of a significant side branch". A significant side branch is a branch that you do not want to lose in the global context of a particular patient (symptoms, location of ischemia, viability, collateralizing vessel, left ventricular function, and so forth) [8]. Treatment of the bifurcation also implies balloon inflation or stent coverage above the ostium of the side branch. Using this definition, the clinical viewpoint is preponderant. It corresponds to what is the most relevant for the patient regardless of the size of the vessel and taking into consideration the physiological role of the side branch rather than its anatomical feature.

Classification of bifurcation lesions have been attempted since 1994. Since then, six major classification systems have been proposed [1,10–14]. A schematic representation of the published classification systems is given on Figure 1.1. Some of these classifications were proposed before the advent of stents and drug-eluting stents [10,11]. These early classifications were not adapted for the

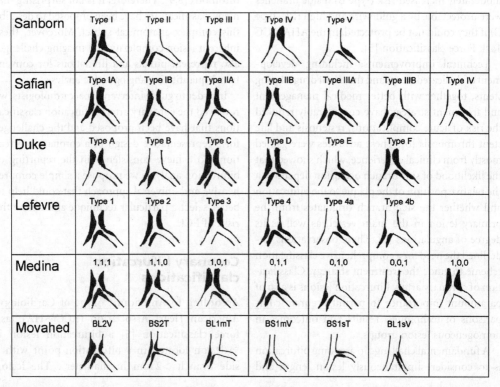

Figure 1.1 Schematic representation of reported classifications of bifurcation lesions according to their morphology. Lefevre classification also takes into consideration side branch angulations (Y- or T-shape). Description of Mohaved classification is given in the text.

contemporary interventional techniques and their rationale was based on results achieved using balloon only, thus not taking into consideration the use of stent(s) and newer treatment strategies such as kissing or crushing. With the use of stent(s), it appeared soon that not only localization of the plaque, but also angulations between branches had an impact on the results and hence may influence the technique used [1,12–14]. All classification systems are based on the presence or absence of a stenosis in each of the three segments that constitute the bifurcation: the main branch proximal to the bifurcation, the main branch distal to the bifurcation and the side branch.

The Sanborn classification [10] describes five types of lesions, it omits situations where the stenosis involves proximal and distal main branch without involvement of side branch, as well as situations without distal main branch stenosis. Balloon dilatation of these lesions usually yielded similar results of non bifurcated lesions, indeed. No description of the bifurcation angle is proposed.

The Safian classification [11] addresses all the possible combinations. Risk of complications or failure is greater in type I lesions followed by type II lesions. Treatment of type III and IV lesions leads to excellent outcomes indistinguishable from low-risk procedures.

The Duke classification [12] is similar to the Safian classification. Lesions involving simultaneously distal main branch and side branch are not described, however. Like the Sanborn and Safian schemes, it ignores the bifurcation angle. This classification first considers stenoses without ostial side branch narrowing (lesions involving the main vessel only: type A, B or C). Lesions involving the side branch are referred to as type D, E or F.

The Lefevre classification [1] considers lesions involving a side branch ≥2.2 mm and take into consideration angulations of the bifurcation as well as the location of the plaque. T-shape lesions refer to bifurcation angle >70°, these lesions are generally perfectly treated using T-stenting, when needed. Conversely, in Y-shape lesions (<70° angle), the risk of a snow-plow effect seems higher and treatment strategy is usually more complex. Types 1, 2 and 4 lesions are similar to Sanborn type I and III, Safian type IA, IB and IIIA and Duke type D, C

classifications. These lesions carry the highest risk of side branch occlusion after stent implantation, particularly when angulations is <70°. In a series of 366 patients treated with stenting, in-hospital major adverse cardiac events were noted respectively in 4.0%, 4.5% and 4.2% of type 1, type 2 and type 4 lesions, versus 2.7% in type 3 and 0% in types 4 A,B lesions [1].

The Medina classification [13] takes the advantage to be the simplest to memorize, even though it provides all the information contained in the others. It consists in recording any narrowing ≥50% in each of the three arterial segments of the bifurcation in the following order: proximal main vessel, distal main vessel and side branch. Presence of a narrowing is coded 1 and absence of a significant stenosis 0. These three figures are separated by commas. This straightforward classification doesn't mentioned bifurcation angle. It has been suggested that the Medina classification should also contain information on lesion length, especially for the side branch, or presence of calcification, in addition to angulations (Y- or T-shape). However, adding these variables would negate the simplicity of the Medina classification. The only parameter that is currently being debated is the lesion length in the side branch, which could have a significant impact on the technique used [6].

A different classification scheme was proposed by Movahed [14] in an attempt to propose a simple algorithm for lesion-specific techniques [15]. The lesion classification begins with the prefix B (for bifurcation) to which four suffixes are added to obtain the final description of the lesion. The first suffix deals with the characteristics of the proximal segment: C = close to bifurcation, N = non-significant side branch, S = small proximal segment, L = large proximal segment (defined as more than two-thirds of the sum of diameters of both branch vessels). The second suffix describes the involvement of bifurcation branches: 1M = only main branch ostium diseased, 1S = only side branch ostium diseased, 2 = both main and side branch ostia diseased. The third suffix describes the angulations of the bifurcation: V = angle <70°, T = angle ≥70°. If the lesion is heavily calcified or involves the left main, a fourth suffix can be added: CA = calcified, LM = left main involvement. Lack of consensus regarding the (evolving) treatment

Table 1.1 Medina class frequency of occurrence

	(1,1,1)	(1,1,0)	(0,1,0)	(0,1,1)	(1,0,0)	(1,0,1)	(0,0,1)
BBC-ONE trial [16]	299(60.0)	45 (9.0)	15 (3.0)	67 (13.5)	24 (4.8)	45 (9.0)	3 (0.6)
Frangos et al. [17]	33 (29.0)	6 (5.3)	26 (22.8)	12 (10.5)	21 (18.4)	8 (7.0)	8 (7.0)
Collins et al. [18]	243 (60.9)	28 (7.0)	52 (13.0)	33 (8.3)	38 (9.5)	n/a	5 (1.2)
Enrico et al. [19]	34 (17.3)	79 (40.3)	45 (23.0)	0 (0.0)	26 (13.3)	1 (0.5)	11 (5.6)
Van Mieghem et al. [20]	5 (10.9)	8 (17.4)	8 (17.4)	2 (4.3)	10 (21.7)	8 (17.4)	5 (10.9)
Total, n (%)	614 (48.6)	166 (13.1)	146 (11.6)	124 (9.8)	119 (9.4)	62 (4.9)	32 (2.5)

strategy of bifurcation lesions limits the widespread utilization of this classification.

Following the second European Bifurcation Club meeting, a consensus emerged to recommend the Medina classification as the "gold standard". Despite limitations underlined above, this binary classification is easy to memorize and to implement in general practice as well as in case record forms. Adding information on angulations, lesion length on side branch, presence of calcification, TIMI flow and vessel size would give a complete description and may be valuable for specific clinical evaluations. For current routine practice and registries, the Medina classification takes advantage to be easily understood and applied by all interventional cardiologists, however.

In some situations, it is not easy to distinguish between the distal main vessel and the side branch when both vessels have the same diameter. The choice may be subjective, but we consider that the side branch is the vessel with the shortest lesion as in most bifurcation stenosis, side branch lesion length is usually short.

Clinical relevance of bifurcation lesion type

Based on recent trials, the five most common Medina classes were (1,1,1), (1,1,0), (0,1,0), (0,1,1) and (1,0,0). These five patterns account for more than 90% of the bifurcations (Table 1.1).

Some bifurcation patterns carry a high risk of snow plow effect or plaque shift. The term "true bifurcation", introduced for many years, refers to lesion types associated with the highest risk of acute complications. These are lesions involving both the main vessel and the side branch. Treatment of theses bifurcation lesions often needs complex

Table 1.2 "Complex" or "true" bifurcation lesions according to classifications systems

System			
Medina	1,1,1	1,0,1	0,1,1
Duke	Type D	Type F	absent
Lefevre	Type 1	absent	Type 4
Safian	Type IA	Type IIA	Type IIIA
Sanborn	Type I	absent	Type III
Movahed	BL(S)2V(T)	BL(S)2V(T)	BL(S)2V(T)

stenting strategies with use of two or more stents, and/or dedicated stents. Based on Table 1.1, "true" bifurcation lesions account for 63% of bifurcated lesions. The definition of "complex" or "true" bifurcation according to the different classifications is given in Table 1.2 (see also Figure 1.1).

Side branch occlusion which was initially thought to be related to plaque shift is mostly related to carina shift. Recent MDCT [21] and IVUS [22] studies have reported that the carina was almost always spared of plaque growth, whereas plaque burden was almost always being present in the proximal vessel. Recognizing that the carina is free of plaque has major implications on interpretation of lesion classification and stenting technique.

Angiographic description and quantification of bifurcation lesions

Classification of coronary bifurcation lesions based on visual evaluation offers the advantage of simplicity, but lacks precision in terms of vessels sizes, angulations and lesion dimensions. These limitations may be overcome by angiographic quantification. Quantitative coronary angiography (QCA) of single lesions is often used to objectively evaluate lesions type and severity. However, because of the fractal nature of coronary bifurcations, lesion shape and complex three-dimensional geometry, QCA assessment of coronary bifurcation lesions is problematic.

Using standard QCA systems, the bifurcation main vessel is considered as a single segment with a single reference diameter function assuming progressive vessel tapering. This is not in line with the fractal geometry and the structure-function scaling laws that govern a coronary tree [23]. It has been shown, indeed, that the coronary tree is an object of fractal geometry governs by the Murray's law [24]. Therefore, the relation between the proximal main vessel (PMV), the distal main vessel (DMV) and side branch (SB) is governed by the following equation: $PMV = 0.67(DMV + SB)$. Current available QCA systems do not use this formula, which leads to an underestimation of the true dimensions of the proximal main vessel or to an underestimation of plaque burden.

Another fundamental challenge in QCA assessment of bifurcations is in acquiring the entire bifurcation lesion without significant foreshortening, geometrical distortion or vessel/side branch overlap. Because of its complex geometry, bifurcation lesion should be assessed in the two best single views. Identification of the projection which displays the widest bifurcation angle is important. Because the PMV is not always in the same plane as the DMV or the SB, this parameter is highly dependent on image acquisition.

Beside reference diameters and vessels angulations and other important morphologic considerations include lesion length on each segment, ostial SB location, extent of coronary calcification, presence of coronary ectasia and irregularity, plaque ulceration, presence of thrombus and flow characteristics, all of which have been shown to have prognostic significance in procedural and long-term outcomes [25,26].

Based on the above mentioned considerations and recommendations of the European Bifurcation Group [9], QCA software with specific algorithm dedicated for bifurcation analysis are currently developed and validated (CAAS 5 Pie Medical Bifurcation Imaging, Maastricht, the Netherlands). Use of dedicated QCA software together with a standard angiographic report of bifurcation analysis will soon provide an objective tool to describe a specific lesion classification and will help to determine treatment strategy as well as to evaluate procedural results. In addition to the visual assessment of lesions morphology, dedicated QCA software should now be recommended for future trials and device comparisons.

Conclusions

Percutaneous coronary angioplasty of coronary artery bifurcation lesions was soon recognized to be associated with an increased risk of procedure-related complications and recurrent ischemia. This observation lead to the development of lesion type classifications, aiming to identify the riskier situations as well as to select the most effective treatment strategy. Since the end of the 1990s, technical evolution of percutaneous techniques and regular use of drug-eluting stents in these situations have dramatically improved both immediate and late results. As such, the role of a classification code is to describe, in a simple and easily understandable manner, the lesions' characteristics in order to allow comparisons between trials and techniques used. Consequently, the Medina classification is now accepted as the universal scheme for the visual assessment of coronary bifurcation lesions. Adding information on angulations and lesion length in the side branch could further improve the information, however.

This classification does not replace QCA measurements, which remain indispensable for an accurate evaluation of plaque morphology and vessels' dimensions. Recent advances and standardization in angiographic analysis software will allow an even more comprehensive assessment of this complex anatomic subset.

References

1 Lefèvre T, Louvard Y, Morice MC, Dumas P, Loubetre C, Benslimane A, Premchand RK, Guillard N, Piéchaud JF. Stenting of bifurcation lesions: Classification, treatment and results. Cathet Cardiovasc Intervent 2000; 49:274–83.

2 Thomas M, Hildick-Smith D, Louvard Y, Albiero R, Darremeont O, Stankovic G, Pan M, Legrand V, De Bruyne B, Lefèvre T. Percutaneous coronary intervention for bifurcation disease. A consensus view from the first meeting of the European Bifurcation Club. EuroInterv 2006;2:149–53.

3 Meier B, Gruentzig AR, King S.B. 3rd, Douglas JS Jr, Hollman J, Ischinger T, Aueron F, Galan K. Risk of side branch occlusion during coronary angioplasty. Am J Cardiol 1984;53:10–14.

4 Al Suwaidi J, Berger PB, Rihal CS, Garratt KN, Bell MR, Ting HH, Bresnahn JF, Grill DE, Holmes Jr. DR. Immediate and long term outcome of intracoronary stent implantation for true bifurcation lesions. J Am Coll Cardiol 2000;35:929–36.

5 Ryan TJ, Faxon DP, Gunnar R.M. *et al.* Guidelines for percutaneous transluminal angioplasty: a report of the American College of Cardiology/American Heart Association Task Force on Assessment of Diagnostic and Therapeutic Cardiovascular Procedures (Subcommittee on Percutaneous Transluminal Angioplasty). Circulation 1998;78:486–502.

6 Stankovic G, Darremont O, Ferenc M, Hildick-Smith D, Lassen JF, Louvard Y, Albiero R, Pan M, Lefèvre T. Percutaneous coronary intervention for bifurcation lesions: 2008 consensus document from the fourth meeting of the European Bifurcation Club. EuroInterv 2009; 5:39–49.

7 Legrand V, Thomas M, Zelisko M, De Bruyne B, reifart N, Steigen T, Hildick-Smith D, Albiero R, Darremont O, Stankovic G, Pan M, Lassen JF, Louvard Y, Lefèvre T. Percutaneous coronary intervention of bifurcation lesions: state-of-the-art. Insights from the second meeting of the European Bifurcation Club. EuroInterv 2007; 3:44–9.

8 Louvard Y, Thomas M, Dzavik V, Hildick-Smith D, Galassi AR, Pan M, Burzotta F, Zelizko M, Dudek D, Ludman P, Sheiban I, Lassen JF, Darremont O, Kastrati A, Ludwig J, Iakovou I, Brunel P, Lansky A, Meerkin D, Legrand V, Brunel P, Medina A, Lefèvre T. Classification of coronary artery bifurcation lesions and treatments: Time for a consensus! Catheter Cardiovasc Interv 2008; 71:175–83.

9 Lansky A, Tuinenburg J, Costa M, Maeng M, Koning G, Popma J, Cristea E, Gavit L, Costa R, Rares A, Van Es GA, Lefevre T, Reiber H, Louvard Y, Morice MC. Quantitative angiographic methods for bifurcation lesions: A consensus statement from the European Bifurcation Group. Catheter Cardiovasc Interv 2009;73:258–66.

10 Spokojny AM, Sanborn TM. Stategic approaches in coronary intervention. Baltimore, MD, Williams and Wilkins, 1996: 288.

11 Popma JJ, Leon MB, Topol EJ. Atlas of interventional cardiology. Philadelphia, PA, W.B. Saunders, 1994: 77.

12 Freed M, Grines C, Safian RD. Bifurcation stenosis. In Freed M, Grines C, Safian RD,eds. The New Manual of interventional Cardiology. Birmingham, MI, Physician Press, 1996: 233–43.

13 Medina A, Suarez de Lezo J, Pan M. A new classification of coronary bifurcation lesions. Rev Esp Cardiol 2006; 59:183–4.

14 Mohaved MR, Stinis CT. A new proposed simplified classification of coronary artery bifurcation lesions and bifurcation interventional techniques. J Invasive Cardiol 2006;18:199–204.

15 Mohaved MR. Coronary artery bifurcation lesion classifications, interventional techniques and clinical outcome. Expert Rev Cardiovasc Ther 2008;6:261–74.

16 Hildick-Smith D, de Belder AJ, Cooter N, Curzen NP, Clayton TC, Oldroyd KG, Bennett L, Holberg S, Cotton JM, Glennon P.E. *et al.* Randomized trial of simple versus complex drug-eluting stenting for bifurcation lesions: the British Bifurcation Coronary Study: old, new and evolving strategies. Circulation 2010;121:1235–43.

17 Frangos C, Noble S, Piazza N, Asgar A, Fortier A, Doucet S, Bonan R. Impact of bifurcation lesions on angiographic characteristics and procedural success in primary percutaneous coronary intervention for ST elevation myocardial infarction. EuroInterv 2010; in press.

18 Collins N, Seidelin PH, Daly P, Ivanov J, Barolet A, Mackie K, Bui S, Schwartz L, Dzavik V. Long-term outcomes after percutaneous coronary intervention of bifurcation narrowings. Am J Cardiol 2008;102:404–410.

19 Enrico B, Suranyi P, Thilo C, Bonomo L, Costello P, Schoepf UJ. Coronary artery plaque formation at CT angiography: morphological analysis and relationship to hemodynamics. Eur Radiol 2009;19:837–44.

20 Van Mieghem CA, Thury A, Meijboom WB, Cademartiri F, Mollet NR, Weustink AC, Sianos G, de Jaegere PP, Serruys PW, de Feyter P. Detection and characterization of coronary bifurcation lesions with 64-slice computed tomography coronary angiography. Eur Heart J 2007;28: 1968–76.

21 van der Giessen AG, Wentzel JJ, Meijboom WB, Mollet NR, van der Steen AF, van de Vosse FN, de Feyter PJ, Gijsen FJ. Plaque and shear stress distribution in human coronary bifurcations: a multislice computed tomographic study. EuroInterv 2009;4:654–61.

22 Oviedo C, Maehara A, Mintz GS, Araki H, Choi SY, Tsujita K, Kubo T, Doi H, Templin B, Lansky A.J. *et al.* Intravascular ultrasound classification of plaque distribution in left main coronary artery bifurcations: Where is the plaque really located? Circ Cardiovasc Interv 2010; 2:105–12.

23 Kassab GS. Scaling laws of vascular trees: Of form and function. Am J Physiol Heart Circ Physiol 2006;290: 894–903.

24 Zhou Y, Kassab GS, Molloi S. On the design of the coronary arterial tree: A generalization of Murray's law. Phys Med Biol 1999;44:2929–45.

25 Ellis SG, Vandormael MG, Cowley M, *et al.* Coronary morphologic and clinical determinants of procedural outcome with angioplasty for multivessel coronary disease. Implication for patient selection. Circulation 1990;82:1193–202.

26 Dzavik VKR, Ivanov J, Ing DJ, Bui S, Mackie K, Ramsamujih R, Barolet A, Schwartz L, Seidelin PH. Predictors of long term outcome after crush stenting of coronary bifurcation lesions: importance of bifurcation angle. Am Heart J 2006;152:762–9.

CHAPTER 2

Provisional side branch stenting for the treatment of bifurcation lesions

Thierry Lefèvre, MD, FESC, FSCAI *and Yves Louvard,* MD, FSCAI
Institut Cardiovasculaire Paris Sud, Massy, France

Background

The treatment of coronary bifurcation lesions forms an integral part of the history of coronary angioplasty [1–4] and kissing balloon inflation was strongly recommended as early as the 1980s. In those days, the two angioplasty balloons were positioned using two separate guiding catheters.

A few studies were carried out on the use of directional or rotational atherectomy and showed relatively disappointing results [5,6]. The advent of stenting resulted in the creativity of interventional cardiologists being challenged. For this reason, many stent implantation techniques were described during the 1990s [7–18]. Among these strategies, the single-stent technique, that is stenting of the main branch (MB) with provisional SB stenting (Figure 2.1), was associated with the most acceptable outcome [19–25].

The development of the DES technology at the dawn of the third millennium brought about a very significant reduction in the risk of restenosis [26] and repeat intervention [27] as shown in Figure 2.2. As a result, surgery for patients with bifurcation lesions in large coronary vessels became obsolete. Simultaneously, the decreased risk of restenosis led certain teams to re-implement techniques that had been discredited in the BMS era [28] and carry out new 'very metallic' strategies [29–34].

Six randomized studies [35–40] as well as various meta-analyses [41–47] comparing dual-stent techniques with provisional SB stenting have demonstrated that complex strategies do not confer any benefit; in addition, they are associated with an increase in the risk of myocardial infarction and probably also in stent thrombosis (Figure 2.3).

Circumstances in which dual-stent strategies are required as a primary option, such as difficult access or long SB lesions are the subject of controversy, as is the choice of the optimal technique in such cases [48]. Implantation of stents dedicated to the treatment of bifurcation lesions, using the provisional SB stenting strategy in a reproducible manner with permanent access to both branches, seems to be associated with satisfactory results. However, there is no formal evidence as yet that these stents are instrumental in simplifying the procedure and improving procedural success

It is important to keep in mind that the main objective is not only to achieve a good mid-term outcome with a low risk of repeat intervention, but also to avoid jeopardizing the SB with potential non Q-wave-myocardial infarction, or compromising the MB by focusing on the achievement of a perfect result in the SB.

Basic principles

Considerable progress has been achieved since the turn of the millennium in the understanding of fundamental aspects of coronary bifurcations in

Bifurcation Stenting, First Edition. Edited by Ron Waksman and John A. Ormiston.
© 2012 Blackwell Publishing Ltd. Published 2012 by Blackwell Publishing Ltd.

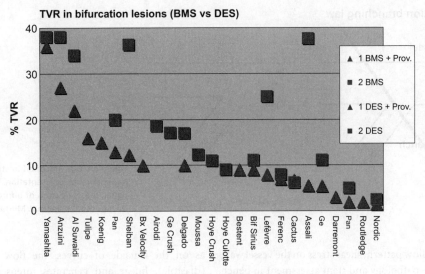

Figure 2.1 Repeat intervention rate after bifurcation stenting with BMS and DES.

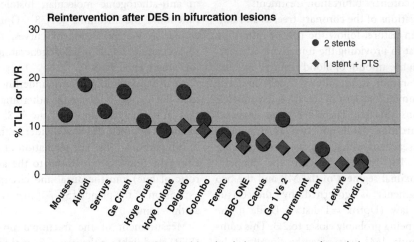

Figure 2.2 Repeat intervention rate with DES using provisional techniques versus complex techniques.

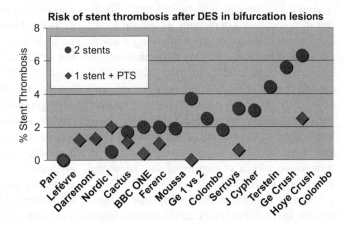

Figure 2.3 Risk of stent thrombosis associated with DES using provisional techniques versus complex techniques.

Bifurcation branching law

Main Vessel

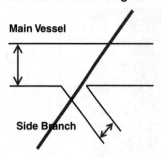

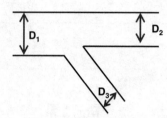

Murray's law: $D_1{}^3 = D_2{}^3 + D_3{}^3$

Finet's law: $D_1 = 0.678\,(D_2 + D_3)$

Figure 2.4 Drawing of bifurcations. Right panel: former representation. Left panel: representation of bifurcations taking into the account Murray's law.

terms of flow pattern, shear stress on the vessel wall, anatomo-pathology and stent assessment in bench tests. Knowledge of these aspects is fundamental for managing coronary bifurcation treatment.

Ramifications of the coronary tree, as all ramifications in nature, follow the rule of minimum energy cost in providing the underlying myocardium with the amount of blood required [49,50]. Coronary ramification follows a self-similarity fractal geometry pattern of iterative, asymmetric bifurcations [51–53]. There are three segments in a bifurcation (and not two as previously thought), each of which has its own reference diameter. The relation between the diameter of the proximal segment of the MB and the two distal segments is governed by the classic Murray's law ($Dprox^3 = Ddist^3 + Dside^3$), the exponent being probably closer to 2.3. This complex formula [54] was recently simplified by Finet [55]: $Dprox = (Ddist + Dside) \times 0.678$ (Figure 2.4). Consequently, the reference diameter of a coronary artery from its ostium to its distal segment does not taper following a linear pattern, but by steps, following the formation of a bifurcation branch. Therefore, the diameter of a coronary vessel is constant between two bifurcations. This makes all conventional quantitative coronary angiography computer programs obsolete, at least in the vicinity of bifurcations. They have been replaced by dedicated software in compliance with a consensus of the European Bifurcation Club [56].

Coronary bifurcation flow has specific characteristics. In the vicinity of the carina (flow divider),

as on the outside of curves, the flow is rapid (diastole), linear and generates intense friction (wall shear stress, WSS) on the vessel wall resulting in anti-atherogenic molecular, histological and functional modifications [57,58]. Opposite the carina, as on the inside of curves, there is a re-circulating, oscillating flow generating low and pro-atherogenic WSS.

Anatomopathologists have underlined the fact that the carina is generally atheroma-free and that atheroma develops in low WSS areas in segments opposite the flow divider in the vicinity of bifurcations [58]. The formation of atheroma alters the flow pattern (distal to the atherosclerotic plaque) and the distal and circumferential expansion of the plaque [59, 60] may reach as far as the carina.

Measurement of the fractional flow reserve (FFR) shed light on the issue of ostial SB stenosis following MB stenting. Although such a lesion may often appear to be angiographically tight, it is in fact seldom significant from a physiological point of view (FFR <0.80). As demonstrated in the article by Koo [61], only 28% of >75% SB stenoses (QCA) are physiologically significant lesions. The reason for this discrepancy between angiographic images and flow has not been thoroughly accounted for: lesion of the SB ostium related to the carina shift phenomenon reshaping a circular ostium into a "slit", which is angiographically visualized from the worst possible angle, phenomenon of slow flow and turbulences hampering adequate contrast filling of the ostium and border effect artifact.

Role of bench testing

The assessment of stents in bench tests has been essential in improving the comprehension of bifurcation stenting [62–65]. The initial bench tests did not comply with Murray's law and stent deployment was filmed inadequately. The tests currently used comply with the laws of branching and stent deployment is digitally recorded either in a micro CT [66] or by rotational acquisition in a cath-lab. The more elaborate bench tests are perfused.

The first benefit of bench testing was to show the distortion generated in the MB stent by the opening of a strut towards the SB, resulting in the projection of struts into the SB ostium and attraction of opposite struts in the main lumen. Various stenting techniques have been simulated in benches, allowing an accurate description of the inherent advantages and disadvantages of each technique as well as a reproduction of complication instances.

Digital simulation is likely to replace bench testing in the near future. Indeed, it is now possible to acquire images of a bifurcation lesion via rotational angiography or 3D reconstruction from orthogonal views of a patient.

The "finite elements" technique allows the reconstruction of a bifurcation by attributing to each element the technical characteristics of the vessel and plaque. It is also possible to reproduce copies of commercially available stents, with their physical properties and simulate their deployment by balloon inflation or the opening of a strut [67].

Definition of a coronary bifurcation lesion

After years of fruitful discussion, the EBC finally reached a consensus: a bifurcation lesion is "a coronary artery narrowing occurring adjacent to, and/or involving the origin of a significant SB". A significant SB is a branch that you do not want to lose in the global context of a particular patient. The prognostic value of an SB occlusion depends on many factors such as size, length, viability of the myocardium perfused by the branch, the collateralizing role of the SB, ventricular function and finally the threshold value defined by the interventional cardiologist himself. Although,

biomarker elevation has been correlated with prognosis, including mortality, the level from which biomarker elevation is likely to influence the outcome is still debated.

Given the relationship between the diameter of a branch and the amount of perfused myocardium, and between the size of the artery and the area under the biomarker curve (when the artery is occluded), it should be possible to determine the minimum diameter at which SB occlusion may influence the outcome, thus providing a more objective definition of "a significant side branch".

Many bifurcation lesion classifications have been proposed [68], most of which need to be memorized, except for the classification established by Medina [69], which has become widely accepted. The EBC suggested that the bifurcations be individually identified using the same codification as the Medina classification, namely 1 (lesion $\geq$ 50%) or 0 in the proximal MB segment, 1 or 0 in the distal SB segment and 1 or 0 in the SB, separated by a coma. Medina classification forms can be filled in after visual assessment or using dedicated QCA software. The three segments of a bifurcation generate three angles: A (approach), between the proximal MB and SB; B (between), between the two distal branches; and C between the proximal and distal MB segments. As Biplane QCA does not provide reliable measurements of these angles, 3D QCA is required.

Angle A defines the difficulty in accessing the SB. This angle, when small, can be significantly increased by the insertion of a guide wire [70]. A small angle B predicts the occurrence of SB occlusion after MB stenting [71].

Definition of treatments

Many techniques have been described in the literature. The MADS classification [68], adopted by the EBC in 2007 is an open classification based on two principles: a definition of "generic" techniques according to the final positioning and aspect of stents at the end of the procedure, and strategic techniques, according to the position of the first stent deployed in the bifurcation.

Variations of generic techniques can subsequently be described according to the manner in which guides and balloons are used.

What is provisional SB stenting?

This strategy was designed to meet the main objectives of bifurcation lesion treatment focusing on the MB whilst ensuring patency of the SB. This strategy consists in deploying a stent from the proximal segment to the distal segment of the MB. In some instances, due to technical (angles), or anatomical reasons (location of the tightest stenosis), or for reasons of myocardial viability, the stent is deployed from the proximal segment of the MB to the SB (inverted provisional).

The advantages of this strategy lie mainly in the "open" nature of this approach, the purpose of which is to perform an optimal treatment of the MB and coronary bifurcation with a single stent whenever possible. When necessary, a second stent can be deployed in the SB using the T or Culotte implantation technique. This procedure can be easily carried out with a 6 F guiding catheter in the majority of cases.

The drawbacks of this technique are, on the one hand, the difficulty in ensuring permanent access to the SB, and on the other hand, potential problems in re-crossing the stent struts towards the SB or even in implanting a second stent in the SB after stenting the MB.

The relative simplicity of the provisional approach requiring a single stent in 80–90% of cases [72] and resulting in similar outcome compared with more complex strategies as demonstrated in randomized studies [35–47], has made this strategy the gold standard of bifurcation treatment even for the left main coronary artery as illustrated by the Syntax data [73]. Indeed, in the treatment of the distal left main, the Syntax study showed that the provisional approach was associated with a lower MACE risk compared to systematic dual-stenting strategies.

How to perform bifurcation stenting using the provisional approach

Coronary angiography allows an appropriate selection of stents to be made and provides the diameter and length of lesions located in the coronary bifurcation. Given the tri-dimensional structure of bifurcations, it is impossible to obtain a plane image of the three bifurcation segments without avoiding the foreshortening effect. Consequently, it is necessary to record several views from various angles in order to obtain a comprehensive picture of the lesion characteristics, to carry out the technical procedure appropriately and assess the procedural outcome.

The SB ostium poses the most frequent technical problems and is associated with poor outcome and occurrence of restenosis. This site is rarely visualized adequately from two orthogonal views and may be explored from a single angle called "the working view". This view allows the visualization of branch division as well as the measurement of angles and assessment of the degree of ostial SB stenosis. This is generally an RAO or LAO view with caudal inclination for the left main coronary artery, an anterior-posterior projection with marked cranial angulation for LAD-diagonal bifurcations, a slight RAO or LAO projection with caudal angulation for circumflex-proximal marginal bifurcations or cranial angulation for dominant distal circumflex coronary arteries and an antero-posterior projection with cranial angulation for distal right coronary arteries.

Role of IVUS

The benefit of IVUS in the treatment of bifurcation lesions is still being evaluated with a randomized study (BLAST) comparing angiography-guided with IVUS-guided coronary bifurcation PCI. IVUS is currently recommended as a guidance tool for complex treatments especially in the left main coronary artery.

One or two guide wires?

Systematic insertion of a guide wire in the SB at the beginning of the procedure is a sign that the operator considers the lesion to be a bifurcation stenosis. There are several advantages associated with the initial insertion of a guide wire in each branch. In addition to ensuring patency of the branch post dilatation, which has never been demonstrated, the wire modifies angle A, thus facilitating guide wire exchange as well as balloon and stent advancement [70]. Furthermore, in cases of occlusion, the guide wire is a good marker of the SB and may be

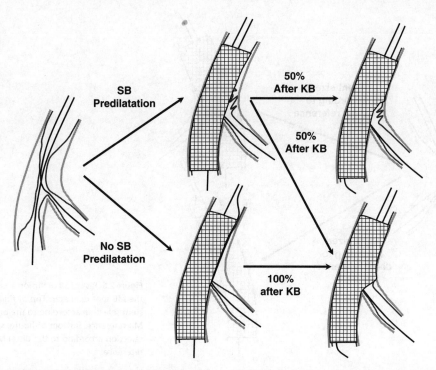

Figure 2.5 Potentially untoward effects of SB predilatation. Top of figure: SB predilatation followed by stenting of the MB and result after kissing balloon inflation according to whether or not the proximal strut has been opened towards the SB. Bottom of figure: no SB predilatation.

rarely used as a "bail-out" strategy in order to re-open the SB with a small balloon advanced outside the stent. Cases of guide rupture have been associated with the use of "jailed" hydrophilic wires or when the radio-opaque distal segment of a wire is "jailed". When treating a coronary bifurcation (a branch that we do not want to lose) our strategy is to begin the procedure with systematic insertion of two guide wires. In the TULIP multicenter study [74], use of only one wire when starting the procedure was a predictor of SB treatment failure and repeat intervention at 6 months.

Should we pre-dilate the lesion or not?

Kissing pre-dilatation is not recommended due to the risk of extensive dissection in unstented segments. Predilatation of the MB may be left to the discretion of the operator according to the type of lesion. However, predilatation of the SB remains a subject of controversy. Our opinion is that it is preferable not to predilate the SB for two reasons.

Firstly, the occurrence of dissection inherent in the enlargement of the lumen of the SB ostium may hinder or prevent access to the SB through the struts of the MB stent, and secondly, the enlargement of the SB lumen increases the likelihood that access to the SB may also be possible through a proximal strut, although access through a distal strut is the only possibility for projecting struts in the SB (Figure 2.5). Certain teams choose to dilate the SB, but generally complete the procedure by stent deployment in the MB without final kissing inflation [37].

Stenting across

Selection of the MB stent is an important step. Although DES allow a reduction in the risk of restenosis and repeat intervention compared with BMS, acceptable rates of restenosis may be obtained with BMS when using only one stent. Stent selection should be made according to the maximal expansion ability of the stent allowing stent apposition on the MB wall and on the SB ostium. The size

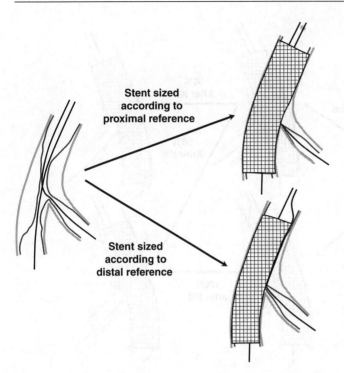

Stent sized
according to
proximal reference

Stent sized
according to
distal reference

Figure 2.6 Risk of SB occlusion according to the MB sent diameter. Top of figure: stent selection according to the proximal MB reference. Bottom of figure: stent selection according to the distal MB reference.

of the stent struts is also an important criterion for the most proximal bifurcations. Stents with uneven struts should be avoided.

The choice of stent diameter for implantation in the MB is crucial. When excessively large (commensurate with the proximal segment), it may significantly increase the risk of SB occlusion by causing the carina to shift (Figure 2.6). Selection of the stent diameter should be made according to the diameter of the main distal segment in compliance with Murray's law. In such cases, the drawback is the inadequate apposition of the stent on the proximal segment, especially when the difference between the diameter of the proximal and distal segments is large (i.e. when the SB is large).

POT (proximal optimization technique)

This technique provides a solution to the problem of under-deployment of the proximal part of the MB stent. It involves the post-dilatation of the proximal segment of the stent in order to match the diameter of the main proximal segment of the bifurcation. It is carried out by inflating a short

balloon along the whole length of the proximal segment. As a result, the original anatomical configuration of the bifurcation is restored in compliance with the branching law (Figure 2.7). It changes also the orientation of the SB ostium, facilitating the insertion of a guide-wire, balloon and, if necessary, a stent in the SB (Figure 2.8), as well as the projection of struts in the SB ostium.

POT is especially useful in large SBs with a marked difference in the diameter of the proximal and distal main segments, which increases the need for implantation of a second stent in the SB. This technique is not useful in small SB which do not require stenting and which are only protected by the presence of a guide wire.

Outcome analysis: when should the SB be treated?

Angiographic assessment of the procedural outcome in the SB ostium is not easy. The degree of angiographic stenosis is higher than when assessment is made by IVUS or FFR. In the case of > 75% residual SB stenosis by angiography, FFR analysis shows that only a minority of lesions are

Proximal Optimization Technique

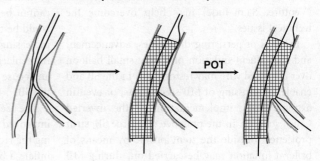

Figure 2.7 Representation of the proximal optimization technique (POT).

< 0.80 [61]. The reasons for this poor angiographic performance are the non-circular shape of the SB ostium and the edge effect generated by angiography. The use of FFR for outcome evaluation in the SB may prove a valid approach.

Should kissing balloon inflation be performed after simple technique?

When POT has not been previously performed, balloon inflation in the SB ostium tends to cause stent distortion in the MB and attraction of the struts opposite the SB in the MB lumen. Kissing balloon inflation (KB) allows SB treatment and apposition of the MB stent struts on the SB ostium, which, when inadequately apposed, generate flow disruption. It also enables correction of stent distortion and correction of inadequate apposition in the MB.

Initial stent diameter and SB ostium orientation

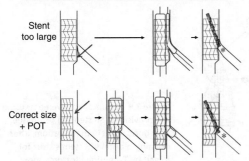

Figure 2.8 Drawing of carina modification brought about by MB stenting. Top: carina modification caused by excessive stent size. Bottom: stent of appropriate size.

However, KB increases procedural complexity and may result in stent ovalization, proximal dissection when balloons are inadequately positioned and even suboptimal deployment of the proximal stent segment. Although final KB is recommended after dual stenting, it remains a controversial issue in the case of single stent implantation. The one-year follow-up results of the NORDIC III trial should provide an answer to this unresolved problem.

The pending issue is not whether KB is the right strategy, but when the SB should be treated. In cases of angiographic slow flow in the SB combined with EKG signs of ischemia and chest pain, SB treatment is unanimously considered as necessary. In large SBs, a poor procedural outcome may result in the occurrence of symptoms and residual ischemia. Absence of cell opening towards the SB may cause serious difficulties in treating restenosis or de novo distal disease. Consequently, although this is not standard practice, it is preferable to systematically open the stent towards the SB when performing PCI of the distal left main.

How to carry out final kissing balloon inflation appropriately?

First of all, it is fundamental to insert a free wire in the SB through the struts of the MB stent and, if possible, in the strut closest to the carina. In order to achieve this, we exchange guide-wires in most cases, although a third wire may also be used. The MB wire, pre-shaped into a long form and secured by the stent, is pulled towards the SB ostium. When guide wire advancement proves difficult, utilization of POT, reshaping of the guide wire, use of a hydrophilic or a more rigid wire with improved torque, or even an orientable micro-catheter (Venture, Saint-Jude) may help overcome the technical issues.

In cases of persisting difficulties, advancement and subsequent inflation of a very small balloon over the jailed wire may restore flow in the SB and enable the crossing of MB stent struts, or even in extreme cases, implementation of the inverted Crush strategy. In the presence of a large SB, strut projection outside the stent profile by means of balloon inflation may be carried out during MB stent implantation.

Following insertion of a free wire in the SB, the jailed wire must be withdrawn proximal to the stent. During this maneuver, the guiding catheter must be closely monitored in order to avoid deep intubation which might cause proximal dissection. In rare occurrences where the guide wire cannot be easily withdrawn, the use and potential inflation of a small balloon may prove efficient.

Once released, the wire, having previously been made into a short and angulated form, should be advanced in the MB if possible with a loop whilst avoiding advancement outside the stent.

Selection of balloons for KB is crucial. The diameter must match that of the two distal branches. The balloons must be sufficiently short to avoid inflation outside the stent in the MB, and in disease-free areas in the SB. In cases where POT has not been performed, KB may optimize the proximal segment of the MB. When the SB lesion cannot be dilated at a reasonable pressure, which could be the result of inadequate stent expansion, increasing the pressure of semi- compliant balloon may enlarge the diameter of the unstented segment and cause dissection requiring stent deployment in the SB.

The use of non-compliant balloons for KB allows improved stent expansion in the MB whilst reducing the risk of dissection in the SB. During KB, we inflate a balloon in the MB first and then the SB balloon in order to achieve strut projection in the ostium. The pressure applied depends on the persistence of a waist on the balloon.

Sequential balloon inflation (side, main, side) has been proposed as an alternative to kissing balloon inflation.

When and how should the SB be stented ?

As for balloon angioplasty treatment, the decision to stent the SB depends on the occurrence of complications as well as the angiographic result assessed from various views (projections), IVUS or FFR analysis, size of the SB and amount of its distributive volume.

Several implantation techniques may be utilized for SB stenting (Figure 2.9). The authors use the provisional T-stenting technique. Contrary to the

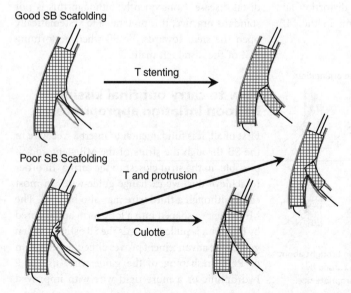

Figure 2.9 Technical achievements using the provisional SB stenting technique. Top: good result in the SB ostium, after opening a distal MB stent's strut followed by T-stenting. Bottom: poor result in the SB ostium (proximal MB stent's strut, treated by TAP (T and protrusion) or Culotte).

systematic T-stenting technique, which starts with stent deployment in the SB, a second stent can be implanted without leaving any gap, especially in instances where the struts of the MB stent cover the SB ostium efficiently (POT, distal insertion of a free wire in the SB. . .). Advancement of the stent towards the SB fails very rarely especially when the proximal segment of the MB stent has been appropriately optimized (1.5% in the BBK study). In order to carry out accurate stenting, it is necessary to have a good angiographic "working view" and to know the relation between the proximal marker of the balloon and the proximal extremity of the stent which vary according to the type of stent used.

In cases where the proximal segment of the SB has not been sufficiently opened by the MB stent, the operator may apply the TAP technique (T and protrusion) or culotte stenting.

Conclusion

Angioplasty of coronary bifurcations has posed technical issues since the beginning of interventional cardiology. The advent of stenting generated the development of various techniques, and the management of coronary bifurcations gradually improved thanks to a better understanding of anatomo-pathology, rheology, branching law, lesion assessment and stenting outcome. Technical strategies have now reached a certain maturity and it has become clear that the provisional SB stenting strategy is the reference technique and the most commonly used worldwide. Though many aspects remain to be addressed, this simple and relatively flexible technique provides excellent short and mid-term results.

References

1 Zack PM, Ischinger T. Experience with a technique for coronary angioplasty of bifurcational lesions. Cathet Cardiovasc Diagn 1984;10:433–43.

2 Pinkerton CA, Slack JD, Van Tassel JW, Ort CM. Angioplasty for dilatation of complex coronary artery bifurcation stenosis. Am J Cardiol 1985;55:1626–8.

3 George BS, Myler RK, Stertzer SH, et al. Balloon angioplasty of bifurcation lesions: the kissing balloon technique. Cathet Cardiovasc Diagn 1986;12:124–38.

4 Meier B, Grüntzig AR, King SB, Ill, et al. Risk of side branch occlusion during coronary angioplasty. Am J Cardiol 1984;53:10–4.

5 Brener SJ, Leya FS, Apperson-Hansen C, Cowley MJ, Califf RM, Topol EJ. A comparison of debulking versus dilatation of bifurcation coronary arterial narrowing (from the CAVEAT I Trial). Coronary angioplasty versus excisional atherectomy trial-I. Am J Cardiol 1996;78: 1039–41.

6 Dauerman HL, Higgins PJ, Sparano AM, et al. Mechanical debulking versus balloon angioplasty for the treatment of true bifurcation lesions. J Am Coll Cardiol 1998;32:1845–52.

7 Colombo A, Gaglione A, Nakamura S, Finci L. "Kissing" stents for bifurcation coronary lesion. Cathet Cardiovasc Diagn 1993;30:327–30.

8 Schampaert E, Fort S, Adelman A, Schwartz L. The V-stent: a novel technique for coronary bifurcation stenting. Cathet Cardiovasc Diagn 1996;39:320–6.

9 Carrie D, Karouny E, Chouairi S, et al. "T"-shaped stent placement: a technique for the treatment of dissected bifurcation lesions. Cathet Cardiovasc Diagn 1996;37: 311–3.

10 Fort S, Lazzam C, Schwartz L. Coronary 'Y' stenting: A technique for angioplasty of bifurcation stenosis. Can J Cardiol 1996;12:678–82.

11 Carison TA, Guarneri EM, Stevens KM, Norman SL, Schatz RA. "T-stenting": the answer to bifurcation lesions? Circulation 1996;94:I-86–I-87.

12 Khoja A, Ozbek C, Bay W, Heisel A. Trouser-like stenting: a technique for bifurcation lesions. Cathet Cardiovasc Diagn 1997;41,2: 192–9.

13 Carrie D, Elbaz M, Dambrin G, et al. Coronary stenting of bifurcation lesions using "T" or "reverse Y" configuration with Wiktor stent. Am J Cardiol 1998;82:1418–21, A8.

14 Chevalier B, Glatt B, Royer T, Guyon P. Placement of coronary stents in bifurcation lesions by the "culotte" technique. Am J Cardiol 1998;82:943–9.

15 Kobayashi Y, Colombo A, Adamian M, Nishida T, Moussa I, Moses JW. The skirt technique: A stenting technique to treat a lesion immediately proximal to the bifurcation (pseudobifurcation). Catheter Cardiovasc Interv 2000;51(3):347–51.

16 Perin MA, Martinez EE, Ambrose JA, et al. A new method for stenting bifurcation lesions with preservation of side-branch access. European J Cardiol 2000.(abs supp); 21:640.

17 Spedicato L, Bonin M, Bernardi G, Gelsomino S, Fioretti PM, Morocutti G. "Side balloon stenting": a novel technique for bifurcation lesions. J Invasive Cardiol 2001;10:684–8.

18 Aroney N. A new technique to guarantee access to the side branch during bifurcational coronary stenting. J Invas Cardiol 2000;12:25–28.

19 Al Suwaidi J, Yeh W, Cohen HA, Detre KM, Williams DO, Holmes DR, Jr., Immediate and one-year outcome in patients with coronary bifurcation lesions in the modern era (NHLBI dynamic registry). Am J Cardiol 2001; 87(10):1139–44.

20 Yamashita T, Nishida T, Adamina M, et al. Bifurcation lesions: two stents versus one stent-immediate and follow-up results. JACC 2000;35:1145–51.

21 Sheiban I, Albiero R, Marsico F, et al. Immediate and long-term results of "T"-stenting for bifurcation coronary lesions. Am J Cardiol 2000;85:1141–44.

22 Pan M, Suarez de Lezo J, Medina A, et al. Simple and complex stent strategies for bifurcated coronary arterial stenosis involving the side branch origin. Am J Cardiol 1999;83:1320–5.

23 Pan M, Suarez de Lezo J, Medina A, et al. A stepwise strategy for the stent treatment of bifurcated coronary lesions. Catheter Cardiovasc Interv 2002;55:50–7.

24 Lefèvre T., Louvard Y., Morice M.C., Dumas P., Loubeyre C., Benslimane A., et al. Stenting of bifurcation lesions: Classification, Treatment, and Results. Cathet Cardiovasc Intervent 2000;49:274–83.

25 Lefevre T, Louvard Y, Morice MC. Bifurcation lesions: we can save both the mother and the child. Catheter Cardiovasc Interv 2001;52:136–7.

26 Louvard Y, Lefèvre T. Coronary bifurcation stenting: state of the heart. In Oxford Textbook of Interventional Cardiology, Oxford University Press, Great Clarendon Street, Oxford, OX2 6DP, 2010; 293–313.

27 Tsuchida K, Colombo A, Lefèvre T, Oldroyd KG, Guetta V, Guagliumi G, et al. The clinical outcome of percutaneous treatment of bifurcation lesions in multivessel coronary artery disease with the sirolimus-eluting stent: insights from the Arterial Revascularization Therapies Study part II (ARTS II). Eur Heart J 2007;28:433–42.

28 Carlier SG, Colombo A, de Scheerder I, et al. Stenting of bifurcational coronary lesions: results of the multicentric European culottes registry. Euro Heart J 2001;22 [Abstr.Suppl]:348.

29 Colombo A, Stankovic G, Orlic D, Corvaja N, Liistro F, Airoldi F, Chieffo A, Spanos V, Montorfano M, Di Mario C. Modified T-stenting technique with crushing for bifurcation lesions: immediate results and 30-day outcome. Catheter Cardiovasc Interv 2003;60(2):145–51.

30 Ge L, Airoldi F, Iakovou I, Cosgrave J, Michev I, Sangiorgi GM, Montorfano M, Chieffo A, Carlino M, Corvaja N, Colombo A. Clinical and angiographic outcome after implantation of drug-eluting stents in bifurcation lesions with the crush stent technique: importance of final kissing balloon post-dilation. J Am Coll Cardiol 2005;46(4): 613–20.

31 Sharma SK, Choudhury A, Lee J, Kim MC, Fisher E, Steinheimer AM, Kini AS. Simultaneous kissing stents (SKS) technique for treating bifurcation lesions in medium-to-large arteries. Am J Cardiol 2004;94(7):913–7.

32 Helqvist S, Jørgensen E, Kelbaek H, Aljabbari S, Thuesen L, Flensted Lassen J, Saunamäki K. Percutaneous treatment of coronary bifurcation lesions: a novel "extended Y" technique with complete lesion stent coverage. Heart 2006;92(7):981–2.

33 Burzotta F, Gwon HC, Hahn JY, Romagnoli E, Choi JH, Trani C, Colombo A. Modified T-stenting with intentional protrusion of the side-branch stent within the main vessel stent to ensure ostial coverage and facilitate final kissing balloon: the T-stenting and small protrusion technique (TAP-stenting). Report of bench testing and first clinical Italian-Korean two-centre experience. Catheter Cardiovasc Interv 2007;70(1):75–82.

34 Galassi AR, Colombo A, Buchbinder M, Grasso C, Tomasello SD, Ussia GP, Tamburino C. Long-term outcomes of bifurcation lesions after implantation of drug-eluting stents with the "mini-crush technique". Catheter Cardiovasc Interv 2007;69(7):976–83.

35 Colombo A, Moses JW, Morice MC, Ludwig J, Holmes DR Jr, Spanos V, Louvard Y, Desmedt B, Di Mario C, Leon MB. Randomized study to evaluate sirolimus-eluting stents implanted at coronary bifurcation lesions. Circulation 2004;109:1244–9.

36 Steigen TK, Maeng M, Wiseth R, Erglis A, Kumsars I, Narbute I, Gunnes P, Mannsverk J, Meyerdierks O, Rotevatn S, Niemelä M, Kervinen K, Jensen JS, Galløe A, Nikus K, Vikman S, Ravkilde J, James S, Aarøe J, Ylitalo A, Helqvist S, Sjögren I, Thayssen P, Virtanen K, Puhakka M, Airaksinen J, Lassen JF, Thuesen LRandomized study on simple versus complex stenting of coronary artery bifurcation lesions: the Nordic bifurcation study. Nordic PCI Study Group. Circulation 2006;114(18):1955–61.

37 Pan M, de Lezo JS, Medina A, Romero M, Segura J, Pavlovic D, Delgado A, Ojeda S, Melián F, Herrador J, Ureña I, Burgos L. Rapamycin-eluting stents for the treatment of bifurcated coronary lesions: a randomized comparison of a simple versus complex strategy. Am Heart J 2004;148(5):857–64.

38 Ferenc M, Gick M, Kienzle RP, Bestehorn HP, Werner KD, Comberg T, Kuebler P, Büttner HJ, Neumann FJ. Randomized trial on routine vs. provisional T-stenting in the treatment of de novo coronary bifurcation lesions. Eur Heart J 2008;29(23):2859–67.

39 Colombo A, Bramucci E, Saccà S, Violini R, Lettieri C, Zanini R, Sheiban I, Paloscia L, Grube E, Schofer J, Bolognese L, Orlandi M, Niccoli G, Latib A, Airoldi F. Randomized study of the crush technique versus provisional side-branch stenting in true coronary bifurcations: the CACTUS (Coronary Bifurcations: Application of the Crushing Technique Using Sirolimus-Eluting Stents) Study. Circulation 2009;119(1):71–8.

40 Hildick-Smith D, De Belder AJ, Cooter N, Curzen NP, Clayton TC, Oldroyd KG, Bennett L, Holmberg S, Cotton JM, Glennon PE, Thomas MR, MacCarthy PA, Baumbach A, Mulvihill NT, Henderson RA, Redwood SR, Starkey IR, and Stables RH. Randomized Trial of Simple Versus Complex Drug-Eluting Stenting for Bifurcation Lesions: The British Bifurcation Coronary Study: Old, New, and Evolving Strategies. Circulation 2010;121:1235–43.

41 Biondi-Zoccai GG, Lotrionte M, Moretti C, et al. A collaborative systematic review and meta-analysis on 1278 patients undergoing percutaneous drug-eluting stenting for unprotected left main coronary artery disease. Am Heart J 2008;155:274–83.

42 Zhang F, Dong L, Ge J. Simple versus complex stenting strategy for coronary artery bifurcation lesions in the drug-eluting stent era: a meta-analysis of randomised trials. Heart 2009;95(20):1676–81.

43 Brar SS, Gray WA, Dangas G, Leon MB, Aharonian VJ, Brar SK, Moses JW. Bifurcation stenting with drug-eluting stents: a systematic review and meta-analysis of randomised trials. EuroIntervention 2009;5(4):475–84.

44 Katritsis DG, Siontis GC, Ioannidis JP. Double versus single stenting for coronary bifurcation lesions: a meta-analysis. Circ Cardiovasc Interv 2009;2(5):409–15.

45 Hakeem A, Khan FM, Bhatti S, Samad Z, Effat MA, Eckman MH, Helmy T, Provisional vs. complex stenting strategy for coronary bifurcation lesions: meta-analysis of randomized trials. J Invasive Cardiol 2009;21(11):589–95.

46 Niccoli G, Ferrante G, Porto I, Burzotta F, Leone AM, Mongiardo R, Mazzari MA, Trani C, Rebuzzi AG, Crea F. Coronary bifurcation lesions: to stent one branch or both? A meta-analysis of patients treated with drug eluting stents. Int J Cardiol 2010;139(1):80–91.

47 Athappan G, Ponniah T, Jeyaseelan L. True coronary bifurcation lesions: meta-analysis and review of literature. J Cardiovasc Med (Hagerstown) 2010;11(2):103–10.

48 Hildick-Smith D, Lassen JF, Albiero R, Lefèvre T, Darremont O, Pan M, Ferenc M, Stankovic G, and Louvard Y. Consensus from the 5th european bifurcation club. Eurointervention 2010;6:34–38.

49 Kassab GS. Functional hierarchy of coronary circulation: direct evidence of a structure-function relation. Am J Physiol Heart Circ Physiol 2005;289(6):H2559–65.

50 Kassab GS. Design of Coronary Circulation: The Minimum Energy Hypothesis. Comput Methods Appl Mech Engrg 2007;196:3033–42.

51 Kalsho G, Kassab GS. Bifurcation asymmetry of the porcine coronary vasculature and its implications on coronary flow heterogeneity. Am J Physiol Heart Circ Physiol 2004;287(6):H2493–500.

52 Kamiya A, Takahashi T. Quantitative assessments of morphological and functional properties of biological trees based on their fractal nature. J Appl Physiol 2007; 102(6):2315–23.

53 Choy JS, Kassab GS. Scaling of myocardial mass to flow and morphometry of coronary arteries. J Appl Physiol 2008;104(5):1259.

54 Murray CD. The physiological principle of minimum work: I. The vascular system and the cost of blood volume. Proc Natl Acad Sci USA 1926;12:207–14.

55 Finet G, Gilard M, Perrenot B, Rioufol G, Motreff P. et al. Fractal geometry of cornary bifurcations: a quantitative coronary angiography and intravascular ultrasoubnd analysis. EuroIntervention 2008;3:490–98.

56 Lansky A, Tuinenburg J, Costa M, Maeng M, Koning G, Popma J, Cristea E, Gavit L, Costa R, Rares A, Van Es GA, Lefèvre T, Reiber H, Louvard Y, Morice MC; European Bifurcation Angiographic Sub-Committee. Quantitative angiographic methods for bifurcation lesions: a consensus statement from the European. Catheter Cardiovasc Interv 2009;73(2):258–66.

57 Asakura T, Karino T. Flow patterns and spatial distribution of atherosclerotic lesions in human coronary arteries. Circ Res 1990;66(4):1045–66.

58 Chatzizisis YS, Jonas M, Coskun AU, Beigel R, Stone BV, Maynard C, Gerrity RG, Daley W, Rogers C, Edelman ER, Feldman CL, Stone PH. Prediction of the localization of high-risk coronary atherosclerotic plaques on the basis of low endothelial shear stress: an intravascular ultrasound and histopathology natural history study. Circulation 2008;117(8):993–1002.

59 Shimada Y, Courtney BK, Nakamura M, Hongo Y, Sonoda S, Hassan AH, Yock PG, Honda Y, Fitzgerald PJ. Intravascular ultrasonic analysis of atherosclerotic vessel remodeling and plaque distribution of stenotic left anterior descending coronary arterial bifurcation lesions upstream and downstream of the side branch. Am J Cardiol 2006;98(2):193–6.

60 Medina A. Is the carena free of plaque in coronary bifurcation lesions?. Personal communication European bifurcation club, Berlin 2009. http://www.bifurc.net

61 Koo BK, Kang HJ, Youn TJ, Chae IH, Choi DJ, Kim HS, Sohn DW, Oh BH, Lee MM, Park YB, Choi YS, Tahk SJ. Physiologic assessment of jailed side branch lesions using fractional flow reserve. J Am Coll Cardiol 2005;46 (4):633–7.

62 Pomerantz RM, Ling FS. Distortion of Palmaz-Schatz stent geometry following side- branch balloon dilation through the stent in a rabbit model. Cathet Cardiovasc Diagn 1997;40:422–6.

63 Ormiston JA, Webster MW, Ruygrok PN, Stewart JT, White HD, Scott DS. Stent deformation following simulated side-branch dilatation: a comparison of five stent designs. Catheter Cardiovasc Interv 1999 Jun;47(2): 258–64.

64 Ormiston JA, Currie E, Webster MW, Kay P, Ruygrok PN, Stewart JT, Padgett RC, Panther MJ. Drug-eluting stents for coronary bifurcations: insights into the crush technique. Catheter Cardiovasc Interv 2004 Nov;63 (3):332–6.

65 Mortier P, Van Loo D, De Beule M, Segers P, Taeymans Y, Verdonck P, Verhegghe B. Comparison of drug-eluting stent cell size using micro-CT: important data for bifurcation stent selection. EuroIntervention 2008; Nov;4(3):391–6.

66 Murasato Y, Horiuchi M, Otsuji Y. Three-dimensional modeling of double-stent techniques at the left main coronary artery bifurcation using micro-focus X-ray computed tomography. Catheter Cardiovasc Interv 2007 Aug 1;70(2):211–20.

67 Mortier P, De Beule M, Van Loo D, Verhegghe B, Verdonck P. Finite element analysis of side branch access during bifurcation stenting. Med Eng Phys. 2009;31(4):434–40.

68 Louvard Y, Thomas M, Dzavik V, Hildick-Smith D, Galassi AR, Pan M, Burzotta F, Zelizko M, Dudek D, Ludman P, Sheiban I, Lassen JF, Darremont O, Kastrati A, Ludwig J, Iakovou I, Brunel P, Lansky A, Meerkin D, Legrand V, Medina A, Lefèvre T. Classification of coronary artery bifurcation lesions and treatments: time for a consensus! Catheter Cardiovasc Interv 2008;71(2): 175–83.

69 Medina A, Suarez de Lezo J, Pan M. A new classification of coronary bifurcation lesions. Rev Esp Cardiol 2006;59:183.

70 Y. Louvard, T. Lefèvre, R. Cherukupalli et al. Favorable effect of the "Jailed Wire" Technique when stenting bifurcation lesions. Am J Cardiol 2003;6(AbstrSupp): 62–5.

71 Louvard Y, Sashikant T, Lefèvre T, Garot P, Darremont O, Brunel P, Morice MC. Angiographic predictors of side branch occlusion during treatment of bifurcation lesions. Catheter Cardiovasc Interv 2005;65:113 (abstr Supp).

72 Lefèvre T, Morice MC, Sengottuvel G. et al. Influence of technical strategies on the outcome of coronary bifurcation stenting. Eurointervention 2005;1:31–37.

73 Morice MC, Serruys PW, Kappetein AP, Feldman TE, Stahle E, Colombo A, Mack MJ, Holmes DR, Torracca L, van Es GA, Leadley K, Dawkins KD, Mohr F. Outcomes in patients with de novo left main disease treated with either percutaneous coronary intervention using paclitaxel-eluting stents or coronary artery bypass graft treatment in the synergy between percutaneous coronary intervention with TAXUS and cardiac surgery. Circulation 2010;121:2645–53.

74 Brunel P, Lefevre T, Darremont O, Louvard Y. Provisional T-stenting and kissing balloon in the treatment of coronary bifurcation lesions: results of the French multicenter "TULIPE" study. Catheter Cardiovasc Interv 2006;68(1):67–73.

CHAPTER 3

The Nordic experience

Niels Ramsing Holm, MD, *Michael Maeng,* MD,
Jens Flensted Lassen, MD, PhD, FESC *and Leif Thuesen,* MD, DMSci

Department of Cardiology, Aarhus University Hospital, Skejby, Denmark

Introduction

Percutaneous coronary intervention (PCI) of coronary bifurcation lesions is associated with increased risk of procedural complications, restenosis and stent thrombosis when compared to PCI of simple lesions [1,2]. Approximately 15–20% of treated lesions are located at bifurcating branches [3]. Thus, PCI operators frequently have to consider the optimal treatment strategy for this complex lesion subset. The Nordic bifurcation studies are a series of randomized, clinical multicenter trials aimed at establishing the optimal strategies for treatment of bifurcation lesions [4–7].

The Nordic PCI Study Group was formed in 2005 at initiation of the first Nordic bifurcation study. The study group constituted the formal body for a Nordic collaboration on training of PCI operators, and for designing and executing a series of multicenter studies regarding treatment of bifurcation lesions. By 2005 there was limited systematic and adequately controlled results available on the optimal treatment of bifurcation lesions. At the founding meeting in Aare, Sweden in 2005, it was decided that the consecutive studies should lead to a study comparing treatment of unprotected left main coronary artery (LMCA) disease by PCI to treatment by coronary artery bypass grafting (CABG). This study was launched in 2009 as the Nordic-Baltic-British left main revascularization study (NOBLE).

The Nordic bifurcation studies

Design

The first four Nordic Bifurcation studies (not including NOBLE) all have the same basic study design. The purpose of the study design was to provide the strongest possible scientific base for addressing the hypothesis of each study. Randomization and low cross over rates are the prevailing concept in comparison of different treatments. The multicenter setting included both high and low volume centers, thereby ensuring the external validity of the results. A single study stent was chosen, the Cypher Select+ (Cordis, Johnson & Johnson, Miami Lakes, Fla. USA), which, at that time, was the best available drug-eluting stent (DES) [8] and to avoid the possible confounding impact of different kinds of DES.

Clinical endpoints

The primary endpoint was a clinical combined endpoint of 6-month major adverse cardiac events (MACE). The composite endpoint consisted of cardiac death, non-procedure related index lesion myocardial infarction (MI), target lesion revascularization (TLR) or definite stent thrombosis (ST) within 6 months. The primary endpoint assessment was scheduled before an angiographic follow-up at 8 months to avoid angiography driven target lesion revascularization influencing the clinical primary endpoint. The individual endpoints of MACE were reported as well. Index lesion myocardial infarction

Bifurcation Stenting, First Edition. Edited by Ron Waksman and John A. Ormiston.
© 2012 Blackwell Publishing Ltd. Published 2012 by Blackwell Publishing Ltd.

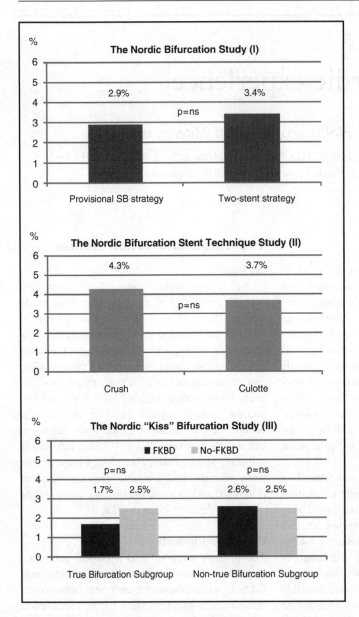

Figure 3.1 Primary endpoints of major adverse cardiac events (MACE) in the first six months. FKBD: final kissing balloon dilatation [4,5,7].

was assessed according to the current definitions and available biomarkers for myocardial injury. The complete definitions are reported in the main articles [4,5].

Although an important marker of procedure complexity and long-term outcome, index lesion MI was not included in the composite of MACE for two reasons: the significance of biomarker release concerning procedure related outcome is incompletely understood; and the interpretation of bio-marker release is problematic in a population with a high prevalence of non-ST elevation myocardial infarction (NSTEMI). This is supported by registry findings that only very substantial increases in biomarker release affects the prognosis [9], but is questioned by more recent findings that marker elevation above upper limit of normal is associated with increased risk of death [10]. All endpoints were adjudicated by independent endpoint committees.

Procedural endpoints

Important markers of procedural complexity are reported in the papers [4,5]. Contrast media has the potential to affect the renal function, especially in patients with kidney failure of different degrees. Fluoroscopy time is strongly related to radiation exposition for the patient and staff, and is an indicator of procedure time. Increased procedure time is mostly a health economic problem but also a marker of increased complexity of the procedure and is related to procedural success and treatment outcome.

Angiographic substudies

Angiographic follow-up at 8 months was performed to obtain detailed information on lesion characteristics. The substudies were predefined to be presented in the main papers along with the primary clinical endpoint to add information on specific lesion subsets and localization of stenoses at follow-up. Quantitative coronary analysis (QCA) was undertaken using pre-PCI, post-PCI and 8-month follow-up angiograms. The angiograms were analyzed using a software dedicated to bifurcating branches, QAngio XA 7.0 and later QAngio XA 7.2 (Medis Medical Imaging Systems, Leiden, The Netherlands)[11].

Approximately three-quarters of the patients in each study had a complete angiographic follow-up. The reason for not including all patients was the extremely long distance to interventional centers in the northern part of Norway, Sweden and Finland. Scientifically, it is important that the follow-up was scheduled at randomization and that there was a stratification on +/− angiographic follow-up in the randomization algorithm. Thus, angiographic follow-up was available in >90% of patients with planned angiographic follow up.

Angiographic segmentation

The bifurcation lesion was divided into three main segments: the proximal main vessel (MV), the distal MV, and the side branch (SB). The segmentation is important to integrate the step-down phenomenon in the lesion assessment and reference function. The reference function was individually constructed for each of the three segments and connected by a smooth transition in the bifurcation core area. Further, the MV was divided into proximal and distal MV. Otherwise, the minimal luminal diameter would be located too often in the distal MV due to the smaller reference diameter of the distal vessel [11]. The three vessel segments were divided into in-stent and edge segments. The edge segments comprised the first 5 mm adjacent to the stented area. The side branch (SB) analysis in the first two Nordic bifurcation studies was treatment specific. The size of the SB segment was dependent on the balloon edge or stent edge. If the SB was not treated, the first 5 mm was defined as both treated segment and edge segment. The SB analysis was simplified in the third Nordic bifurcation study by reporting only the results of the first 5 mm of the SB irrespective of the treatment. This was possible, because few patients received a SB stent.

Angiographic endpoints

Reference diameters at pre-PCI were used as baseline lesion characteristics. Minimal luminal diameter (MLD) and diameter stenosis (DS) % ((MLD/reference diameter)*100) was reported for each in-stent segment, edge segment and in the third Nordic-Baltic bifurcation study, for the ostial 5 mm of the SB. For each in-stent segment the lumen late loss was calculated.

The Nordic bifurcation study (I)

Randomized study on simple versus complex stenting of coronary artery bifurcation lesions

The first Nordic Bifurcation study was a comparison of stenting the main vessel and optional stenting of the SB versus stenting of both the main vessel and the SB in coronary bifurcation lesions. This first large randomized multicenter study of basic techniques for stenting bifurcation lesions using DES was performed by 28 centers in Norway, Sweden, Finland, Latvia and Denmark.

Background

At the beginning of the DES era, it was the general opinion that two-stent techniques were superior to the one-stent technique. Despite the fact that two-stent techniques were associated with increased procedure complexity [2], DES was believed to overcome the problems with the exceedingly high TLR rates of bare metal stents in these treatments [12].

Small-scale studies and clinical experience showed that stenting across a SB was feasible [13]. In a fraction of cases the SB would close or substantial residual SB stenosis persist, often as SB ostial pinching. It was also an experience that closure of especially smaller SBs might be clinically silent with little or no impact on ejection fraction. A strategy of stenting the MV and only stenting the SB in case of SB closure or impaired flow was proposed. This strategy is known and referred to as the provisional SB stenting strategy or the simple one-stent strategy. The expected advantages of the simple strategy were simpler and shorter procedures and that only one stent had to be deployed in the majority of cases reducing the risks associated with multiple stents and strut layers.

Aim
The aim of first Nordic Bifurcation study was to compare the simple one-stent strategy with a strategy of stenting both the MV and the SB.

Patients
A total of 413 patients were included in the main study and 307 of these had a prescheduled angiographic follow-up in the angiographic substudy. Patients were eligible for inclusion, if their bifurcation lesion was located in bifurcations with MV ≥ 2.5 mm and SB ≥ 2.0 mm. Patients with ST-elevation myocardial infarction and severely ill patients were not included.

Stenting techniques
The study lesion was pre-dilated and/or post-dilated at the discretion of the operator. Operators were instructed to avoid pre-dilatating MV areas not to be covered by stent.

The recommended treatment principles in the two treatment groups
The simple strategy comprised: (1) wiring both the MV and the SB, and (2) stenting the MV jailing the SB wire. If thrombolysis in myocardial infarction (TIMI) flow 3 was achieved, the procedure was terminated. If SB flow was impaired, balloon dilation was performed. If TIMI flow was 0 after balloon dilation a stent was inserted in the SB and final kissing balloon performed (FKBD).

The complex strategy comprised any two-stent technique at the operators discretion. FKBD was mandatory independent of the applied technique.

Results
The 6-month MACE rate was very low and similar for the two groups (complex 3.4% vs simple 2.9% (p = ns)) (Figure 3.1). Procedure related myocardial infarction could be evaluated in 279 patients where elevation of >3 times the upper limit of normal was seen in 18% of patients in the complex group versus 8% in the simple group (p = 0.011). No patients in the simple one-stent group had ST compared with one patient in the complex group. TLR rates were equally low (1.9%) in both groups. These excellent clinical results seem durable based on the reports of 14- [6] and 60-month outcome (not published).

Procedural characteristics
As expected, significant difference in indices of procedural complexity between the simple and the complex group was found. Procedure time was 62 ± 51 vs 76 ± 40 (p < 0.0001), fluoroscopy time 15 ± 9 vs 21 ± 10 (p < 0.0001) and contrast volume 233 ± 93 vs 283 ± 117 (p < 0.0001) in the simple and complex groups, respectively.

In the simple group, about one-third had FKBD and only 4.3% had a SB stent. Procedural success was 97%. In the complex group, 50% were treated by the crush technique, 21% by culotte, and 24% were treated by other two-stent techniques. In the complex group, 4% did not receive a SB stent and the procedural success was 94%.

Angiographic results
Angiographic follow-up after 8 months showed excellent results for both proximal and distal MV in both groups. Late lumen loss was very low in proximal MV (0.00 ± 0.55 vs 0.10 ± 0.60 (ns)) and in distal MV (0.04 ± 0.47 vs 0.10 ± 0.50 (ns)) for the simple and complex groups respectively. These results were also reflected in very low and equal rates of binary restenosis (≥50% DS) for the entire main vessel.

Side branch results (Figure 3.2) showed that the residual SB stenosis in the simple one-stent group improved slightly as assessed by average diameter stenosis (34 ± 23% post-PCI to 31 ± 22% at

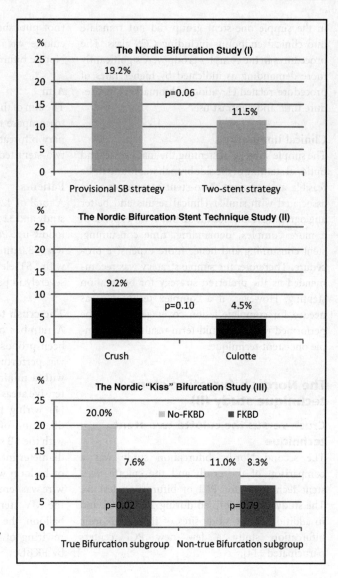

Figure 3.2 Eight-month angiographic binary restenosis; diameter stenosis ≥50%. FKBD: final kissing balloon dilatation [4,5,7].

follow-up (FU)) and by a negative late lumen loss at −0.04 ± 0.52 mm. In the complex group, a significant better result was found with an average diameter stenosis at FU of 24 ± 21% but with a significantly increased late lumen loss (0.20 ± 0.57) as compared to the simple one-stent group. These results reflect that SB stenoses after MV stenting often improve over time. Stented SBs, however, have higher late lumen loss and higher rate of restenosis than stented MVs. These results may reflect late stent recoil and the problems of multiple stent layers in the SB ostium and inability to re-

cross a jailed SB for FKBD in some patients causing suboptimal results.

The differences in SB results could not be detected in the clinical results where 9.2% in the simple group vs 8.6% in the complex group had Canadian Cardiovascular Society (CCS) score ≥2 at 6-month FU.

Conclusion
No differences were found in 6-months clinical outcome between the two strategies. The higher average SB diameter stenosis at angiographic FU

in the simple one-stent group did not translate into clinical endpoints including CCS class. The procedures in the complex group were significantly more demanding as indicated by higher rates of procedure-related elevation of biomarkers, procedure time and contrast use.

Clinical implications

The simple strategy of stenting the main vessel and optional stenting of the side branch was found to be feasible and efficient. Two-stent techniques were associated with similar clinical results and better angiographic results for the SB but at the expense of a more complex, demanding, time consuming, stent consuming and hence more expensive procedure. Therefore, the simple strategy was recommended as the preferred strategy for bifurcation stenting. However, if a complex technique was needed for complete lesion coverage it could be performed with same mid-term results as the simple one-stent technique.

The Nordic bifurcation stent technique study (II)

Crush versus the culotte two-stent technique

The second Nordic bifurcation study was a comparison of the crush and the culotte two-stent techniques for PCI of bifurcation lesions. The study was performed during 2005–2008 and in addition to the study sites of the first Nordic bifurcation study a few new PCI centers participated [14].

Background

Various two-stent techniques for bifurcation lesions were proposed and to some degree evaluated in bench models and *in vivo*. Expert and scientific momentum pointed to the crush [15,16] and the culotte [17] techniques for complete lesion coverage [4] including the proximal part of the SB ostium, which was often left uncovered using the T-technique [18,19]. Experiences with the crush and culotte techniques were reported in a number of smaller series but no clear picture of one prevailing technique had been established. The two techniques were used at the operators discretion in the first Nordic bifurcation study with comparable results

(not published). The study comparing crush and culotte was initiated before the results of the first Nordic bifurcation study were known.

Aim

The aim of the second Nordic bifurcation study was to compare the outcome after treatment of coronary bifurcation lesions by the crush and culotte two-stent techniques.

Patients

A total of 424 patients were included in the main study and 324 of these had a complete angiographic follow-up. Patients were eligible, if MV diameter was ≥ 3.0 mm and SB diameter ≥ 2.5 mm. Patients with ST-elevation myocardial infarction and severely ill patients were not included.

The crush technique

A number of variations of this technique have been proposed [15,20–22]. The crush technique was performed according to Colombo *et al.* [15] with a minimal crush modification to avoid extensive areas of multiple layers of stent struts [21]: (1) wiring the MV and SB; (2) optional predilatation of MV and/or SB; (3) stenting of SB with the SB stent protruding through half the MV diameter into the MV where an un-inflated stent or balloon was placed; (4) SB stent balloon and wire was removed; (5) the SB stent was crushed by the MV stent or balloon; (6) when crushed by balloon the MV stent was deployed; and (7) rewiring of the double jailed SB and finalizing by FKBD.

The culotte technique

The culotte two-stent technique was performed as proposed by Chevalier *et al.* [17]. The MV first strategy was chosen to ensure SB patency. The procedure was as follows: (1) wiring the MV and SB; (2) optional predilatation of MV and/or SB; (3) stenting of the MV; (4) rewiring of the jailed SB through MV stent; (5) optional predilation of SB ostium for opening of stent struts; (6) stenting of SB through MV stent, the proximal end of SB stent positioned in the proximal MV (7) rewiring of the jailed MB; (8) optional predilation of the ostium of the distal MV; and (9) finalizing with FKBD.

Results

The 6-month MACE rates were 4.3% for crush vs 3.7% for culotte (ns) (Figure 3.1). These low rates were comparable to the result of the complex group in the first Nordic Bifurcation study (3.4%). No differences were found in any of the individual MACE components or procedural markers of procedural complexity. The crush technique was however associated with higher percentage of procedure-related increase in biomarkers of myocardial damage as compared with the culotte technique.

Procedural characteristics

A marked difference was found in the success of performing FKBD. This important step in a two-stent bifurcation treatment [23] was carried out in 85% after crush vs 92% (p = 0.03) of patients after culotte. However, no difference between crush and culotte in procedural success (residual stenosis <30% and TIMI flow III in MV and SB at the end of index procedure) was found. Other markers of procedural complexity; procedure time, fluoroscopy time and use of contrast volume showed no difference between the two two-stent techniques and compared well to results of the complex group in the first Nordic Bifurcation study.

Angiographic results

No differences in angiographic outcome were detected for both the proximal and distal MV. Lumen late loss was very low and rates of binary restenosis were below 2%. In the SB the LLL was similar and comparable to the results obtained in the complex group in the first Nordic bifurcation study. In-stent SB binary restenosis was found in 9.8% after crush stenting vs 3.8% after culotte stenting (p = 0.04%) (Figure 3.2) but the difference was insignificant in the entire in-segment bifurcation lesion; crush 12.1% vs culotte 6.6% (p = 0.1).

Conclusion

The crush and the culotte two-stent techniques were associated with equal and low rates of 6-month MACE. The trend of higher rate of 8-month SB binary restenosis in the crush group was not detectable in clinical endpoints (including CCS class). Procedural markers of complexity showed no differences, except that FKBD could be performed in more cases in the culotte group. The larger challenges of performing FKBD in crush might be explained by the difficulty of rewiring the SB and advancing a balloon through the two strut layers jailing the SB ostium.

Clinical implications

The simple one-stent strategy is the preferred strategy in PCI of bifurcation lesions. The crush and the culotte two-stent techniques can both be used with excellent and similar short- and midterm results when complete coverage of a bifurcation lesion is needed.

The Nordic-Baltic bifurcation study (III)

Final kissing balloon dilatation in simple stenting of bifurcation lesions

After establishing the simple one-stent strategy as the preferred strategy for PCI of most coronary bifurcation lesions the next question was; how simple should the simple strategy be? The debated step was the FKBD, which was known to have pros and cons.

Background

It has been suggested that opening up the jailed SB ostium by balloon dilatation or FKBD might improve the acute SB result as well as midterm outcome [24]. Further, advantages of FKBD might include better strut apposition at the SB ostium and facilitate future SB access [18,25]. Disadvantages might be a more complex and demanding procedure and SB dilatation without subsequent stent coverage possibly inducing neointimal growth. Furthermore, FKBD might distort the proximal main vessel and necessitate a subsequent post-dilatation of the proximal MV.

Aim

The aim was to settle if the simple one-stent strategy should always be finalized by a kissing balloon dilatation [7].

Patients

A total of 477 patients were included in study and 326 of the patients had complete follow-up in the angiographic substudy. The diameters of the bifurcating vessels had to be MV ≥2.5 mm and SB

≥2.25 mm. Patients with ST-elevation myocardial infarction and severely ill patients were not included.

Procedure

The study lesion was predilated at the discretion of the operator. Operators were instructed to avoid predilatation of MV areas not to be covered by stent. The procedural algorithm was as follows: (1) wiring of both MV and SB; (2) optional predilatation of stenosed areas of the MV; (3) optional therapeutically dilatation (using adequately sized balloon or cutting balloon) of significant SB stenoses; (4) followed by MV stenting, jailing the SB wire; And (5) if there was TIMI 3 flow in the SB after MV stenting, the patient was randomized to +/− FKBD. If the patient was randomized to the no-FKBD group, the procedure was terminated, even if server ostial pinching was present. In the FKBD-group, the SB was re-wired through the MV stent, and simultaneous FKBD performed. In case of SB TIMI flow <3 after FKBD, a stent was deployed in the SB.

Results

The primary endpoint of 6-month MACE occurred in 2.1% in the FKBD arm vs 2.5% (p = 1.00) in the no-FKBD arm. Procedure related myocardial infarction could be evaluated in 350 patients and an increase of >3 times the upper limit of normal was seen in 6.3% of patients in both study groups. One patient in both groups experienced an ST. TLR rates were equally low; 1.3% vs 1.7% (p = 1.00) after FKBD and no-FKBD, respectively.

Angiographic results

In the MV, restenosis occurred in 3.1% and 2.5% (p = 0.68) in the FKBD and no-FKBD groups, respectively. In the SB segment, the rates were 7.9% vs 15.4% (p = 0.039). At follow-up no patients in the FKBD group had a ≥75% diameter SB binary (re)stenosis as compared to four patients (2.5%) in the no-FKBD group (p = 0.06). MV and SB late lumen loss were similar for the treatment groups.

True and non-true bifurcation subgroups

Clinical endpoint rates in true and non-true bifurcation lesions were low and similar (Figure 3.1).

Hence, possible differences in the clinical outcome between the two treatment groups were not detectable in patients with and without a true bifurcation lesion. In the true bifurcation lesion subgroup, FKBD reduced SB (re)-stenosis significantly as compared with no-FKBD (Figure 3.2). In the subgroup of non-true bifurcation lesions, no difference in clinical or angiographic outcome between FKBD and no-FKBD was found.

Procedural characteristics

The markers of higher procedural complexity were significantly influenced, when FKBD was added to the procedure. Procedure time was 61 ± 28 vs 47 ± 22 (p < 0.0001), fluoroscopy time 16 ± 12 vs 11 ± 10 (p < 0.0001) and contrast volume 235 ± 97 vs 200 ± 92 in the FKBD and no-FKBD group respectively.

In the no-FKBD group 1.7% had SB post dilatation or FKBD and no one was stented. In the FKBD group FKBD was performed in 97.1% of cases and 1.3% had a SB stent. Difficulties in SB rewiring was the dominant reason for lack of success in the few cases, where FKBD was not performed.

Conclusion

Excellent and similar midterm results were achieved whether FKBD was performed or not. However, the superior SB results in true bifurcation lesions after FKBD as compared to no-FKBD might over time become clinical relevant and justify the more complex FKBD procedure in this subgroup.

Clinical implications

The simple stenting technique nearly halved the number of stents used to treat bifurcation lesions and reduced procedure time, fluoroscopy time and use of contrast media in comparison to the two-stent strategy [4]. The third Nordic bifurcation study showed that these markers of procedural complexity could be further reduced by MV stenting without FKBD. Therefore, midterm results in the third and the first Nordic Bifurcation study seem to justify the simple MV vessel stenting strategy without FKBD, at least in bifurcation lesion with no significant SB stenosis. If FKBD is needed, the resulting distortion of the proximal MV apparently does not induce restenosis.

The Nordic bifurcation study (IV)

Randomized study on simple versus complex stenting of coronary artery bifurcation lesions with significant side branches

After the first Nordic bifurcation study the question was raised whether the results were applicable to true bifurcation lesions with significant lesion in large SBs. It is a widespread expert opinion that this subset of bifurcation lesions should be treated using two-stent stent techniques.

The fourth Nordic bifurcation study is aimed at comparing a simple one-stent strategy with a two-stent strategy (with preference for the culotte technique) for true bifurcation lesions with server lesions in large SBs.

The study setup is like the previous Nordic Bifurcation studies featuring 6-month clinical and 8-month angiographic follow-up. An optical coherence tomography single center substudy was added to provide further insight in acute and follow-up results at stent strut level. Patients are eligible for inclusion if the true bifurcation lesion is located in vessels measuring $MV \geq 3.0$ mm and $SB \geq 2.75$ mm. Left main bifurcation lesions may be included in the study

The Nordic-Baltic-British left main revascularisation study (NOBLE)

This randomized multicenter comparison of PCI and CABG for treatment of unprotected left main coronary artery (LMCA) disease is performed in centres in the Nordic and Baltic countries plus centres in United Kingdom. Inclusion of the estimated 1200 patients was initiated in 2009.

Background

CABG has been the preferred treatment for unprotected LMCA disease. After introduction of DES, a number of registry studies [26–28] have found no difference in outcome of unprotected LMCA disease treated with PCI or CABG. Actually, the Korean Main Compare [29] registry pointed to a small advantage for PCI as compared to CABG.

The "Synergy between percutaneous coronary intervention with TAXUS and cardiac surgery (SYNTAX) trial" [30] was a large scale study comparing PCI with CABG in patients with multivessel diease with or without LM affection. LM patients were included in a predefined substudy; "Outcomes in patients with de novo left main disease treated with either percutaneous coronary intervention using paclitaxel-eluting stents or coronary artery bypass graft treatment in the SYNTAX trial" (SYNTAX LMCA) [31]. The substudy included 705 patients with left main disease. PCI was not non-inferior to CABG in the main study assessed by the one-year rate of MACCE (death, myocardial infarction, stroke and new revascularization). The difference made the results of the LMCA substudy difficult to interpret, although the rate of MACCE was similar for PCI and CABG in this subset of patients. The one-year rate of revascularisation was higher for PCI (11.8%) as compared with CABG (6.5% ($p = 0.02$)) but CABG was associated with a significantly higher number of strokes (0.3% vs 2.7% (0.009)) compared to PCI.

The limitations of SYNTAX LMCA were the substudy design and the use of a paclitaxcel eluting stent, which is associated with increased risk of late stent thrombosis, myocardial infarction and death [32–34]

The NOBLE study was designed to overcome these limitations by a dedicated LM study design and use of a second generation DES.

Aim

The aim of the NOBLE study is to compare clinical outcome after revascularization of unprotected LM disease by either PCI or CABG.

Study design

NOBLE is a randomized multicenter trial with an open labelled design. Patients should be eligible for treatment by CABG and by PCI, have a significant LMCA lesion and a maximum of three additional simple lesions. Additional complex lesions are exclusion criteria. The primary endpoint is the combined endpoint of death, stroke, non-index procedure related MI and new revascularization (PCI or CABG) within 2 years.

Perspective

PCI of unprotected LMCA disease is established as an alternative to CABG. The mixed results in previous trials can be explained by various shortcomings in study designs. NOBLE is designed to establish, if state of the art PCI is equivalent to CABG for patients with LM disease

Patient level meta-analysis collaboration

Several meta-analyses of the six largest RCTs comparing simple and complex stenting techniques have been published [35–37] providing a uniform result comparable to the conclusion of the first Nordic bifurcation study. Limited new information has emerged from these meta-analyses based on published data.

Simple vs complex strategies

The two largest multicenter RCTs comparing simple and complex stenting techniques for coronary bifurcation lesions are the British bifurcation coronary – old new and evolving strategies (BBC ONE) [38] and the Nordic bifurcation study (I) [4]. To provide further insight into the differences between the two strategies for various subgroups, a patient level meta-analysis was performed and the results were presented at the EuroPCR 2010.

Crush vs culotte

Another patient level meta-analysis comparing patients treated with the crush or the culotte techniques in BBC ONE [38] and in the first two Nordic Bifurcation studies [4,5] was also presented at EuroPCR 2010. These meta-analyses provide new information on outcomes for lesion specific subgroups.

Recommended strategies for treatment of bifurcation lesions

The simple one-stent strategy is the preferred strategy for most bifurcation lesions. After stenting of the MV, FKBD should be performed in true bifurcation lesions. In case of servere ostial pinching and/or TIMI flow <3 after MV stenting, FKBD should be performed independent of SB disease. The SB should be stented if TIMI flow <3 despite FKBD using the provisional T- or the culotte technique. Recommendations to use a simple one-stent strategy or a complex two-stent technique in true bifurcation lesions with a significant

lesion in a large SB await the results from the fourth Nordic bifurcation study.

Future studies from the Nordic PCI study group

The studies from the Nordic PCI study group have focused on treatment of left main and bifurcation lesions. Future studies from this group will focus on different stent platforms and the use of dedicated bifurcation stents. When biodegradable stents will be commercially available, these stents may have the potential of changing completely existing strategies and recommendations for bifurcation lesion treatment.

Very low clinical event rates have been characteristic for the Nordic bifurcation studies and for other recently published RCT using DES in treatment of coronary bifurcation lesions. Therefore, it may be relevant to shift the focus from a primary clinical endpoint to surrogate endpoints like imaging or physiological evaluation.

Future perspectives

The Nordic PCI study group organization has proven efficient in performing large-scale multicenter studies on complex PCI techniques. Although a decline in the incidence of symptomatic atherosclerotic coronary heart disease is expected in a portion of the developed countries, the world wide increase in life expectancy, in population size, but also in the incidence of diabetes mellitus will cause the need for a continuous pursue of optimal PCI techniques with respect to clinical outcome and healthcare costs.

In a clinical perspective, bifurcation lesions used to be associated with unfavourable outcome and CABG was often advocated in these patients. The excellent midterm clinical results of modern bifurcation treatment using DES make catheter based interventions first choice in most patients with coronary bifurcation lesions.

References

1 Al Suwaidi J, Yeh W, Cohen HA, Detre KM, Williams DO, Holmes DR, Jr. Immediate and one-year outcome in patients with coronary bifurcation lesions in the

modern era (NHLBI dynamic registry). Am J Cardiol 2001;87:1139–44.

2 Yamashita T, Nishida T, Adamian MG, Briguori C, Vaghetti M, Corvaja N, Albiero R, Finci L, Di MC, Tobis JM, Colombo A. Bifurcation lesions: two stents versus one stent – immediate and follow-up results. J Am Coll Cardiol 2000;35:1145–51.

3 Meier B, Gruentzig AR, King SB, III, Douglas JS, Jr., Hollman J, Ischinger T, Aueron F, Galan K. Risk of side branch occlusion during coronary angioplasty. Am J Cardiol 1984;53:10–14.

4 Steigen TK, Maeng M, Wiseth R, Erglis A, Kumsars I, Narbute I, Gunnes P, Mannsverk J, Meyerdierks O, Rotevatn S, Niemela M, Kervinen K, Jensen JS, Galloe A, Nikus K, Vikman S, Ravkilde J, James S, Aaroe J, Ylitalo A, Helqvist S, Sjogren I, Thayssen P, Virtanen K, Puhakka M, Airaksinen J, Lassen JF, Thuesen L. Randomized study on simple versus complex stenting of coronary artery bifurcation lesions: the Nordic bifurcation study. Circulation 2006;114:1955–61.

5 Erglis A, Kumsars I, Niemela M, Kervinen K, Maeng M, Lassen JF, Gunnes P, Stavnes S, Jensen JS, Galloe A, Narbute I, Sondore D, Mäkikallio T, Ylitalo A, Christiansen EH, Ravkilde J, Steigen TK, Mannsverk J, Thayssen P, Hansen KN, Syvänne M, Helqvist S, Kjell N, Wiseth R, Aaroe J, Puhakka M, Thuesen L. Randomized comparison of coronary bifurcation stenting with the crush versus the culotte technique using sirolimus eluting stents. Circ Cardiovasc Intervent 2009;2:27–34.

6 Jensen JS, Galloe A, Lassen JF, Erglis A, Kumsars I, Steigen TK, Wiseth R, Narbute I, Gunnes P, Mannsverk J, Meyerdierks O, Rotevatn S, Niemela M, Kervinen K, Nikus K, Vikman S, Ravkilde J, James S, Aaroe J, Ylitalo A, Helqvist S, Sjogren I, Thayssen P, Virtanen K, Puhakka M, Airaksinen J, Thuesen L. Safety in simple versus complex stenting of coronary artery bifurcation lesions. The nordic bifurcation study 14-month follow-up results. EuroIntervention 2008;4:229–33.

7 Niemela M, Kervinen K, Erglis A, Holm NR, Maeng M, Christiansen EH, Kumsars I, Jegere S, Dombrovskis A, Gunnes P, Stavnes S, Steigen TK, Trovik T, Eskola M, Vikman S, Romppanen H, Makikallio T, Hansen KN, Thayssen P, Aberge L, Jensen LO, Hervold A, Airaksinen J, Pietila M, Frobert O, Kellerth T, Ravkilde J, Aaroe J, Jensen JS, Helqvist S, Sjogren I, James S, Miettinen H, Lassen JF, Thuesen L. Randomized comparison of final kissing balloon dilatation versus no final kissing balloon dilatation in patients with coronary bifurcation lesions treated with main vessel stenting: the Nordic-Baltic Bifurcation Study III. Circulation 2011;123:79–86.

8 Galloe AM, Thuesen L, Kelbaek H, Thayssen P, Rasmussen K, Hansen PR, Bligaard N, Saunamaki K,

Junker A, Aaroe J, Abildgaard U, Ravkilde J, Engstrom T, Jensen JS, Andersen HR, Botker HE, Galatius S, Kristensen SD, Madsen JK, Krusell LR, Abildstrom SZ, Stephansen GB, Lassen JF. Comparison of paclitaxel- and sirolimus-eluting stents in everyday clinical practice: the SORT OUT II randomized trial. JAMA 2008;299:409–16.

9 Stone GW, Mehran R, Dangas G, Lansky AJ, Kornowski R, Leon MB. Differential impact on survival of electrocardiographic Q-wave versus enzymatic myocardial infarction after percutaneous intervention: a device-specific analysis of 7147 patients. Circulation 2001;104:642–7.

10 Andron M, Stables RH, Egred M, Alahmar AE, Shaw MA, Roberts E, Albouaini K, Grayson AD, Perry RA, Palmer ND. Impact of periprocedural creatine kinase-MB isoenzyme release on long-term mortality in contemporary percutaneous coronary intervention. J Invasive Cardiol 2008;20:108–12.

11 Lansky A, Tuinenburg J, Costa M, Maeng M, Koning G, Popma J, Cristea E, Gavit L, Costa R, Rares A, Van Es GA, Lefevre T, Reiber H, Louvard Y, Morice MC. Quantitative angiographic methods for bifurcation lesions: a consensus statement from the European Bifurcation Group. Catheter Cardiovasc Interv 2009;73:258–66.

12 Kastrati A, Mehilli J, Pache J, Kaiser C, Valgimigli M, Kelbaek H, Menichelli M, Sabate M, Suttorp MJ, Baumgart D, Seyfarth M, Pfisterer ME, Schomig A. Analysis of 14 trials comparing sirolimus-eluting stents with bare-metal stents. N Engl J Med 2007;356:1030–9.

13 Pan M, de Lezo JS, Medina A, Romero M, Segura J, Pavlovic D, Delgado A, Ojeda S, Melian F, Herrador J, Urena I, Burgos L. Rapamycin-eluting stents for the treatment of bifurcated coronary lesions: a randomized comparison of a simple versus complex strategy. Am Heart J 2004;148:857–64.

14 Erglis A, Kumsars I, Niemela M, Kervinen K, Maeng M, Lassen JF, Gunnes P, Stavnes S, Jensen JS, Galloe A, Narbute I, Sondore D, Makikallio T, Ylitalo K, Christiansen EH, Ravkilde J, Steigen TK, Mannsverk J, Thayssen P, Hansen KN, Syvanne M, Helqvist S, Kjell N, Wiseth R, Aaroe J, Puhakka M, Thuesen L. Randomized comparison of coronary bifurcation stenting with the crush versus the culotte technique using sirolimus eluting stents: the Nordic stent technique study. Circ Cardiovasc Interv 2009;2:27–34.

15 Colombo A, Stankovic G, Orlic D, Corvaja N, Liistro F, Airoldi F, Chieffo A, Spanos V, Montorfano M, Di Mario C. Modified T-stenting technique with crushing for bifurcation lesions: immediate results and 30-day outcome. Catheter Cardiovasc Interv 2003;60:145–51.

16 Hoye A, Iakovou I, Ge L, Van Mieghem CA, Ong AT, Cosgrave J, Sangiorgi GM, Airoldi F, Montorfano M, Michev I, Chieffo A, Carlino M, Corvaja N, Aoki J,

Rodriguez Granillo GA, Valgimigli M, Sianos G, van der Giessen WJ, de Feyter PJ, van Domburg RT, Serruys PW, Colombo A. Long-term outcomes after stenting of bifurcation lesions with the "rush" technique: predictors of an adverse outcome. J Am Coll Cardiol 2006;47:1949–58.

17 Chevalier B, Glatt B, Royer T, Guyon P. Placement of coronary stents in bifurcation lesions by the "culotte" technique. Am J Cardiol 1998;82:943–9.

18 Ormiston JA, Webster MW, El Jack S, Ruygrok PN, Stewart JT, Scott D, Currie E, Panther MJ, Shaw B, O'Shaughnessy B. Drug-eluting stents for coronary bifurcations: bench testing of provisional side-branch strategies. Catheter Cardiovasc Interv 2006;67:49–55.

19 Burzotta F, Gwon HC, Hahn JY, Romagnoli E, Choi JH, Trani C, Colombo A. Modified T-stenting with intentional protrusion of the side-branch stent within the main vessel stent to ensure ostial coverage and facilitate final kissing balloon: the T-stenting and small protrusion technique (TAP-stenting). Report of bench testing and first clinical Italian-Korean two-centre experience. Catheter Cardiovasc Interv 2007;70:75–82.

20 Chen SL, Zhang JJ, Ye F, Chen YD, Patel T, Kawajiri K, Lee M, Kwan TW, Mintz G, Tan HC. Study comparing the double kissing (DK) crush with classical crush for the treatment of coronary bifurcation lesions: the DKCRUSH-1 Bifurcation Study with drug-eluting stents. Eur J Clin Invest 2008;38:361–71.

21 Galassi AR, Colombo A, Buchbinder M, Grasso C, Tomasello SD, Ussia GP, Tamburino C. Long-term outcomes of bifurcation lesions after implantation of drug-eluting stents with the "mini-crush technique". Catheter Cardiovasc Interv 2007;69:976–83.

22 Ormiston JA, Currie E, Webster MW, Kay P, Ruygrok PN, Stewart JT, Padgett RC, Panther MJ. Drug-eluting stents for coronary bifurcations: insights into the crush technique. Catheter Cardiovasc 2004; Interv 63:332–6.

23 Ge L, Airoldi F, Iakovou I, Cosgrave J, Michev I, Sangiorgi GM, Montorfano M, Chieffo A, Carlino M, Corvaja N, Colombo A. Clinical and angiographic outcome after implantation of drug-eluting stents in bifurcation lesions with the crush stent technique: importance of final kissing balloon post-dilation. J Am Coll Cardiol 2005;46:613–20.

24 Korn HV, Yu J, Ohlow MA, Huegl B, Schulte W, Wagner A, Wassmer G, Gruene S, Petek O, Lauer B. Interventional therapy of bifurcation lesions: a TIMI flow-guided concept to treat side branches in bifurcation lesions – a prospective randomized clinical study (Thueringer bifurcation study, THUEBIS study as pilot trial). Circ Cardiovasc Interv 2009;2:535–42.

25 Ferenc M, Gick M, Kienzle RP, Bestehorn HP, Werner KD, Comberg T, Kuebler P, Buttner HJ, Neumann FJ. Randomized trial on routine vs. provisional T-stenting in the treatment of de novo coronary bifurcation lesions. Eur Heart J 2008;29:2859–67.

26 Makikallio TH, Niemela M, Kervinen K, Jokinen V, Laukkanen J, Ylitalo I, Tulppo MP, Juvonen J, Huikuri HV. Coronary angioplasty in drug eluting stent era for the treatment of unprotected left main stenosis compared to coronary artery bypass grafting. Ann Med 2008;40:437–43.

27 Chieffo A, Morici N, Maisano F, Bonizzoni E, Cosgrave J, Montorfano M, Airoldi F, Carlino M, Michev I, Melzi G, Sangiorgi G, Alfieri O, Colombo A. Percutaneous treatment with drug-eluting stent implantation versus bypass surgery for unprotected left main stenosis: a single-center experience. Circulation 2006;113:2542–7.

28 Lee MS, Kapoor N, Jamal F, Czer L, Aragon J, Forrester J, Kar S, Dohad S, Kass R, Eigler N, Trento A, Shah PK, Makkar RR. Comparison of coronary artery bypass surgery with percutaneous coronary intervention with drug-eluting stents for unprotected left main coronary artery disease. J Am Coll Cardiol 2006;47:864–70.

29 Seung KB, Park DW, Kim YH, Lee SW, Lee CW, Hong MK, Park SW, Yun SC, Gwon HC, Jeong MH, Jang Y, Kim HS, Kim PJ, Seong IW, Park HS, Ahn T, Chae IH, Tahk SJ, Chung WS, Park SJ. Stents versus coronary-artery bypass grafting for left main coronary artery disease. N Engl J Med 2008;358:1781–92.

30 Serruys PW, Morice MC, Kappetein AP, Colombo A, Holmes DR, Mack MJ, Stahle E, Feldman TE, van den Brand M, Bass EJ, Van DN, Leadley K, Dawkins KD, Mohr FW. Percutaneous coronary intervention versus coronary-artery bypass grafting for severe coronary artery disease. N Engl J Med 2009;360:961–72.

31 Morice MC, Serruys PW, Kappetein AP, Feldman TE, Stahle E, Colombo A, Mack MJ, Holmes DR, Torracca L, Van Es GA, Leadley K, Dawkins KD, Mohr F. Outcomes in patients with de novo left main disease treated with either percutaneous coronary intervention using paclitaxel-eluting stents or coronary artery bypass graft treatment in the Synergy Between Percutaneous Coronary Intervention with TAXUS and Cardiac Surgery (SYNTAX) trial. Circulation 2010;121:2645–53.

32 Kaltoft A, Jensen LO, Maeng M, Tilsted HH, Thayssen P, Bottcher M, Lassen JF, Krusell LR, Rasmussen K, Hansen KN, Pedersen L, Johnsen SP, Soerensen HT, Thuesen L. Two-year clinical outcomes after implantation of coronary sirolimus- and paclitaxel-eluting stents and bare metal stents in western Denmark. J Am Coll Cardiol 2008;53:658–64.

33 Daemen J, Kukreja N, van Twisk PH, Onuma Y, de Jaegere PP, van DR, Serruys PW. Four-year clinical follow-up of the rapamycin-eluting stent evaluated at Rotterdam Cardiology Hospital registry. Am J Cardiol 2008;101:1105–11.

34 Stettler C, Wandel S, Allemann S, Kastrati A, Morice MC, Schomig A, Pfisterer ME, Stone GW, Leon MB, de Lezo JS, Goy JJ, Park SJ, Sabate M, Suttorp MJ, Kelbaek H, Spaulding C, Menichelli M, Vermeersch P, Dirksen MT, Cervinka P, Petronio AS, Nordmann AJ, Diem P, Meier B, Zwahlen M, Reichenbach S, Trelle S, Windecker S, Juni P. Outcomes associated with drug-eluting and bare-metal stents: a collaborative network meta-analysis. Lancet 2007;370:937–48.

35 Katritsis DG, Siontis GC, Ioannidis JP. Double versus single stenting for coronary bifurcation lesions: a meta-analysis. Circ Cardiovasc Interv 2009;2:409–15.

36 Zhang F, Dong L, Ge J. Simple versus complex stenting strategy for coronary artery bifurcation lesions in the drug-eluting stent era: a meta-analysis of randomised trials. Heart 2009;95:1676–81.

37 Hakeem A, Khan FM, Bhatti S, Samad Z, Effat MA, Eckman MH, Helmy T. Provisional vs. complex stenting strategy for coronary bifurcation lesions: meta-analysis of randomized trials. J Invasive Cardiol 2009;21:589–95.

38 Hildick-Smith D, de Belder AJ, Cooter N, Curzen NP, Clayton TC, Oldroyd KG, Bennett L, Holmberg S, Cotton JM, Glennon PE, Thomas MR, Maccarthy PA, Baumbach A, Mulvihill NT, Henderson RA, Redwood SR, Starkey IR, Stables RH. Randomized trial of simple versus complex drug-eluting stenting for bifurcation lesions: the British Bifurcation Coronary Study: old, new, and evolving strategies. Circulation 2010;121:1235–43.

CHAPTER 4

Crush and mini-crush

Alfredo R. Galassi, MD, FACC, FESC, FSCAI,

Salvatore Davide Tomasello, MD, PhD,

Luca Costanzo, MD *and Giombattista Barrano,* MD

Department of Internal Medicine and Systemic Disease, Catheterization Laboratory and Cardiovascular
Interventional Unit, Cannizzaro Hospital, University of Catania, Catania, Italy

The decision to implant two stents from the beginning of the procedure, in a "intention to treat" fashion, depends on various factors such as the size of the side branch and the respective extension of myocardium supplied by it. Indeeed, data from a swine heart model, indicates a quantitative relationship between both side branch diameter and length, and the size of any resulting myocardial infarction [1]. In addition, it is important to evaluate if the disease involves only the ostium of the side branch or it extends into the proximal segment of the vessel; this last condition will more likely demand for a second stent as suggested by Colombo (Figure 4.1) [2]. In this regards, an important distinction is also to divide bifurcation into, true bifurcation and false bifurcation. According to the Medina classification [3] they are, respectively, *true bifurcation:* Medina 1.1.1, 1.0.1, 0.1.1; *false bifurcation:* Medina 1.1.0, 1.0.0, 0.1.0, 0.0.1. (Figure 4.2).

The crush technique

The crush technique was originally introduced by Antonio Colombo as a 2-stent technique aimed to optimize side branch ostium scaffolding and drug delivery to the side branch, common sites of stent restenosis [5,6]. According to the consensus of the European Bifurcation Club and the MADS classification [7] the classical crush technique is included in the "S" family bifurcation, characterized by the deployment of the side branch stent first. However, a modification of the crush technique was included in "A" family, in which the main vessel stent is implanted first allowing provisional (elective) deployment of the side branch stent, "the provisional crush". In such a condition an internal crush (formerly known as reversed crush) is going to be performed (8–9).

The crush technique could determine some procedural benefits in comparison with T-stenting technique. Indeed, in the T-stenting technique the positioning of the side branch stent is difficult to perform precisely under fluoroscopic imaging. Therefore, the side branch stent often either does not cover fully the side branch ostium, or the stent struts protrude excessively into the main vessel, making subsequent deployment of a stent within the main vessel difficult or even impossible; this may prolong and complicate the whole PCI procedure.

The "original and standard" crush technique is presented in Figure 4.3 [5]. Both branches are wired and alternatively dilated or in a kissing fashion technique (A). A first stent is advanced into the side branch but not expanded and a second stent is advanced into the main branch to fully cover the bifurcation (B). The side-branch stent is retracted into the main branch for 2–3 mm. The proximal marker of the side-branch stent must be situated in the main branch at a distance of few millimeters

Bifurcation Stenting, First Edition. Edited by Ron Waksman and John A. Ormiston.
© 2012 Blackwell Publishing Ltd. Published 2012 by Blackwell Publishing Ltd.

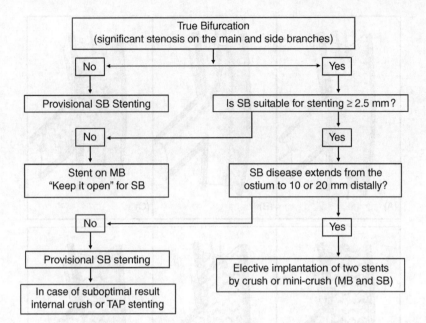

Figure 4.1 Bifurcation treatment algorithm. This approach to bifurcation stenting is based on morphologic assessment of atherothrombotic disease, and the size of the side branch (diameter and length). MB = main branch; SB = side branch. (Adapted from Latib and Colombo [4]). Reprinted from JACC: Cardiovascular Interventions; Bifurcation Disease: What Do We Know, What Should We Do?; Azeem Latib, Antonio Colombo; Vol 1; 3; 2008 with permission from Elsevier.

(4–5 mm) proximally to the carina of the bifurcation, in a similar fashion to the culottes technique [10]. At the same time, it is important to position correctly the stent in the main branch covering the entire lesion and ensuring that it is in the appropriate position, because following expansion of the stent in the side branch, it could be difficult to move and reposition the stent in the main branch in any direction. When the side-branch stent is appropriately positioned the balloon is inflated and the stent is deployed (C). After stent implantation, the proximal part of this stent will clearly protrude in the main vessel. The delivery balloon is removed from the side branch and a contrast injection is performed to ensure that no distal dissection is present and no additional stents are needed in the side branch. It is possible at this time to advance another stent in the side branch in

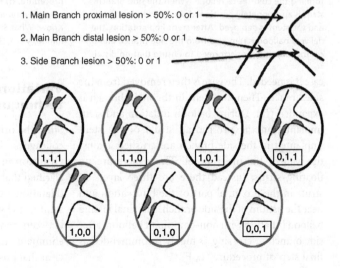

Figure 4.2 Medina Classification. In this classification, a binary value (1,0) is given to each of the 3 components of a bifurcation (main branch proximal, main branch distal, and the side branch) according to whether each of these segments is compromised (1) or not (0). Black circles = true bifurcations; Grey circles = false bifurcations. Reprinted from JACC: Cardiovascular Interventions; Bifurcation Disease: What Do We Know, What Should We Do?; Azeem Latib, Antonio Colombo; Vol 1; 3; 2008 with permission from Elsevier.

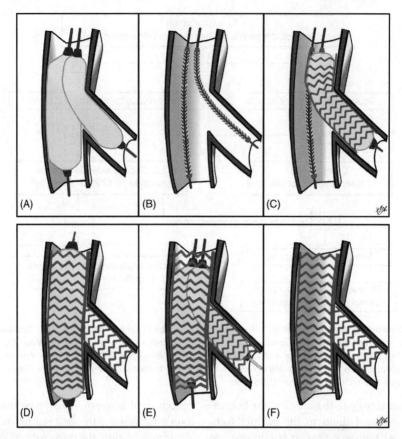

Figure 4.3 A cartoon scheme of the crush technique. (a) Both branches are wired and dilated alternatively or in a kissing balloon fashion; (b) First stent is advanced into the side branch but not expanded and a second stent is advanced into the main branch to fully cover the bifurcation; (c) The stent in the side branch is positioned protruding 3–4 mm in the main branch, in a similar fashion to the procedure employed by the operator when performing the culottes technique. When the side-branch stent is appropriately positioned the balloon is inflated and the stent is deployed. After stent implantation, the delivery balloon is removed from the side branch and a contrast injection is performed to ensure that no distal dissection is present and no additional stents are needed in the side branch; (d) Then, the stent in the main branch is expanded; during balloon inflation and stent implantation the protruding struts of the stent implanted in the side branch are crushed against the wall of the main vessel; (e) Afterwards, the side branch are re-crossed in order to perform final kissing balloon inflation with non-compliant balloon, which is highly recommended as the final step of procedure; (f) Final result. Reprinted from JACC: Cardiovascular Interventions; Bifurcation Disease: What Do We Know, What Should We Do?; Azeem Latib, Antonio Colombo; Vol 1; 3; 2008 with permission from Elsevier.

case it is needed. The wire is then removed from the side branch. Then, the stent in the main branch is expanded (D). During balloon inflation and stent implantation the protruding struts of the stent implanted in the side branch are crushed against the wall of the main vessel. Thus, there are no floating struts; instead there are three layers of struts in the proximal part of the bifurcation and near the ostium of the side branch. The final kissing balloon inflation with non-compliant balloon, after side branch re-crossing, is highly recommended as final step of procedure (E, F).

Variations of the standard crush technique

Since the original publication from Colombo and colleagues [5], the bifurcation phantom by Ormiston and colleagues on the crush technique [6] clarified that simultaneous side- and main-branch dilatation (kissing balloons) fully expanded the stent in the side-branch ostium, widened the gaps between stent struts covering the side branch, and eliminated the main branch distortion. It was also clear that post-dilatation of the main branch with a balloon of narrower diameter than the deploying balloon might have caused main-branch stent distortion [6]. Other experimental work on standard crush in pigs, during those years, underlined the possibility that despite final kissing balloon inflation side-branch stent was left narrowed at the site of stent overlap, creating a metal mass, which could promote the development of thrombosis [11]. Furthermore, post-procedure analysis with intravascular ultrasound (IVUS) imaging showed in the majority of cases a side-branch stent underexpansion, with the smallest minimal stent area frequently found at the ostium site [12]. Moreover, incomplete stent apposition in the crush area was common [12]. This was the reason why many researchers were searching for new refinements of

the crush technique to improve both clinical outcomes and angiographic restenosis at follow-up.

From 2005, the "double kissing", "double crushing" or "sleeve technique" was proposed to improve final kissing balloon inflation with technical methods that are different from the steps used in the classical crush [13–15]. The main advantage of this modified approach, described by Jim and colleagues, is to simplify the re-crossing of the side branch following the initial crush of the protruding segment of the side branch stent into the main branch, splitting the final kissing balloon inflation procedure into two steps, so that the wire and balloon have to cross only one layer of stent struts each time [14]. Figure 4.4 describes the procedure. Although, this approach avoids manipulations

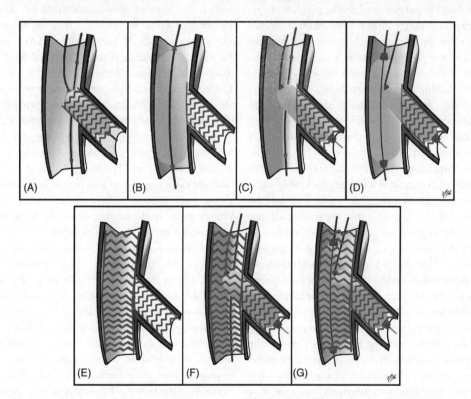

Figure 4.4 A cartoon scheme of the Sleeve technique. (a) Firstly, the stent on the side branch is positioned with the proximal segment of the stent protruding into the main vessel. A balloon is already loaded in the main vessel covering the protruding stent segment once the side branch stent is implanted; (b) Balloon inflation in the main vessel is then accomplished, crushing the side branch stent against the main vessel wall; (c) Rewiring of the side branch through its own stent strut is followed by balloon dilatation of the side branch ostium; (d) First kissing balloon inflation of the

bifurcation is performed and a new sleeve has been reconstructed; (e) At this stage stenting of the main vessel is accomplished; (f) A second rewiring of the side branch stent through the main vessel stent strut is followed by second balloon dilatation of the side branch ostium; (g) Finally, a second final kissing balloon inflation of the bifurcation is performed. Reprinted from JACC: Cardiovascular Interventions; Bifurcation Disease: What Do We Know, What Should We Do?; Azeem Latib, Antonio Colombo; Vol 1; 3; 2008 with permission from Elsevier.

and/or positioning of two bulky stents simultaneously, it has the likely drawback of being a more cumbersome and prolonged procedure. One year later, in the first technique report, Jim and colleagues describes the technical feasibility (100%) of the sleeve technique in 41 consecutive patients [16].

Another report from Collins and Dzavik [17] in 2006 described a modified balloon crush approach in 10 patients with coronary bifurcation lesions. This modification of the balloon crush technique entails the addition of re-dilating the side branch stent (notably, not kissing balloon inflation) following the balloon crush, while the remaining steps were similar to classical balloon crush.

In many ways all these previously described techniques are similar to the "step crush technique" that Colombo [18] has reported in the past when utilizing a 6-Fr guiding catheter, with a main difference due to the performance of re-crossing, balloon inflation, and kissing inflation before the implantation of a stent into the main branch. However, "double kissing", "double crushing", "sleeve technique" and "modified balloon crushing" all require a second crossing into the side branch and further final kissing inflation as compared to the step crush technique described by Colombo [18–19]. After the first description by Colombo and Stankovitc [18], the step crush technique has been reported in some anecdotal cases by Lim and Dzavik [20] and by Sianos et al. [8]. In their study they confirmed that each stent might have been easily advanced and deployed separately when using a 6 French guiding catheter, which did not allow the contemporary position of the two stents. Thus, a stent is advanced in the side branch protruding into the main branch 4–5 millimeters, as described by Colombo et al. [5]; a balloon is then placed within the main vessel across the side branch, ensuring that it fully covers the segment of the side branch stent protruding into the main vessel. Secondly, the stent on the side branch is deployed, the balloon removed, and the wire, may or not may be left in place, performing or not jailing wire technique. The main branch balloon is then inflated, to crush the protruding side branch and removed thereafter. Finally, a stent is advanced in the main branch covering the side branch and the crushed portion of the first stent and deployed. The next steps are similar to the crush technique and involve re-crossing of the side branch, side branch dilatation, and final kissing balloon

dilatation. Despite the results of bifurcations lesion being excellent in these few cases, no IVUS and angiographic follow up were performed in any of these cases [8,20].

Internal crush technique for "provisional crush" approach

From a technical point of view, it is important to decide beforehand whether or not to use two stents. Using the provisional T strategy, the operator is restricted to adopt a technique where the side branch is stented through the main vessel stent. This technique has an inborn risk of missing coverage of the side branch ostium or protruding into the main vessel. Thus this problem can only be solved by use of provisional internal crush (formerly known as "reverse crush technique") [8,9,18] or the T And Protrusion (TAP) technique [21] The technical result might be better in a two-stent technique if the side branch is stented first, resulting in a satisfying result in main vessel, but also a more complex procedure than a provisional approach where side branch stent is not needed.

A provisional internal crush [8,9,18] and TAP technique [21] are included to the "A" family, of the MADS classification [7]. Indeed, in these techniques the main vessel stent is deployed first allowing provisional (elective) deployment of the side branch stent. Both techniques can be performed utilizing a 6 French guiding catheter.

The provisional internal crush technique was described by Colombo [18] as outlined in Figure 4.5. In the original bench work of provisional side-branch stenting, Ormiston and colleagues showed that after standard internal crush, the final kissing balloon clearly caused distortion [22]. This effect was shown despite kissing balloon was able to retain or improve the expansion of the side branch stent at the ostium. Indeed, the distorted portions of stents at the distal margin of the ostium were pushed into the main vessel lumen potentially causing obstruction. Considering these findings, Ormiston and colleagues have suggested to repair main-branch distortion using sequential side- and main branches post-dilatation with an appropriately sized balloon [22]. Furthermore, some improvement in technique result might also occur in case of smaller retraction of the side-branch stent, by employing the "so called" mini-crush

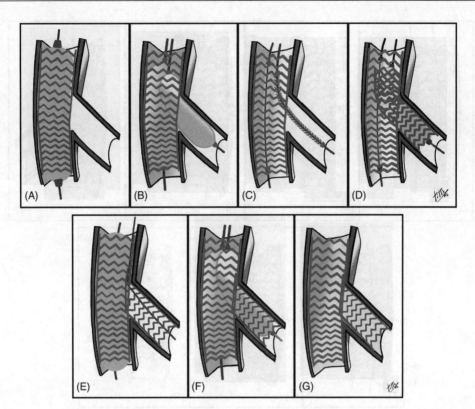

Figure 4.5 A cartoon scheme of the internal crush technique. (a) Firstly a stent is deployed in the main branch; (b) A balloon dilatation with kissing inflation towards the side branch is performed; (c) In case of unsatisfactory result, the procedure is continued by placing a second stent into the side branch and left in position without being deployed. A balloon sized according to the diameter of the main branch is advanced in the main branch and positioned at the level of the bifurcation, paying attention to stay inside the stent previously deployed in the main branch; (d) The stent in the side branch is retracted about 2–3 millimeters into the main branch and deployed; (e) The crush of side branch stent is performed by balloon positioned into the main vessel; (f) Recross of the side branch is performed in order to accomplish final kissing balloon; (g) Final result. Reprinted from JACC: Cardiovascular Interventions; Bifurcation Disease: What Do We Know, What Should We Do?; Azeem Latib, Antonio Colombo; Vol 1; 3; 2008 with permission from Elsevier.

technique [23–25]. Provisional side-branch stenting, which results from the need to crush the side branch stent internally has been systematically examined by Rashdan and colleagues in 156 patients [26]. These authors described this technique as "carina modification by stenting" and confirm the high procedural success rate (99%) with low major adverse coronary events at medium-term follow up. However, no systematic angiographic follow up was performed except for those clinically driven revascularized patients, thus providing no information on the real restenosis rate achieved on both main and side branches.

As already explained, in the case of a provisional approach that may require stenting of the side branch, the TAP technique may be used. This technique, described by Burzotta and colleagues [21], is a modification of T-stenting where the side branch stent protrudes slightly into the main branch to ensure complete coverage of the ostium without deformation of the stent or malapposed struts. In this regard, this technique should not be strictly defined among crushing techniques. The TAP technique appears to be a simple and practical alternative to the internal crush technique to cross over to stenting the side branch when needed (Figure 4.6). The main advantage of this approach is the fact that there is no need to re-cross the side branch with the wire when applying the internal crush or to risk a small gap between the main branch stent and the side branch stent when using the T technique. On the other hand, the risk of an excess of stent protrusion remains one of the main limitation of the TAP technique; indeed, this occurrence will demand

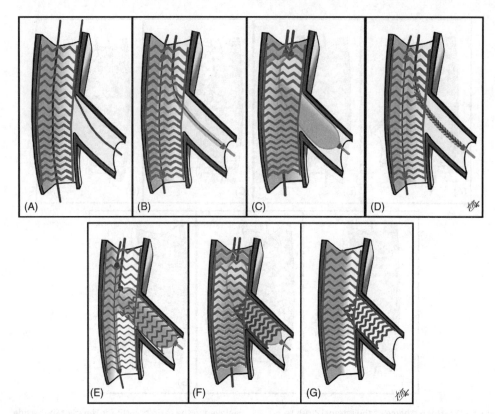

Figure 4.6 A cartoon scheme of the T And Protruding technique. (a) The stent on the main vessel is positioned with a jailed guidewire into the side branch and then deployed; (b) Rewiring of the side branch by guidewire and balloon; (c) Kissing balloon is performed; (d) In case of unsatisfactory results, the procedure is continued by placing an uninflated balloon catheter into the main vessel, which will be used for the final kissing balloon, and a stent of the appropriate length and size into the side branch. The position of the side branch stent is adjusted to fully cover the proximal (or "upper") part of the side branch ostium; (e) The side branch stent is inflated while the main vessel balloon is kept uninflated in the main vessel; (f) Finally the balloon of the stent is slightly pulled back and final kissing balloon is performed by inflating simultaneously the side branch stent's balloon and the main vessel balloon; (g) Final result; protruding side branch stent struts are reoriented by kissing balloon inflation resulting in a small single stent struts neocarina. Reprinted from JACC: Cardiovascular Interventions; Bifurcation Disease: What Do We Know, What Should We Do?; Azeem Latib, Antonio Colombo; Vol 1; 3; 2008 with permission from Elsevier.

immediate correction by an internal crush while the presence of a very minimal stent protrusion could possibly be tolerated. The lack of systematic IVUS evaluation in the original study does not permit to determine whether insufficient stent expansion or excessive stent protrusion might be associated with the risk of stent thrombosis [21].

The mini-crush technique

The mini-crush technique is presented in Figure 4.7 [24,25]. The bifurcation lesion is preferably a true bifurcation lesion. (A). Initially both branches are wired and because of the general complexity of the lesion, alternatively dilated or pre-dilated in a kissing balloon fashion. A stent is advanced into the side branch and a balloon is advanced into the main branch to fully cover the bifurcation (B). The side-branch stent is retracted into the main branch for approximately 1–2 mm. Generally, the proximal marker of the side branch stent is located in contact with the wire of the main vessel balloon, as seen in two different orthogonal projections (B), thus providing uniform minimal crushing; as this method uses the wire where the main vessel balloon is loaded as an indicator for the positioning of the side branch stent, it is an objective and standardized method, and there is no

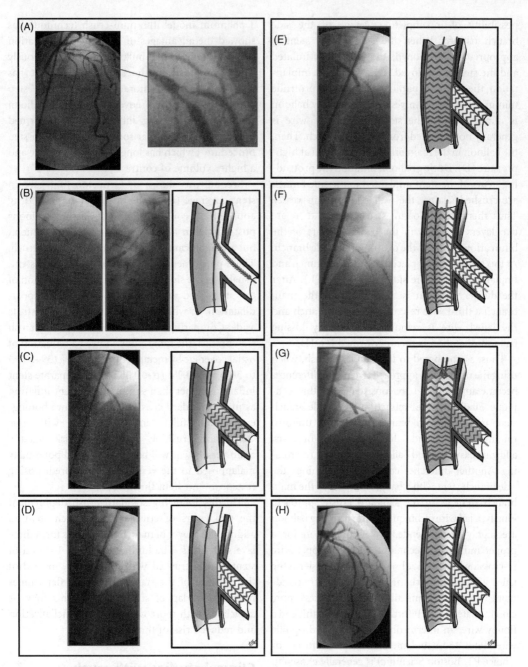

Figure 4.7 A cartoon scheme (right side) with corresponding angiograms (left side) showing a case of mini-crush technique. (a) Antero-posterior cranial angiograms show narrowing stenosis of mid left anterior descending involving the ostium and proximal part of a big diagonal branch. Left side: angiogram, right side: magnification; (b) Positioning of side branch stent after advancing of a balloon into main branch; it is essential to check the position of side branch stent in at least two projections before the deployment; the stent should be placed 1–2 mm out of the side branch ostium before its deployment; (c) The side branch stent is deployed; (d) A balloon is inflated at high pressure in the main branch in order to obtain the complete crush of stent struts protruding into the main branch; (e) Main branch stent deployment; (f) Re-crossing of the side branch stent by a third wire; jail wire technique is applied and it is removed after the side branch re-crossing is performed; (g) Final kissing balloon; (h) Final result. Reprinted from JACC: Cardiovascular Interventions; Bifurcation Disease: What Do We Know, What Should We Do?; Azeem Latib, Antonio Colombo; Vol 1; 3; 2008 with permission from Elsevier.

possibility of incomplete coverage of the side branch ostium. When the side-branch stent is appropriately positioned, the balloon is inflated and the stent is deployed (C). After stent implantation, the proximal part of this stent will protrude minimally in the main vessel. The delivery balloon is removed from the side branch. The wire is generally not removed from the side branch. Then, the balloon in the main branch is expanded at high-pressure (D). During balloon inflation the protruding struts of the stent implanted in the side branch are crushed against the wall of the main vessel. Thus, there are no floating struts; instead there are two layers of struts in the proximal part of the bifurcation and near the ostium of the side branch. At this stage a stent is placed in the main branch and implanted, jailing the side branch wire (E). After the delivery balloon is removed from the main branch a third wire re-crosses the side branch and the jailed wire is removed (F). Finally kissing balloon dilatation is then performed (G, H).

Thus, as compared to the standard crush, when using the mini-crush approach two main differences become apparent and are consistent with this technique. Firstly, a minor retraction of the side branch stent into the main branch provides a uniform minimal crushing and reduces the overlap of struts, allowing easy wire and balloon side branch re-crossing. Another difference consists of "crushing" the side branch stent with a balloon instead of the main branch stent as in the standard crush approach. Finally, a jail wire technique and final kissing balloon are highly recommended as an obligation for a proper mini-crush technique; indeed, proper wire re-crossing into the side branch might be easier as the jailed wire might trace the side branch entry (landmark wire) and permit the third wire access more closely related to the bifurcation carina. To this end a floppy wire, an intermediate wire or a hydrophilic wire (Pilot 150, Guidant, Temecula, California or Choice PT, Boston Scientific) is generally chosen to re-cross into the side branch.

Comparison of the mini-crush and classical crush techniques

There are three reasons to prefer using the mini-crush technique rather than the classical crush technique. Firstly, as shown by Ormiston [27] in

a phantom model, the mini-crush technique has showed the advantages of avoiding manipulation or positioning of two bulky stents simultaneously when compared to the standard crush. It has also be shown to be more feasible than the "step crush technique". Moreover, re-crossing, balloon inflations and kissing inflations are performed only once, in comparison with the "two-step procedure", which has longer procedural time and a higher volume of contrast [13–16].

Secondly, as shown by Ormiston [27] gaps in stent coverage (and thus in scaffolding and drug application) could occur with kissing balloons post-dilatation after standard crush deployment, but are significantly less common with mini-crush. These phenomena occur in the side branch stent, usually on the side opposite the crushed portion of the stent, and are caused by side branch post-dilatation, in which the balloon pushes the struts aside. Comparing standard crush with mini-crush side-branch, the same study showed a reduction of ostial coverage by metal struts from 47% (39–53%) to 36% (31–40%) (p < 0.002). Also, separate stent inflations rather than simultaneous stent inflation as in the standard crush may favor more homogenous and full stent apposition; with this "ballooning crushing" there is less risk that the main vessel stent will be deformed and potentially malapposed to the vessel wall, thus predisposing restenosis and stent thrombosis.

Thirdly, following standard crush deployment the two layers of crushed side branch stent in addition to a layer of main branch struts form three layers of struts. The limited length of 1–2 mm of stent that is crushed with mini-crush, instead of the 3–4 mm of the standard crushed determines minimal overlap of struts; indeed, this may be associated with more complete endothelialization and reduced risk of thrombosis [27].

Clinical studies with crush technique vs single stent techniques

In a small randomized study, Colombo et al. [28] compared the crush technique with the provisional T strategy. On angiographic follow up, there was no significant difference between these two groups. However, it must be underlined that among a total number of 85 patients recruited, due to a high crossover rate, about the 73% of patients ultimately received a two-stent strategy.

The lack of routine final kissing balloon inflation in the crush stent group, the importance of which was demonstrated the following year [29], limited significantly the benefit of the crush technique [5]. Ge et al. compared the crush technique and the systematic T-stent techniques in a non-randomized assessment of 181 patients, two-thirds of whom had crush stenting [30]. Ostial side-branch restenosis and target-vessel revascularization at 1 year were both more common in the T-stent group. Long-term outcomes of the crush have shown its safety profile during the same years [31,32]. Nonetheless, despite the excellent patency rates of the main vessel, the need for revascularization at the ostium of the side branch was not fully eliminated as shown by a restenosis rate of 9.6% in the study by Hoye et al. [31] and by a TLR of 8.7% in the study by Moussa et al. [32]. Steigen et al. undertook a randomized comparison of main vessel stenting versus stenting of both branches in "The Nordic Bifurcation study" [33]. A low rate of MACE was seen in both groups at 6-month follow-up (2.9% versus 3.4%, respectively), despite the fact that two-stents group of patients were treated by different techniques such as (crush, coulotte, or other techniques at discretion of the operator), TLR was extremely low (1.9%). The combined angiographic end point was the significant restenosis (>50% diameter stenosis) of the main vessel and/or occlusion of the side branch and apparently this outcome was similar for the two arms of treatment. However, in this series restenosis rate in the side branch was significantly higher in patients treated with a single stent (19.2%) as compared to those of using a double stent strategy (10.9%).

More recently in the CACTUS study (coronary bifurcations: application of the crushing technique using sirolimus-eluting stents) [34], 350 patients with coronary bifurcations were randomized to crush or provisional T-stenting with implantation of sirolimus stents. Kissing balloon inflations were mandate in both groups and were achieved in 92% and 90%, respectively. Six-month MACE was similar in the two groups (16% versus 15%), and there was also no difference in the rate of angiographic restenosis in either the main and

the side branch in these subset of patients 92% with true bifurcations lesions. Finally the BBC ONE study recently published by Hildick-Smith et al. [35] provides a good illustration. This large multicenter trial randomized 500 patients to a simple (stepwise T-provisional stenting) or a complex (crush or culotte) treatment strategy. This study highlights that a complex procedure involving the use of a systematic two-stent technique results in higher rates of in-hospital and 9-month major adverse cardiovascular events. Despite the fact that the two-stent strategy involved a mixture of two techniques (crush or culotte), the difference between the two-stent and single-stent strategy was largely driven by peri-procedural myocardial infarction; indeed, in the BBC study biomarker data formed part of the primary end point. Although peri-procedural myocardial infarction may be important as an adverse prognostic indicator [36], not all studies have reached the same conclusion in this respect [37]. Furthermore, although the recruitment criteria in BBC were broad, the long recruitment period (21 centers for 3 years), and the unexpectedly low use of side branch stent (2.8%) in patients assigned to the simple treatment strategy imply that these cases were highly selected despite being randomized. Thus, the strategy on the side branch was quite similar to "Keep it open" and there was no specific attempt to optimize the angiographic result on the side branch. Thus, the concern is that patients with lesions at highest risk may not have been included in BBC ONE trial.

All, these randomized studies of stenting of both branches by the crush technique [28–35] failed to demonstrate superiority over main vessel stenting and balloon dilatation with provisional stenting of the side branch. Thus, based on these results, routine usage of two stents is actually not recommended. However, as recently stated, it holds true that it might be impossible to carry out randomized trials in bifurcation lesions as each patient's anatomy may favor a particular technique, but trial patients overall will be heterogeneous [38] and still a remarkable subgroup of patients with bifurcation lesions (with larger side-branches and/or large myocardium at risk supplied by the side branch and/or more diseased vessels and/or with suboptimal result of the side branch) may be treated with double stenting even if the intention is to try to avoid it.

Clinical studies with minicrush technique vs single stent techniques

A previous meta-analysis studied the single-stent strategy in comparison with the double-stent strategy in false and true coronary bifurcations, revealing important heterogeneity and publication bias, especially for side branch restenosis [39]. In this study, significant publication bias for the clinical endpoints of early and late MI, target vessel revascularization and late stent thrombosis were also detected. Niccoli and colleagues [39] acknowledged the fact that the heterogeneity of the techniques and the lack of information on the individual outcomes might have diluted the potential advantages associated with universal use of a unique technique in the two-stent strategy. Indeed, the problems of study design and reporting have limited our progress in the treatment of true coronary bifurcation lesions and on the other hand all too often data from single center series are inappropriately discounted [23].

Going back to the refinement of the crush technique after some anecdotal cases many authors have shown the outcome of crush technique optimization in various studies performed on consecutive patients. One of the earlier studies is the one presented by our group [24] who described the mini-crush technique in a consecutive group of 45 patients. Using this technique, excellent in-hospital outcomes were shown with low MACE (15.5%) and restenosis rates especially at the side branch (2%). Following this approach it seems that there is reduced risk that the main-vessel stent will be deformed and potentially unapposed to the vessel wall and thus predispose to restenosis or stent thrombosis of the side branch, as further suggested by Ormiston and colleagues by bench studies [6,22].

Soon after this study, Chen and colleagues [15] from Nanjing Medical College in China confirmed the good results of the sleeve technique described by Jim *et al.* one year before in the original study [14] and by the same author in 2007 in 41 consecutive patients [16]. In this report, 44 consecutive patients

treated by double kissing (DK) crush technique were compared to 44 consecutive patients treated by the classical crush technique. Although results were confined to 30 days only, those patients treated by DK crush were characterized by a bigger minimum luminal diameter at the side branch ostium $(3.01 \pm 0.13 \text{ mm}$ vs $2.74 \pm 0.12 \text{ mm}$, respectively, $p < 0.01$) and a smaller degree of residual stenosis at the ostial side branch as compared to the classical crush cases $(7.3 \pm 8.6\%$ vs $17.4 \pm 11.2\%$, respectively, $p < 0.05$).

The same authors, one year later, confirmed further similar results of the sleeve technique in a randomized study where 155 patients treated by DK crush were compared to 156 patients treated by classical crush [40]. Clinical follow up was available in 100% and angiographic follow up in 82% patients at 8-month follow up. The overall restenosis was 20.3% in DK crush significantly lower than 35.9% found in the classical crush ($p < 0.01$). Cumulative 8-month MACE was 11.4% in DK crush as compared to 19.7% in the classical crush ($p < 0.02$) when in all cases final kissing balloon inflation was performed. Also the incidence of stent thrombosis was significantly lower in DK crush (1.7%) as compared to classical crush 3.2% ($p < 0.05$).

The concept of crushing a small segment of the side branch stent in the mini-crush technique was also assessed in a large consecutive series of patients with bifurcation lesions and compared to a provisional treatment strategy [25]. The results of this study showed that despite having angiographic markers associated with poorer outcomes, patients treated with the mini-crush technique trended toward a better clinical outcome (with a 21% reduction in cumulative major adverse cardiac events (mini-crush: 20.6%, provisional 26%, $p = \text{NS}$) and showed a better angiographic outcome. Indeed, binary angiographic restenosis at the side branch was significantly reduced by 60% in the mini-crush group (8.5%) when compared with restenosis rates in patients treated with a provisional strategy (21.2%) ($p < 0.01$). Similar results were obtained by Yang and colleagues [41] who employed the minicrush technique in a group of 52 consecutive patients with bifurcation lesions (Medina 1,1,1 in 89.2%). The incidences of MACE and TLR at 9-month follow up were 11.8% and

7.8%, respectively. The in-stent restenosis rate was 14.9% (side branch ostium 10.6%) with a focal pattern in most of the cases.

Conclusions

Side branching stenting may be required in approximately one-third of bifurcations. The main indications for two-stent techniques are represented by the size of the side branch, the respective amount of myocardium supplied by it, and the extension of the atherosclerotic disease beyond the ostium of the side branch.

Indeed, the most unanswered question is whether, in the case of angiographic stenosis being >50% on both branches (true bifurcation lesion), elective stenting of both branches provides greater benefits than the simpler approach of stenting only the main branch, with additional stenting on the side branch, in case of an unsatisfactory result at that site. However, as recently stated by Latib and Colombo [4], bifurcations vary not only in morphology (plaque burden, location of plaque, angle between branches, diameter of branches, bifurcation site), but also in the dynamic changes in anatomy that happen during treatment, because of plaque shift and/or dissection. Thus, pre-treatment evaluation to decide whether to use a two-stent technique or a single stent technique might be rather difficult to perform.

The *crush technique*, which uses the contemporary placement of two stents, has the advantage of assuring the immediate patency of both branches. However, restenosis on the side branch might be due to stent underexpansion with the smallest minimum stent area at the side branch ostium. The *double kiss crush technique (sleeve technique* or *modified balloon crushing)* might be a more cumbersome technique although the increase in the number of steps might be rewarded with a shorter time needed to re-cross into the side branch. The *internal crush* has the advantage of allowing an opportunity for provisional side branch stenting, but may be more laborious in the case of requiring an additional stent in the side branch; furthermore, final kissing balloon dilatation clearly causes stent distortion. The *TAP technique* appears to be a simple and practical approach to cross-over to stent the side branch when needed. However, the risk of an excess of stent protrusion in the main branch remains the main limitation and possibly increases the risk of thrombosis. The *mini-crush technique,* designed to provide complete coverage of the ostium of the side branch while minimizing the length of the crushed segment by single balloon dilatation, might be the best option in patients with complex bifurcation anatomy in which the side branch is heavily affected by atherosclerotic disease, but this technique calls for careful procedural planning and should only be performed by experienced operators.

There are other important technical factors that may contribute to optimizing outcomes when performing crush or mini-crush techniques, such as high-pressure, side branch inflation, the use of non-compliant balloons, selection of correct balloon size for final kissing inflation, and the use of IVUS. Finally, it should be taken into consideration the fact that stenting of bifurcation lesions with DES is associated with an increased risk of stent thrombosis, but this risk is not the greater when crush or minicrush versus single-stent stategy is used. However, final kissing balloon is highly recommended as a final step to improve the result of bifurcation treatment in all cases of crush or mini-crush techniques.

References

1 Hildick-Smith D, Lassen JF, Albiero R, *et al.* Consensus of the 5th European Bifurcation club. EuroIntervention 2010;6:34–8.

2 Colombo A. Stenting bifurcations: the last frontier for fantasy in coronary interventions. Catheter Cardiovasc Interv 2006;67:410–11.

3 Medina A, Suarez de Lezo J, Pan M. A new classification of coronary bifurcation lesions. Rev Esp Cardiol 2006; 59:183.

4 Latib A, Colombo A. Bifurcation disease: what do we know, what should we do? I Am Coll Cardiol Intv 2008;1:218–26.

5 Colombo A, Stankovic G, Orlic D, *et al.* Modified T-stenting technique with crushing for bifurcation lesions: immediate results and 30-Day outcome. Catheter Cardiovasc Interv 2003;60:145–51.

6 Ormiston JA, Currie E, Webster MWI, *et al.* Drug-eluting stents for coronary bifurcations: insight into the "crush" technique. Catheter Cardiovasc Interv 2004;63:332–6.

7 Louvard Y, Thomas M, Dzavik V, *et al.* Classification of coronary artery bifurcation lesions and treatments: time for a consensus! Catheter Cardiovasc Interv 2008;71:175–83.

8 Sianos G, Vaina S, Hoye A, Serruys PW. Bifurcation stenting with drug eluting stents: Illustration of the crush technique. Catheter Cardiovasc Interv 2006;67:839–45.

9 Porto I, van Gaal W, Banning A. "Crush" and "reverse crush" technique to treat a complex left main stenosis. Heart 2006;92:1021.

10 Chevalier B, Glatt B, Royer T, Guyon P. Placement of coronary stents in bifurcation lesions by the "culotte" technique. Am J Cardiol 1998;82:943–9.

11 Murasato Y, Suzuka H, Kamezaki F. Vascular endoscopic and macroscopic observations after crush stenting of coronary artery bifurcations in pigs. Catheter Cardiovasc Interv 2005;66:237–43.

12 Costa RA, Mintz GS, Carlier S.G. et al. Bifurcation coronary lesions treated with the "crush" technique: an intravascular ultrasound analysis. J Am Coll Cardiol 2005;46:599–605.

13 Chen SL, Ye F, Zghang J.J. et al. DK crush technique: modified treatment of bifurcationm lesions in coronary artery. Chin Med J 2005;118:1746–50.

14 Jim MH, Hwa H, Miu R, Chow WH. Modified crush technique with double kissing balloon inflation (sleeve technique): a novel technique for coronary bifurcation lesions. Catheter Cardiovasc Interv 2006:67;403–9.

15 Chen SL, Zhang J, Ye F, et al. DK crush (double-kissing and double crush) technique for treatment of true coronary bifurcation lesions: illustrations and comparison with classic crush. J Invasive Cardiol 2007;19:189–93.

16 Jim MH, Ho H, Chan AO, Chow W. Stenting of coronary bifurcation lesions by using modified crush technique with double kissing balloon inflation (sleeve technique): immediate procedure result and short-term clinical outcomes. Catheter Cardiovasc Interv 2007; 69; 969–75.

17 Collins N, Dzavik V. A modifiedballoon crush aproach improves side branch access and side branch stent apposition during crush stenting of coronary bifurcation lesions. Catheter Cardiovasc Interv 2006;68:365–71.

18 Stankovic G. Lesion specific stenting; chapter 3: pp 34–54. From Colombo's Tip and Tricks with Drug-Eluting Stents. Colombo A and G Stankovic. Taylor & Francis, London, 2005.

19 Colombo A. Stenting bifurcations: the last frontier for fantasy in coronary interventions, Catheter Cardiovasc Interv 2006; 67; 410–1.

20 Lim PO, Dzavik V. Balloon crush: Treatment of bifurcation lesions using the crush stenting technique as adapted for transradial approach of percutaneous coronary interventions. Catheter Cardiovasc Interv 2004;63:412–16.

21 Burzotta F, Gwon H, Hahn J. et al. Modified T-stenting with intentional protrusion of the side-branch stent within the main vessel stent to ensure ostial coverage and facilitate final kissing balloon: the T-stenting and small protrusion technique (TAP-stenting). Report of bench testing and first clinical Italian-Korean two-centre experience. Catheter Cardiovasc Interv 2007; 70; 75–82.

22 Ormiston JA, Webster MWI, Jack SE, et al. Drug-eluting stents for coronary bifurcations: bench testing of provisional side-branch strategies. Catheter Cardiovasc Interv 2006;67:49–55.

23 Kaplan A. Percutaneous coronary intervention treatment of bifurcation lesions. A work in progress. JACC Cardiovasc IntvIntv 2009;2:195–6.

24 Galassi AR, Colombo A, Buchbinder M. Long term outcome of bifurcation lesions after implantation of drug-eluting stents with the "Mini-Crush Technique". Catheter Cardiovasc Interv 2007;69:976–83.

25 Galassi AR, Tomasello SD, Capodanno D, Barrano G, Ussia GP, Tamburino C. Mini-Crush versus T-Provisional techniques in bifurcation lesions: clinical and angiographic long-term outcome after implantation of drug eluting stents. JACC Cardiovasc Intv 2009;2:185–94.

26 Rashdan IA, Amin H. Carina modification T stenting, a new bifurcation stenting technique: clinical and angiographic data from the first 156 consecutive patients. Catheter Cardiovasc Interven 2009;74:683–90.

27 Ormiston JA, Webster MWI, Webber B, Stewart JT, Ruygrok PN, Hatrick RI. The "crush" technique for coronary artery bifurcation stenting: insight from micro-computed tomographic imaging of bench deployments. JACC Cardiovasc Intv 2008;1:351–7.

28 Colombo A, Moses J, Morice MC, et al. The randomized study to evaluate sirolimus–eluting stents implanted in coronary bifurcation lesions. Circulation 2004;109: 1244–9.

29 Ge I, Airoldi F, Iakovou I, et al. Clinical and angiogarphic outcome after implantation of drug-eluting stents in bifurcation lesions with the crush stent technique: importance of final kissing balloon post-dilatation. J Am Coll Cardiol 2005;46:613–20.

30 Ge I, Ikavou I, Cosgrave J, et al. Treatment of bifurcation lesions with two stents: one year angiographic and clinical follow-up of crush versus T stenting. Heart 2006;92:371–6.

31 Hoye A, Iakovou j, Ge L, et al. Long-term outcomes after stenting of bifurcation lesions with the "crush technique". J Am Coll Cardiol 2006; 47; 1949–58.

32 Moussa I, Costa RA, Leon MB, et al. A prospective registry to evaluate sirolimus-eluting stents implanted at coronary bifurcation lesions using the "crush technique". Am J Cardiol 2006;97:1317–21.

33 Steigen TK, Maeng M, Wiseth R, et al. Ramdomized study on simple versus complex stenting of coronary artery bifurcation lesions: the Nordic Bifurcation Study. Circulation 2006;114:1955–61.

34 Colombo A, Bramucci E, Saccà S, *et al.* Randomized study of the crush technique versus provisional side-branch stenting in true coronary bifurcations: the CACTUS (Coronary bifurcations: Application of the Crushing Technique Using Sirolimus-eluting stents) study. Circulation 2009;119:71–8.

35 Smith DH, Belder AJ, Cooter N, *et al.* Randomized of simple versus complex drug-eluitng stenting for bifurcation lesions: the British Bifurcation Coronary Study: old, new and evolving strategies. Circulation 2010;121:1235–43.

36 Andron M, Stables RH, Egred M, *et al.* Impact of periprocedural creatine kinase–MB isoenzyme release on long-term mortality in contemporary percutaneous coronary intervention. J Invasive Cardiol 2008;20:108–12.

37 Stone GW, Mehran R, Dangas G, Lansky AJ, Kornowski R, Leon MB. Differential impact on survival of electrocardiographic Q-waves versus enzymatic myocardial infarction after percutaneous intervention: a device specific analysis of 7147 patients. Circulation 2001;104:642–7.

38 Thomas M, Hildick-Smith D, Louvard Y, *et al.* Percutaneous coronary intervention for bifurcation disease. A consensus view from the first meeting of the European Bifurcation Club. EuroIntervention 2006;2:149–53.

39 Niccoli G, Ferrante G, Porto I, *et al.* Coronary bifurcation lesions: to stent one branch or both? A meta analysis of patients treated with drug eluting stents. Int J Cardiol 2010; 139:80–91.

40 Chen SL, Zhang JJ, Ye F, *et al.* Study Comparing the double kissing (DK) crush with classical crush for the treatment of coronary bifurcation lesions: the DKCRUSH-1 Bifurcation Study with drug eluting stents. Eur J Clin Invest 2008;38:361–71.

41 Yang HM, Tahk SJ, Woo S, *et al.* Long term clinical and angiographic outcomes after implantation of sirolimus-eluting stents with a "modified mini-crush" technique in coronary bifurcation lesions. Catheter Cardiovasc Interven 2009;74:76–84.

CHAPTER 5

Simultaneous kissing stent technique: A contemporary review

Joseph M. Sweeny, MD *and Samin K. Sharma,* MD, FACC

Cardiac Catheterization Laboratory of the Cardiovascular Institute, Mount Sinai Hospital, New York, NY, USA

Introduction

Coronary artery bifurcations develop atherosclerotic plaque in regional areas of turbulent blood flow and high shear stress [1]. These technically challenging lesions account for 15–20% of the total number of percutaneous coronary interventions (PCI) performed. While the coronary arterial system is composed of multiple bifurcation points, a true coronary bifurcation lesion consists of >50% diameter obstruction of both the main vessel (MV) and of the side branch (SB) vessel in an inverted "Y" fashion.

When treated percutaneously, coronary bifurcations have historically suffered a lower rate of procedural success, higher procedural costs, longer hospitalization, and higher clinical and angiographic restenosis [2–6]. As a result, the treatment of these lesions represents an ongoing challenge to the interventional cardiologist. Numerous technological advances in stent design, selective use of a two-stent technique, acceptance of a suboptimal side branch result and various percutaneous techniques (high pressure post-dilatation, kissing balloon inflation and intravascular ultrasound) have together led to an increase in the number of successfully treated bifurcation lesions with excellent long-term outcomes.

The practice of stenting coronary bifurcations has largely favored a provisional one-stent approach. However, this strategy does have a number of limitations and therefore an in-depth understanding of the dedicated two-stent strategy is necessary. The simultaneous kissing stent (SKS) technique is one type of dedicated two-stent strategy that will be reviewed.

Bifurcation classification

No two coronary bifurcation lesions are alike and no single strategy can be used on every bifurcation [2]. This is largely due to the myriad anatomical variations (location of plaque, plaque burden, angle between branches, site of the bifurcation, size of branches, etc) as well as potential dynamic changes in anatomy that can occur during treatment (i.e. dissection or carinal shift).

Coronary bifurcations have been previously classified according to both the angulation between the MV and the SB and to the particular location and distribution of the plaque: (1) "Y-angulation", when the angulation is <70°, or (2) "T-angulation", when the SB angulation is >70°. Access to the SB is usually more difficult with "T-angulation" but plaque shifting is often minimal and precise stent placement in the ostium is more straightforward compared to the "Y-angulation". Currently, there are six major bifurcation lesion classifications described in the literature (Sanborn, Lefèvre, Safian, Duke, Medina and Movahed). Many

Bifurcation Stenting, First Edition. Edited by Ron Waksman and John A. Ormiston.

© 2012 Blackwell Publishing Ltd. Published 2012 by Blackwell Publishing Ltd.

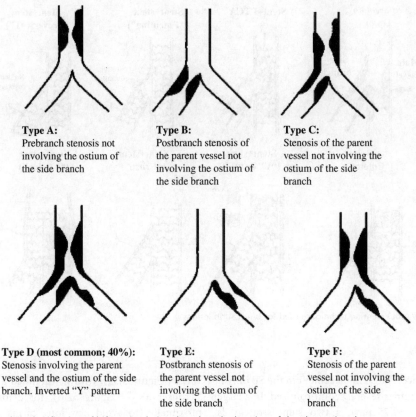

Type A:
Prebranch stenosis not
involving the ostium of
the side branch

Type B:
Postbranch stenosis of
the parent vessel not
involving the ostium of
the side branch

Type C:
Stenosis of the parent
vessel not involving the
ostium of the side
branch

Type D (most common; 40%):
Stenosis involving the parent
vessel and the ostium of the side
branch. Inverted "Y" pattern

Type E:
Postbranch stenosis of
the parent vessel not
involving the ostium of
the side branch

Type F:
Stenosis of the parent
vessel not involving the
ostium of the side
branch

Figure 5.1 Duke's classification of bifurcation lesions based on the location of the obstructive plaque.

of these classifications are similar in describing a bifurcation, (e.g. Duke) (Figure 5.1) [2], but most of these underestimate plaque distribution as well as plaque burden when compared to intravascular ultrasound, and furthermore do not take into account to the fate of the SB on dilatation of the MV [7].

Interventional stenting techniques for bifurcations

Overall, there has been momentum towards treating bifurcation lesions with a provisional one-stent approach as opposed to a dedicated two-stent technique. This shift has been largely based on recent meta-analyses and randomized controlled trials suggesting lower risks of major adverse cardic events (MACE) with a provisional stent technique [13,15], as well as shorter procedure time

and less radiation exposure [14]. However, the one stent strategy does have a number of limitations such as maintaining access to the side branch, jailing the SB ostium or difficulty rewiring the SB and therefore an in-depth understanding of the dedicated two-stent strategy is necessary for any operator who wishes to successfully treat complex coronary bifurcations.

When deciding on a two versus one stent approach, the most important initial question is whether the SB is large enough (>2.75 mm) and is supplying a sufficient territory of myocardium to justify stent implantation. If the SB is small (<1.5 mm) and supplies a small area of myocardium, a stent can usually be placed in the MV, across the SB ostium. In the medium size SB (2–2.75 mm) a strategy of "keep-it-open" (KIO) with predilatation using a cutting balloon (or a non-compliant balloon) and leaving the jailed SB

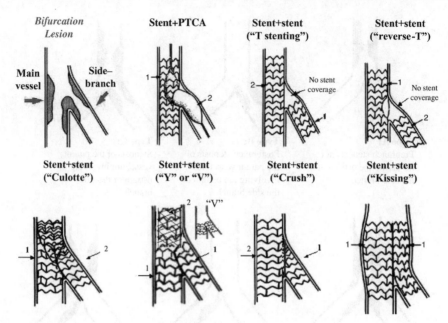

Figure 5.2 Various stenting techniques used for bifurcation lesions.

wire in place, and stent placement in the SB only if the SB ostium is severely compromised. In a large sized SB (>2.75 mm), a two stent strategy is preferred especially if the SB is angulated (>50°), has long lesions beyond the ostium and if there is significant dissection after predilatation. Various two-stent techniques have emerged in the DES era to provide a systematic approach to stenting large sidebranch vessels (Figure 5.2) [8–12,16].

The simultaneous kissing stent (SKS) technique and its variations were developed to obviate the need for recrossing stent struts, prevent stent deformation and assure stent coverage of the SB ostium [19].

Simultaneous kissing stents (SKS) and "V" stenting techniques

The "V" technique consists of the delivery and implantation of two stents together. In this technique one stent is advanced into the SB, the other into the MV, and the two stents touch each other, forming a small proximal stent neocarina (<2 mm). When the stent neocarina extends a considerable length (≥3 mm) into the MV, this technique is termed simultaneous kissing stents or

"SKS" (Figure 5.3a), with its modified alternative "Trouser SKS" (Figure 5.3b), for a long lesion proximally (to avoid new long carina) [17–19]. The type of lesion we consider most suitable for this technique is a very proximal lesion such as a bifurcation lesion of distal left main and other bifurcation with moderate-to-large side-branch (>2.75 mm) and vessel portion proximal to bifurcation free of significant disease (Figure 5.3c).

The selection of the size of the guiding catheter takes place after the decision to treat the side branch. With a successful deployment of one-stent using a provisional stent technique, a 6-F guiding catheter can be used. However, it is not uncommon for a complex bifurcation to involve simultaneous insertion of two balloons or two stents making the choice of guiding catheter paramount. With current low-profile balloons, it is possible to insert two balloons inside a large-lumen 6-F guiding catheter. However, the SKS technique cannot be performed unless a guiding catheter of at least 7-F with an internal diameter of 0.081 inches (2.06 mm) is used.

SKS technique

See Figures 5.3a and 5.3c. This involves using two appropriately sized stents (1:1 stent-to-artery

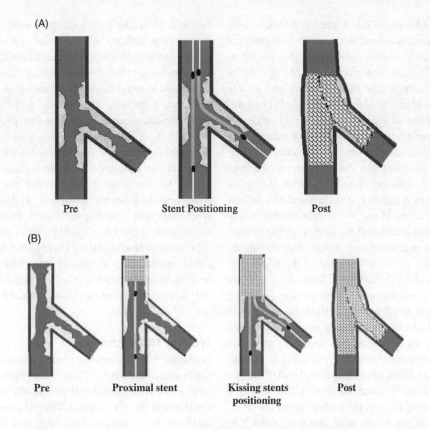

(A)

Pre   Stent Positioning   Post

(B)

Pre   Proximal stent   Kissing stents   Post
                               positioning

(C)   SKS for LAD-D2 Bifurcation with 8-Mo Angiographic Follow-UP

Mid-LAD 90-95% obstruction;   BMW Guidewires in mid-LAD and LAD-D2
LAD-D2 70-80% obstruction

3.0/28.0 mm Cypher in mid-LAD & 2.5/13.0 mm Cypher   Follow-up cath at 8-mo with LAD
in LAD-D2 via SKS technique, with 0% residual stenosis   no restenosis, D2 <30% lesion

Figure 5.3 (a) Simultaneous kissing stents technique; (b) Trouser SKS technique; (c) Angiographic results in a SKS cases.

ratio), one for the MV and one for the SB, with an overlap of the two stents in the proximal segment of the MV (stent sized 1:1 to the MV after the bifurcation). The proximal part of the MV should be able to accommodate the two stents and its size should be approximately two-thirds of the aggregate diameter of the two stents (for example, for two 3.0 mm stents in left anterior descending artery and left circumflex artery, the proximal MV (left main in this case) size should be ≈4 mm). Stent lengths are selected visually to cover the entire length from distal end of the SB and MV lesions to proximal end in the MV. Atheromatous plaque modification and debulking using a cutting balloon or rotablator atherectomy, with or without balloon angioplasty, of the MV and/or of the SB, is performed as clinically indicated. Both MV and SB are wired and lesions >80% stenosis are dilated by appropriate sized balloons. Then two stents are advanced one by one, initially to the SB followed by one to the MV. After this step, both stents are pulled simultaneously back to the bifurcation making a "V" and then into the proximal part of the MV to configure a "Y", with the stem of the "Y" in the MV, allowing for complete coverage of the proximal end of the lesion, with one arm of the Y in distal MV (covering the distal end of the MV lesion) and the other arm in the SB (covering the distal end of SB lesions). The proximal overlapping part of the stents is kept as short as possible but long enough to cover the proximal end of the MV lesion. Once the position of the stents is confirmed and proximal stent markers are aligned, stents are deployed with simultaneous inflation at 10–12 atm, for 10–20 seconds and then simultaneously deflated. This is followed by a second dilatation of the MV stent at 16–20 atmospheres, for 10–20 seconds to fully expand the MV stent struts, while the other SB stent balloon remains deflated in the SB stent. Then a third dilatation of the SB stent at 14–20 atmospheres for 10–20 seconds is performed to allow full expansion of the SB stent struts, while the other MV stent balloon remains deflated in the MV stent. This is then followed by a fourth and final simultaneous inflation and deflation at 10–12 atmospheres for 10–20 seconds to form the uniform carina of the fully expanded kissing stents. Deflated stent balloons are withdrawn simultaneously. In cases of stent under expansion, two high-pressure

balloons of similar length (may be different diameters however) are advanced for simultaneous kissing balloon dilatations. In case of distal dissection, prolonged low-pressure balloon dilatation is performed to avoid the need for stenting. In cases of proximal dissection, two-balloon (one in each stent) simultaneous dilatation at low pressure is done. If there is a need to place a stent at the proximal segment of a vessel treated with an SKS, there are two options: (1) a stent is placed proximally, leaving a small gap between the kissing stents and the proximal stent, and (2) the kissing stent technique is converted into a crush technique, with the stent in the MV compressing the other stent (one arm of the V) in the SB. A wire will then cross the struts into the SB, and a balloon will be inflated toward the SB. After wire removal from the SB, the proximal stent will be advanced toward the MV.

Trouser SKS technique

See Figure 5.3b. In cases that involve a long lesion in the proximal part of MV, before the bifurcation, a large stent is first deployed proximally over the guidewire in the MV. This is followed by wiring the side-branch via the proximal stent and then advancing the two stents through the MV stent to the distal MV and the SB, and deployed as described above ("trouser-and-seat" pattern).

Clinical studies

The SKS technique obviates the need for recrossing a stent strut and reducing stent deformation and has been shown to provide excellent short and long-term results when compared to the conventional stenting strategy for medium-to-large coronary bifurcation lesions.

Animal studies [20] as well clinical retrospective analyses [18,19,21] of the SKS technique have deemed this to be a feasible and safe stenting technique in large bifurcations. Sharma et al. studied 200 consecutive patients who underwent stenting of 202 true de novo bifurcation lesions (Duke type D) using sirolimus-eluting stents (Cypher® stent, Cordis Corp, a Johnson & Johnson Co) and found a high procedural success rate for both the MV and SB, an in-hospital mortality and 30-day MACE of 3 and 5% respectively as well as a low TLR

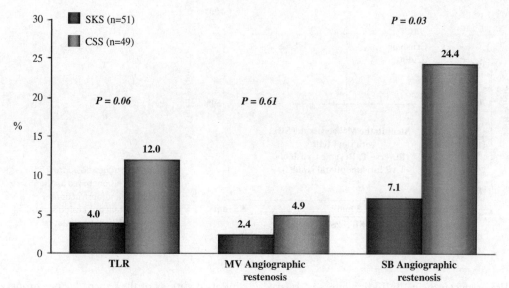

Figure 5.4 8-month MV and SB restenosis and target lesion revascularization rates in both SKS and CSS groups.

rate of 4% at 9-month follow-up [18]. Similarly, the SKS-PRECISE trial involved 100 large bifurcation lesions randomly assigned in a 1:1 fashion to receive either a conventional stenting strategy (CSS) or a simultaneous kissing stent (SKS) [17]. Those patients treated with SKS had a trend towards better procedural angiographic success on the SB intervention when compared to the CSS treated group and at 8-month follow-up there was a lower SB restenosis rate with SKS compared with CSS respectively (7.1 vs 24.4%, p = 0.04). Furthermore, in this study, there were no recorded incidences of stent thrombosis or significant differences in MACE rates between the two techniques (Figure 5.4).

These preliminary studies have established the SKS technique as an effective and safe stenting strategy for medium-to-large bifurcation lesions.

Lesion preparation and adjunct pharmacotherapy

Plaque removal before stent implantation, using directional atherectomy in non-calcified lesions and rotational atherectomy in calcified lesions, has been described in bifurcations. However, encouraging results of many single-center experiences have not been reproduced in large-scale randomized trials. Rotational atherectomy for heavily

calcified bifurcation vessels is essential for lesion dilatation and facilitation of SKS stent delivery and expansion. In most catheterization laboratories, the use of this procedure is <5% of all interventions. When utilized in bifurcation interventions, rotablation is typically performed only on the MV, but occasionally also on the SB depending on the degree of calcification. Therefore, lesion preparation with rotational atherectomy of a heavily calcified lesion can substantially facilitate SKS stent delivery and symmetrical stent expansion with more homogeneous drug delivery after DES implantation.

Techniques using plaque modification by cutting balloon (BSC, Inc., MA) or AngioSculpt balloon (AngioScore Inc., Fremont, CA) have reported the beneficial combination of stenting preceded by atherotomy. In bifurcation lesions, in which there is a large fibrotic plaque at the ostium of the SB, the use of the cutting balloon as a sole device or as a pre-dilatation strategy before stenting seems reasonable [22]. Currently, we suggest the use of a cutting balloon in moderately calcific and fibrotic lesions. Symmetric SKS stent expansion, avoidance of SB recoil and stent compression are all hypotheses for the use of these devices.

Unfractionated heparin to keep the ACT ≈ 250 s or Bivalirudin (ACT > 300 s) are the usual antithrombotic therapies used in complicated PCIs.

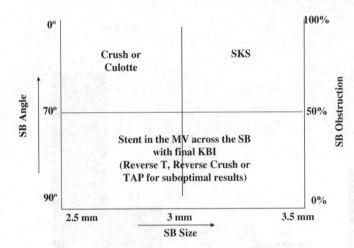

Figure 5.5 Suggested approach for large bifurcation lesions based on the SB size, angulation and obstruction.
SKS = simultaneous kissing stents;
KBI = kissing balloons inflation.

Use of glycoprotein IIb/IIIa inhibitors is reserved for thrombus-containing lesions, when multiple stents or overlapping stents are implanted on both branches. These agents are typically administered when the final result at the SB seems suboptimal and for other procedural complications such as dissection or slow-flow. Aspirin 162–325 mg loading dose or 81–162 mg maintenance dose is recommended and Clopidogrel 600-mg loading dose is routinely used in most catheterization laboratories, followed by 75 mg daily for 1–3 years after DES implantation [23]. The duration of combined thienopyridine and aspirin treatment after stent implantation varies according to the length of the stent implanted, the type of stent used, and the

clinical conditions of the patient (acute coronary syndrome or diabetes mellitus).

Conclusions and future directions

Treating bifurcation lesions is challenging but a simple algorithm based on the SB size, stenosis and angulation can be used (Figure 5.5). The SKS technique using two DES is a well-described stenting technique ideally suited for medium-to-large bifurcation lesions. When treating bifurcation lesions, close attention must be directed towards choosing a guiding catheter large enough to accommodate two balloons and two stents. A wire should be placed in the SB especially if there is

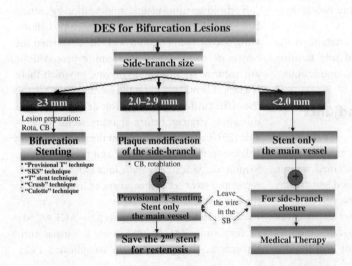

Figure 5.6 Proposed interventional algorithm for approaching bifurcation lesions.

disease at the ostium or with a problematic take-off. The general consensus is to try to keep the procedure safe and simple. When the SB is not severely diseased, implantation of a stent in the MV and provisional stenting in the SB is the preferred strategy. However, implantation of two stents using the SKS technique is appropriate and recommended when both branches are large (>2.75 mm) and significantly diseased (>50% diameter stenosis) and are suitable for stenting. Preliminary clinical studies involving the SKS technique are emerging but randomized controlled trials comparing the SKS technique to other dedicated two-stents strategies are required.

In conclusion, an algorithm for bifurcation lesions treatment based on side branch size has been proposed (Figure 5.6).

References

1 Hahn C, Schwartz M. Mechanotransduction in vascular physiology and atherogenesis. Nat Rev Mol Cell Bio 2009;10:53–62.

2 Louvard Y, Thomas M, Dzavik V, Hildick-Smith D, Galassi A, Pan M, et al. Classification of coronary artery bifurcation lesions and treatments: time for a consensus! Catheter Cardiovasc Interv 2008;71:175–83.

3 Dauerman H, Higgins P, Sparano A, Gibson CM, Garber GR, Carrozza JP, Jr. Kuntz RE, Laham RJ, Shubrooks SJ, Jr. Baim DS, Cohen DJ. Mechanical debulking versus balloon angioplasty for the treatment of true bifurcation lesions. J Am Coll Cardiol 1998;32:1845–52.

4 Al Suwaidi J, Berger P, Rihal C, Garratt KN, Bell MR, Ting HH, Bresnahan JF, Grill DE, Holmes DR. Immediate and long-term outcome of intracoronary stent implantation for true bifurcation lesions. J Am Coll Cardiol 2000; 35:929–36.

5 Yamashita T, Nishida T, Adamian M, Briguori C, Vaghetti M, Corvaja N, Albiero R, Finci L, Di Mario C, Tobis JM, Colombo A. Bifurcation lesions: two stents versus one stent – immediate and follow-up results. J Am Coll Cardiol 2000;35:1145–51.

6 Pan M, Suarez de Lezo J, Medina A, Romero M, Hernández E, Segura J, Castroviejo JR, Pavlovic D, Melian F, Ramírez A, Castillo JC. Simple and complex stent strategies for bifurcated coronary arterial stenosis involving the side-branch origin. Am J Cardiol 1999;83:1320–5.

7 Movahed MR. Coronary artery bifurcation lesion classifications, interventional techniques and clinical outcome. Expert Rev Cardiovasc Ther. 2008;6:261–74.

8 Kobayashi Y, Colombo A, Akiyama T, Reimers B, Martini G, di Mario C. Modified "T" stenting: a technique for kissing stents in bifurcational coronary lesions. Cathet Cardiovasc Diag 1998;43:323–6.

9 Chevalier B, Glatt B, Royer T, Guyon P. Placement of coronary stents in bifurcation lesions by the "culotte" technique. Am J Cardiol 1998;82:943–9.

10 Brueck M, Scheinert D, Flaschskampf F, Daniel WG, Ludwig J. Sequential vs. Kissing Balloon Angioplasty for Stenting of Bifurcation Coronary Lesions. Cathet Cardiovasc Intervent 2002;55:461–6.

11 Cervinka P, Foley D, Sabaté M, Costa MA, Serrano P, Ligthart JMR, Serruys PW. Coronary bifurcation stenting using dedicated bifurcation stents. Cathet Cardiovasc Intervent 2000;49:105–11.

12 Colombo A, Stankovic G, Orlic D, Corvaja N, Liistro F, Airoldi F, Chieffo A, Spanos V, Montorfano M, Di Mario C. Modified T-stenting technique with crushing for bifurcation lesions: Immediate results and 30-day outcome. Cathet Cardiovasc Intervent 2003;60:145–51.

13 Zhang F, Dong L, Ge J. Simple versus complex stenting strategy for coronary artery bifurcation lesions in the drug-eluting stent era: a meta-analysis of randomized trials. Heart 2009;95:1676–81.

14 Steigen T, Maeng M, Wiseth R, Erglis A, Kumsars I, Narbute I. et al. Randomized study on simple versus complex stenting of coronary artery bifurcation lesions. The Nordic Bifurcation Study. Circulation 2006;114; 1955–61.

15 Hildick-Smith D, de Belder AJ, Cooter, N, et al. Randomized trial of simple versus complex stenting for bifurcation lesions. The British Bifurcation Coronary Study: Old, New, and Evolving Strategies. Circulation 2010;121:1235–43.

16 Erglis A, Kumsars I, Niemela M, Kervinen K, Maeng M, Lassen J. et al. Randomized comparison of coronary bifurcation stenting with the crush versus the culotte technique using sirolimus eluting stents. (NORDIC Bifurcation II Study). Circ Cardiovasc Intervent 2009; 2:27–34.

17 Sharma S, Labana S, Krishnan P, Suleman J, Kim M, Moreno P, Mareş A, Kini A. A randomized Pilot Trial for Treatment of Large Bifurcation Lesions with Simultaneous Kissing Stents: PRECISE-SKS Trial. Circulation 2008;118:II–S901.

18 Sharma S, Ahsan C, Lee J, Kim M, Fisher E, Steinheimer A, Kini A. Simultaneous kissing stents (SKS) technique for treating bifurcation lesions in medium-to-large size coronary arteries. Am J Cardiol 2004;94:913–17.

19 Sharma SK. Simultaneous kissing drug-eluting stent technique for percutaneous treatment of bifurcation lesions in large-size vessels. Catheter Cardiovasc Interv 2005;65:10–16.

20 Morton AC, Siota A, Arnold ND, *et al.* Simultaneous Kissing Stent Technique to treat left main stent bifurcation disease. Catheter Cardiovasc Interv 2007;69:209–15.

21 Kim YH, Park DW, Suh IW, *et al.* Long-term outcome of simultaneous kissing stenting technique with sirolimus-eluting stent for large bifurcation coronary lesions. Catheter Cardiovasc Interv 2007;70:840–6.

22 Dahm J, Dorr M, Scholz E, Ruppert J, Hummel A, Staudt A, Felix S. Cutting-balloon angioplasty effectively facilitates the interventional procedure and leads to a low rate of recurrent stenosis in ostial bifurcation coronary lesions: a subgroup analysis of the NICECUT Multicenter registry. International Journal of Cardiology 2008;124: 345–50.

23 Pan M, Suárez de Lezo J, Medina A, *et al.* Drug-eluting stents for the treatment of bifurcation lesions: a randomized comparison between paclitaxel and sirolimus stents Am Heart J 2007;153:15–17.

CHAPTER 6

Stenting for left main coronary artery bifurcation lesions

Seung-Jung Park, MD, PhD *and Young-Hak Kim,* MD, PhD
University of Ulsan College of Medicine, Asan Medical Center, Seoul, Korea

Introduction

The percutaneous coronary approach with coronary stents has been shown to be feasible for patients with unprotected LMCA stenosis [1]. Moreover, DES, together with advances in periprocedural and post-procedural adjunctive pharmacotherapies, have improved outcomes of PCI for these complex coronary lesions [2–9]. In fact, compared with bare-metal stenst, DES reduced the incidence of angiographic restenosis and subsequently the need of repeat revascularization [2–4].

However, in spite of the great benefit of DES, bifurcation location in the unprotected LMCA remains an ongoing challenge. Besides the technical complexity of stenting, bifurcation location has been reported to be an important predictor for late restenosis or stent thrombosis compared with non-bifurcation location [5,10–14]. For instance, a two-stent strategy, in which stents are implanted in both the main branch (MB) and the side branch (SB) for bifurcations with SB stenosis, is likely to result in a high incidence of restenosis and repeat revascularization compared with single-stent strategy, implanting the stent in the MB alone for bifurcations without SB stenosis [11,12]. Therefore, according to the initial plan of bifurcation treatment, a "provisional stenting", as opposed to a "routine SB stenting" with two-stent treatment, is often used as based on single-sent treatment for the MB alone. However, due to a lack of randomized studies comparing single-versus two-stent strategies, the selection of bifurcation stenting technique is generally made by the individual lesion morphology.

In this chapter, the technical steps and outcomes of stenting for unprotected LMCA bifurcation stenosis will be reviewed.

Selection of stenting strategy

When selecting appropriate stenting strategy, plaque distribution and the anatomy of coronary vasculature should be the primary consideration. With regard to plaque distribution, the MEDINA classification is now the most widely applied. In that classification, lesions with plaque location in the MB alone, such as MEDINA class 1.1.0., or 1.0.0., are usually treated by provisional stenting technique. By contrast, lesions with plaque involving the MB and SB, which are "true" bifurcation lesions, are more likely to result in SB deterioration following the MB stenting, with the provisional stenting approach (Table 6.1). Figure 6.1 is an example of a patient treated with provisional stenting, in which a single-stent was placed in the LMCA crossing the left circumflex artery (LCX). In this case, the angiographic plaque distribution in the MB and SB was ascertained by intravascular ultrasound (IVUS) examination. However, as shown in Figure 6.2, a patient with bifurcation LMCA disease involving the ostia of the LCX and left anterior

Bifurcation Stenting, First Edition. Edited by Ron Waksman and John A. Ormiston.
© 2012 Blackwell Publishing Ltd. Published 2012 by Blackwell Publishing Ltd.

Table 6.1 Favorable or unfavorable anatomical features for provisional stenting in the treatment of unprotected left main coronary artery stenosis

	Anatomical features
Favorable	• Significant stenosis at the ostial LCX with MEDINA classification 1.1.0. or 1.0.0. • Large size of LCX with ≥2.5 mm in diameter • Right dominant coronary system • Narrow angle with LAD • No concomitant disease in LCX • Focal disease in LCX
Unfavorable	• Insignificant stenosis at the ostial LCX with MEDINA classification 1.1.1., 1.0.1., or 0.1.1 • Diminutive LCX with <2.5 mm in diameter • Left dominant coronary system • Wide angle with LAD • Concomitant disease in LCX • Diffuse disease in LCX

LAD: left anterior descending artery; LCX: left circumflex artery

descending arteries was treated with elective double stenting technique.

The size of the SB, whether it is large enough to have sufficient ischemic territory thereby justifying a stenting irrespective of bifurcation pattern, should be considered when selecting the stenting streategy. Although a consensus about the significant SB size has not been reached, it is recommended that the SB diameter >2.5 mm (generally LCX) is worth being protected during the procedure or follow-up in LMCA intervention. Therefore, if LCX has the diameter of >2.5 mm and significant stenosis of >50%, the SB stenting is planned during PCI for LMCA bifurcation lesion. When the coronary bifurcations are classified according to the angle between the MB and SB, a Y-angulation less than 70 degrees allows easier wire access to the SB than a wider angle. However, precise stent placement at the ostial SB in Y-angulation is difficult due to a narrow angle between the MB and SB. In contrast, T-angulation, in which the angle between the MB and SB is greater than 70 degrees, provides more difficult SB access but, technically easier complete SB coverage with a stent.

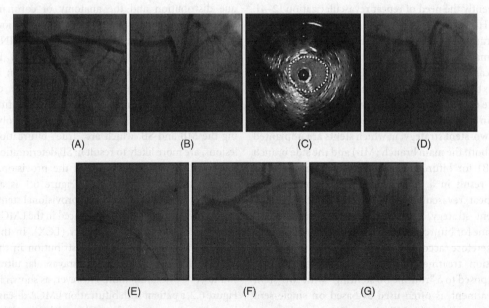

(A)   (B)   (C)   (D)

(E)   (F)   (G)

Figure 6.1 Provisional stenting for a 69-year-old man with normal ejection fraction. (a) and (b) baseline angiograms; (c) IVUS image at the ostial LCX (dotted white circle); (d) angiogram after provisional stenting with a 3.5 × 28 mm Xience everolimus-eluting stent (Abbott Vascular, Santa Clara, CA) in the LMCA-LAD overlapped with a stent in the middle LAD; (e) kissing-balloon inflation after highpressure balloon dilation with a 4.5 × 8 mm non-compliant balloon; (f) and (g) final angiograms after kissing-balloon inflation with two 3.5 × 15 mm non-compliant balloons.

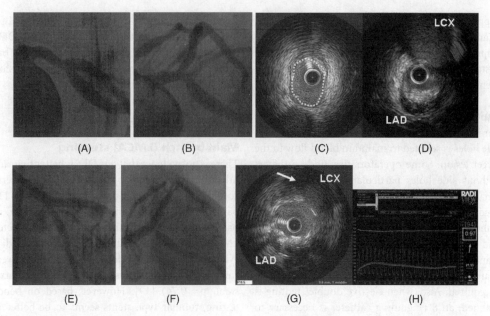

Figure 6.2 Provisional stenting for a 54-year-old woman with normal ejection fraction. (a) and (b) baseline angiograms; (c) baseline IVUS image showing normal ostial LCX (dotted white circle); (d) baseline IVUS images showing diseased ostial LAD and normal ostial LCX; (e) and (f) final angiograms after provisional stenting with a 3.5 × 33 mm Cypher sirolimus-eluting stent (Cordis Corp, Johnson & Johnson, Warren, NJ); (g) final IVUS image from LAD showing normal-looking ostial LCX (arrow); (h) fractional flow reserve (FFR) after hyperemia in the LCX, in which FFR of 0.97 indicates normal blood flow.

Periprocedural preparation

Lesion preparation

In general, the elements of patient preparation before the procedure are dependent on the clinical risk profile of the patient and the anatomic complexity of the lesion. Optimal antithrombotic therapy is, of course, required in all patients but we do not use IIbIIIa receptor antagonists routinely. In addition, elective use of hemodynamic support is also necessary. Although femoral approach is now widely used in LMCA interventions, few studies have reported the feasibility of the radial approach [15,16]. During radial intervention, a 6 Fr or 7 Fr guiding catheter is commonly used due to the small caliber of radial artery. However, when a complex procedure is required, a femoral approach allowing use of a large guiding catheter or hemodynamic support device is recommended.

Hemodynamic support

Hemodynamically unstable patients undergoing LMCA PCI need pharmacological- and/or device-based hemodynamic support. Old age, myocardial infarction, cardiogenic shock and decreased left ventricular ejection fraction are common clinical conditions requiring elective or provisional hemodynamic support. The frequency of elective use of IABP with LMCA PCI varies widely. Recently, a study in 219 elective LMCA interventions evaluated to role of intra-aortic balloon pump (IABP) [17]. An elective IABP was used in a broad range of patients undergoing LMCA bifurcation interventions, including patients with unstable angina, patients with left ventricular ejection fraction <40%, patients with critical right coronary artery disease, and when debulking devices are used. In this study, although the patients receiving elective IABP had a more complex clinical risk profile, the rate of procedural complications was lower than those not receiving an IABP (1.4% vs 9.3%, p = 0.032). Therefore, elective IABP use should be strongly considered for high-risk patients (those with multivessel disease, complex LMCA anatomy, low ejection fraction or unstable presentation). Other, more potent, hemodynamic support devices such as the Tandem-Heart (CardiacAssist, Pittsburgh, Pennsylvania) or the Impella Recover LP 2.5 System (Impella Cardio-Systems, Aachen, Germany) may allow safe treatment of exceedingly high-risk patients.

Guide selection

For LMCA interventions, a guiding catheter with side holes is selected to maintain blood flow to the target lesion. Some operators use guide catheters without side holes particularly in patients with renal insufficiency to reduce the amount of contrast used. Selection of the size and shape of the guiding catheter is based on the complexity of procedure and lesion morphology. When debulking is planned (rotational or directional atherectomy), a large caliber guiding catheter with strong support is required. Also, when elective double stenting is planned, an 8 Fr guiding catheter is necessary to facilitate stent delivery and optimize visualization. In terms of back-up force, an XB (extra-backup) or EBU (extra back up) catheter has stronger back-up support than a JL (Judkins left) catheter. However, caution needs to be exercised when using catheters with strong support due to the possibility of damage to the LMCA. Thus, in the majority of LMCA interventions using provisional stenting, an 8 Fr JL guiding catheter is used.

Role of debulking

In the bare-metal stent era, debulking coronary atherectomy (DCA) before stenting had been used widely in an attempt to reduce restenosis by reducing plaque burden. However, the role of DCA has diminished after the introduction of DES due to the dramatic reduction of restenosis. Nonetheless, a study of 99 patients with LMCA lesions suggested a viable role for DCA even in the DES era [18]. Of interest, DCA in the MB and SB for the LMCA stenoses allowed single-stenting in 60 out of 63 LMCA bifurcation stenoses. Surprisingly, there were no serious adverse events at 1-year follow-up. This study indicates that DCA may have a role in treatment of LMCA bifurcation lesions to optimize the success of the provisional stenting strategy. DCA was used to remove the plaque in the LMCA that was inhibiting the advancement of the wire into left anterior descending artery. Also, rotational atherectomy remains a

valuable technique in severely calcified LMCA lesions. Therefore, although data is limited, DCA or rotational atherectomy still play a limited, but important, role, primarily to reduce plaque shift and facilitate stent expansion.

Stenting procedure

Main branch (LMCA) stenting

There is no evidence that one DES is better than any other in terms of reducing procedural or long-term complications. In a registry that evaluated 110 patients treated with either sirolimus- (N = 55) or paclitaxel- (N = 55) eluting stents for unprotected LMCA stenosis, cumulative major adverse cardiac events at a median follow-up of 660 days were similar (22% in sirolimus stent vs 29% in paclitaxel stent, p = 0.74) [19]. However, based on bench testing, tubular type stents seems to be better in achieving optimal lesion coverage in the SB and a stronger radial force in the LMCA than the coil or hybrid type stents [20]. In the provisional approach, the main branch (LMCA) stent should be directed towards the left anterior descending artery. In cases where the ostial LCX is heavily diseased, elective double stenting should be considered.

Treatment for the side branch

Provisional treatment of the SB (usually LCX) with either balloon angioplasty or stenting is reserved for use in cases with suboptimal results or complications. Despite the controversy, neither balloon angioplasty nor final kissing balloon inflation are routinely performed after MB stenting. As shown in Figure 6.2, angiographic narrowing at the ostial LCX is often caused by the MB stent strut, not by plaque shift. Therefore, to avoid unnecessary barotraumas at the ostial LCX, kissing-balloon inflation is selectively performed in lesions having true narrowing after MB stenting as shown in Figure 6.1. Regarding the type of guidewire, a standard wire is mostly successful in re-crossing to the LCX. However, when a standard wire fails to advance due to wide angle or severe stenosis, hydrophilic coated wire or an intermediate type of stiffer wire is useful to facilitate re-cross. In the case of no success, a small sized over-the-wire balloon, a fixed-wire balloon, or a double lumen catheter can improve support of wire in crossing the stent strut.

Provisional stenting of the LCX artery is selectively used when a suboptimal result or significant dissection occurs after kissing-balloon inflation. As a bail-out procedure, "provisional T-stenting" and "reverse Crush technique" are used. The "provisional T stenting" is a strategy of T stenting in the LCX with the second stent after MB stenting. Final kissing-balloon dilatation after T stenting is a mandatory step for optimal final result. The "reverse Crush" is a variation of Crush technique, in which provisional LCX stenting with T-shape configuration after MB stenting is performed. However, after removal of the LCX wire and balloon, the LCX stent is crushed with the MB balloon. The final step of a kissing-balloon inflation after sequential high pressure in both branches with non-compliant balloons is also mandatory for successful result [21,22]. Furthermore, in both provisional SB stenting strategies, only minimal protrusion of LCX stent into the MB is required [23]. However, an attempt should also be made to avoid incomplete lesion coverage.

The two-stenting technique includes "crush stenting", "T-stenting", "Culotte stenting", and "simultaneous kissing stenting", which were illustrated in the previous chapter. Although several randomized studies comparing single-stent versus two-stent techniques for bifurcation coronary lesions [24,25], have been published, the optimal stenting strategy for LMCA bifurcation lesions has not been determined yet. However, the current consensus is that the two-stent strategy does not have long-term advantages compared with single-stent strategy. Therefore, a systemic treatment of two-stent strategy for all LMCA bifurcation lesions is not justified. Instead, a provisional stenting strategy should be considered as the first line of treatment for LMCA bifurcations without significant SB stenosis.

Role of intravascular ultrasound

Intravascular ultrasound (IVUS) is a useful modality to help in selecting treatment strategies as well as optimizing stent deployment and outcomes even in the DES era [26–28]. Although one study reported that the clinical impact of IVUS-guided stenting for LMCA with DES did not show significant clinical long-term benefit compared with angiography-guided procedure [29], this study was retrospective

and underpowered. The information gathered by IVUS may be crucial for optimal stenting procedure in unprotected LMCA stenosis. Angiography has a limitation in assessing the true luminal size of LMCA because the LMCA is often short and lacks a normal segment for comparison. Therefore, the severity of LMCA disease is often underestimated by the misinterpretation of a normal segment adjacent to focal stenosis. Discrimination of pseudo-obstruction of the SB is another advantage of IVUS examination. The ostial LCX often looks to be falsely compromised by various artifacts including the device, coronary spasm, calcification or stent strut. In addition to the actual assessment of LMCA lesion before procedure, use of IVUS is very helpful to get an adequate expansion of DES, to prevent stent inapposition, and to achieve full lesion coverage with DES. A recent registry study provides evidence that IVUS-guidance may decrease long-term risk of restenosis or late mortality [30,31].

Role of fractional flow reserve

Physiologic flow assessment is a novel method to assess reliably the functional flow in the SB. In a study comparing the discrepancy between angiographic severity and fractional flow reserve (FFR) of the SB for 94 coronary bifurcations, there was a weak correlation between the two measurements [32]. Of interest, only 27% of lesions with ≥75% angiographic stensosis had significant flow impairment as determined by FFR <0.75. Based on this finding, FFR is occasionally measured when the functional severity of SB stenosis is not adequately assessed by morphological analysis.

Antiplatelet therapy

Although the reported incidence of stent thrombosis in DES treatment for LMCA lesions was very low [33], a fear of stent thrombosis remains a major concern to prevent more generalized use of DES. Therefore, a careful administration of antiplatelet agents is a very important treatment to prevent the occurrence of stent thrombosis. In fact, premature discontinuation of clopidogrel was strongly associated with stent thrombosis in several studies [13,34]. Therefore, as generally recommended, dual antiplatelet therapy including aspirin and clopidogrel (or ticlopidine) should be maintained to 1 year. If the patients seem to be at high risk, a high loading dose (600 mg) or lifelong administration of clopidogrel needs to be considered. Furthermore, during the procedure, elective or provisional use of glycoprotein IIb/III inhibitor may play a role in reducing procedure-related thrombotic complications. In some institutions of Asian countries, adjunctive administration of cilostazol has been used for the purpose of reducing thrombotic complications [35]. However, the additive role of glycoprotein IIb/IIa inhibitor, cilostzol, low molecular weight heparin, direct thrombin inhibitor or other new drugs in DES treatment for LMCA lesions needs to be investigated in future studies. Until more evidence is available, the most optimal combination of antithrombotic drugs must be used before, during and after the procedure to avoid thrombotic complications for high-risk patients. Although the features of high risk are not well delineated, off-label use of DES, such as with diabetes mellitus, multiple stenting, long DES, chronic renal failure, or presentation with myocardial infarction, is a good index of high-risk procedure [36].

Conclusion

Bifurcation involvement in the unprotected LMCA is a frequent occurrence that challenges the PCI with DES. However, the provisional stenting strategy is a very simple and effective method to achieve excellent procedural and long-term outcomes in patients with normal or diminutive LCX. Even in the lesions with significant SB stenosis, a complex two-stent strategy can successfully treat the lesions if a careful evaluation of the lesion is performed with angiography and IVUS. Future devices, such as the new dedicated LMCA bifurcated stent, may improve the technical feasibility and clinical prognosis of provisional LMCA stenting.

References

1 Park SJ, Mintz GS. Left Main Stem Disease. Seoul, Informa Healthcare, 2006.

2 Park SJ, Kim YH, Lee BK, Lee SW, Lee CW, Hong MK, Kim JJ, Mintz GS, Park SW. Sirolimus-eluting stent implantation for unprotected left main coronary artery stenosis: comparison with bare metal stent implantation. J Am Coll Cardiol 2005;45(3):351–6.

3 Chieffo A, Stankovic G, Bonizzoni E, Tsagalou E, Iakovou I, Montorfano M, Airoldi F, Michev I, Sangiorgi MG, Carlino M, Vitrella G, Colombo A. Early and mid-term results of drug-eluting stent implantation in unprotected left main. Circulation 2005;111(6):791–5.

4 Valgimigli M, van Mieghem CA, Ong AT, Aoki J, Granillo GA, McFadden EP, Kappetein AP, de Feyter PJ, Smits PC, Regar E, Van der Giessen WJ, Sianos G, de Jaegere P, Van Domburg RT, Serruys PW. Short- and long-term clinical outcome after drug-eluting stent implantation for the percutaneous treatment of left main coronary artery disease: insights from the Rapamycin-Eluting and Taxus Stent Evaluated At Rotterdam Cardiology Hospital registries (RESEARCH and T-SEARCH). Circulation 2005;111(11):1383–9.

5 Price MJ, Cristea E, Sawhney N, Kao JA, Moses JW, Leon MB, Costa RA, Lansky AJ, Teirstein PS. Serial Angiographic Follow-Up of Sirolimus-Eluting Stents for Unprotected Left Main Coronary Artery Revascularization. J Am Coll Cardiol 2006;47(4):871–7.

6 Palmerini T, Marzocchi A, Marrozzini C, Ortolani P, Saia F, Savini C, Bacchi-Reggiani L, Gianstefani S, Virzi S, Manara F. Comparison between coronary angioplasty and coronary artery bypass surgery for the treatment of unprotected left main coronary artery stenosis (the Bologna Registry). Am J Cardiol 2006;98(1):54–9.

7 Lee MS, Kapoor N, Jamal F, Czer L, Aragon J, Forrester J, Kar S, Dohad S, Kass R, Eigler N, Trento A, Shah PK, Makkar RR. Comparison of coronary artery bypass surgery with percutaneous coronary intervention with drug-eluting stents for unprotected left main coronary artery disease. J Am Coll Cardiol 2006;47(4):864–70.

8 Kim YH, Dangas GD, Solinas E, Aoki J, Praise H, Kimura M, Franklin-Bond T, Dasgupta NK, KIrtan AJ, Moussa I, Lansky AJ, Collins M, Stone GW, Leon MB, Moses JW, Mehran R. Effectiveness of drug-eluting stent implantation for patients with unprotected left main coronary artery stenosis. Am J Cardiol 2008;101(6):801–806.

9 Buszman PE, Kiesz SR, Bochenek A, Peszek-Przybyla E, Szkrobka I, Debinski M, Bialkowska B, Dudek D, Gruszka A, Zurakowski A, Milewski K, Wilczynski M, Rzeszutko L, Buszman P, Szymszal J, Martin JL, Tendera M. Acute and late outcomes of unprotected left main stenting in comparison with surgical revascularization. J Am Coll Cardiol 2008;51(5):538–45.

10 Chieffo A, Park SJ, Valgimigli M, Kim YH, Daemen J, Sheiban I, Truffa A, Montorfano M, Airoldi F, Sangiorgi G, Carlino M, Michev I, Lee CW, Hong MK, Park SW, Moretti C, Bonizzoni E, Rogacka R, Serruys PW, Colombo A. Favorable long-term outcome after drug-eluting stent implantation in nonbifurcation lesions that involve unprotected left main coronary artery. A multicenter registry. Circulation 2007;116(2):158–62.

11 Valgimigli M, Malagutti P, Rodriguez-Granillo GA, Garcia-Garcia HM, Polad J, Tsuchida K, Regar E, Van der Giessen WJ, de Jaegere P, De Feyter P, Serruys PW. Distal left main coronary disease is a major predictor of outcome in patients undergoing percutaneous intervention in the drug-eluting stent era: an integrated clinical and angiographic analysis based on the rapamycin-eluting stent evaluated at Rotterdam Cardiology Hospital (RESEARCH) and taxus-stent evaluated at Rotterdam Cardiology Hospital (T-SEARCH) registries. J Am Coll Cardiol 2006;47(8):1530–7.

12 Kim YH, Park SW, Hong MK, Park DW, Park KM, Lee BK, Song JM, Han KH, Lee CW, Kang DH, Song JK, Kim JJ, Park SJ. Comparison of simple and complex stenting techniques in the treatment of unprotected left main coronary artery bifurcation stenosis. Am J Cardiol 2006;97(11):1597–601.

13 Iakovou I, Schmidt T, Bonizzoni E, Ge L, Sangiorgi GM, Stankovic G, Airoldi F, Chieffo A, Montorfano M, Carlino M, Michev I, Corvaja N, Briguori C, Gerckens U, Grube E, Colombo A. Incidence, predictors, and outcome of thrombosis after successful implantation of drug-eluting stents. JAMA 2005;293(17):2126–30.

14 Alfonso F, Suarez A, Perez-Vizcayno MJ, Moreno R, Escaned J, Banuelos C, Jimenez P, Bernardo E, Angiolillo DJ, Hernandez R, Macaya C. Intravascular ultrasound findings during episodes of drug-eluting stent thrombosis. J Am Coll Cardiol 2007;50(21):2095–7.

15 Cheng CI, Wu CJ, Fang CY, Youssef AA, Chen CJ, Chen SM, Yang CH, Hsueh SK, Yip HK, Chen MC, Fu M, Hsieh YK. Feasibility and safety of transradial stenting for unprotected left main coronary artery stenoses. Circ J 2007;71(6):855–61.

16 Ziakas A, Klinke P, Mildenberger R, Fretz E, Williams MB, Della Siega A, Kinloch RD, Hilton JD. Comparison of the radial and femoral approaches in left main PCI: a retrospective study. J Invasive Cardiol 2004;16(3): 129–32.

17 Briguori C, Airoldi F, Chieffo A, Montorfano M, Carlino M, Massimo Sangiorgi G, Morici N, Michev I, Iakovou I, Biondi-Zoccai G, Colombo A. Elective versus provisional intraaortic balloon pumping in unprotected left main stenting. Am Heart J 2006;152(3):565–72.

18 Tsuchikane EAT, Tamai H, Igarashi Y, Kawajiri K, Ozawa N, Nakamura S, Oku K, Kijima M, Hamazaki Y. The efficacy of pre drug eluting stent debulking by directional atherectomy for bifurcated lesions: a multicenter prospective registry (PERFECT Registry). J Am Coll Cardiol 2007; 49 (Suppl 2) (9): 15B.

19 Valgimigli M, Malagutti P, Aoki J, Garcia-Garcia HM, Rodriguez Granillo GA, van Mieghem CAG, Ligthart JM, Ong ATL, Sianos G, Regar E. Sirolimus-eluting versus paclitaxel-eluting stent implantation for the percutaneous treatment of left main coronary artery disease: A combined RESEARCH and T-SEARCH long-term analysis. J Am Coll Cardiol 2006;47(3):507–14.

20 Ormiston JA, Webster MW, Ruygrok PN, Stewart JT, White HD, Scott DS. Stent deformation following simulated side-branch dilatation: a comparison of five stent designs. Catheter Cardiovasc Interv 1999;47(2): 258–64.

21 Ormiston JA, Webster MW, El Jack S, Ruygrok PN, Stewart JT, Scott D, Currie E, Panther MJ, Shaw B, O'Shaughnessy B. Drug-eluting stents for coronary bifurcations: bench testing of provisional side-branch strategies. Catheter Cardiovasc Interv 2006;67(1): 49–55.

22 Ge L, Airoldi F, Iakovou I, Cosgrave J, Michev I, Sangiorgi GM, Montorfano M, Chieffo A, Carlino M, Corvaja N, Colombo A. Clinical and angiographic outcome after implantation of drug-eluting stents in bifurcation lesions with the crush stent technique: importance of final kissing balloon post-dilation. J Am Coll Cardiol 2005;46(4): 613–20.

23 Burzotta F, Gwon HC, Hahn JY, Romagnoli E, Choi JH, Trani C, Colombo A. Modified T-stenting with intentional protrusion of the side-branch stent within the main vessel stent to ensure ostial coverage and facilitate final kissing balloon: the T-stenting and small protrusion technique (TAP-stenting). Report of bench testing and first clinical Italian-Korean two-centre experience. Catheter Cardiovasc Interv 2007;70(1):75–82.

24 Colombo A, Moses JW, Morice MC, Ludwig J, Holmes DR, Jr., Spanos V, Louvard Y, Desmedt B, Di Mario C, Leon MB. Randomized study to evaluate sirolimus-eluting stents implanted at coronary bifurcation lesions. Circulation 2004;109(10):1244–9.

25 Steigen TK, Maeng M, Wiseth R, Erglis A, Kumsars I, Narbute I, Gunnes P, Mannsverk J, Meyerdierks O, Rotevatn S, Niemela M, Kervinen K, Jensen JS, Galloe A, Nikus K, Vikman S, Ravkilde J, James S, Aaroe J, Ylitalo A, Helqvist S, Sjogren I, Thayssen P, Virtanen K, Puhakka M, Airaksinen J, Lassen JF, Thuesen L. Randomized study on simple versus complex stenting of coronary artery bifurcation lesions: the Nordic bifurcation study. Circulation 2006;114(18):1955–61.

26 Sano K, Mintz GS, Carlier SG, de Ribamar Costa Jr J, Qian J, Missel E, Shan S, Franklin-Bond T, Boland P, Weisz G, Moussa I, Dangas GD, Mehran R, Lansky AJ, Kreps EM, Collins MB, Stone GW, Leon MB, Moses JW. Assessing intermediate left main coronary lesions using intravascular ultrasound. Am Heart J 2007;154(5): 983–88.

27 Mintz GS. Features and parameters of drug-eluting stent deployment discoverable by intravascular ultrasound. Am J Cardiol 2007;100(8, Supplement 2): S26–S35.

28 Mintz GS, Weissman NJ. Intravascular Ultrasound in the Drug-Eluting Stent Era. J Am Coll Cardiol 2006; 48(3):421–9.

29 Agostoni P, Valgimigli M, Van Mieghem CAG, Rodriguez-Granillo GA, Aoki J, Ong ATL, Tsuchida K, McFadden EP, Ligthart JM, Smits PC, de Jaegere P, Sianos G, Van der Giessen WJ, De Feyter P, Serruys PW. Comparison of early outcome of percutaneous coronary intervention for unprotected left main coronary artery disease in the drug-eluting stent era with versus without intravascular ultrasonic guidance. Am J Cardiol 2005;95(5):644–7.

30 Roy P, Steinberg DH, Sushinsky SJ, Okabe T, Slottow TLP, Kaneshige K, Xue Z, Satler LF, Kent KM, Suddath WO, Pichard AD, Weissman NJ, Lindsay J, Waksman R. The potential clinical utility of intravascular ultrasound guidance in patients undergoing percutaneous coronary intervention with drug-eluting stents. Eur Heart J 2008;29(15):1851–7.

31 Hong MK, Kim YH, Kim WJ, Suh J, Jung IH, Kim JH, Lee SW, Lee CW, Kim JJ, Park SW, Park SJ. Impact of intravascular ultrasound guidance on long-term clinical outcomes in patients undergoing percutaneous coronary intervention for unprotected left main disease. J Am Coll Cardiol 2008; 51 (Suppl 2): B7.

32 Koo BK, Kang HJ, Youn TJ, Chae IH, Choi DJ, Kim HS, Sohn DW, Oh BH, Lee MM, Park YB, Choi YS, Tahk SJ. Physiologic assessment of jailed side branch lesions using fractional flow reserve. J Am Coll Cardiol 2005;46(4):633–7.

33 Chieffo A, Park S-J, Meliga E, Sheiban I, Lee MS, Latib A, Kim Y-H, Valgimigli M, Sillano D, Magni V, Zoccai GB, Montorfano M, Airoldi F, Rogacka R, Carlino M, Michev I, Lee C-W, Hong M-K, Park S-W, Moretti C, Bonizzoni E, Sangiorgi GM, Tobis J, Serruys PW, Colombo A. Late and very late stent thrombosis following drug-eluting stent implantation in unprotected left main coronary artery: a multicentre registry. Euro Heart J 2008;29(17):2108–15.

34 Park DW, Park SW, Park KH, Lee BK, Kim YH, Lee CW, Hong MK, Kim JJ, Park SJ. Frequency of and risk factors for stent thrombosis after drug-eluting stent implantation during long-term follow-up. Am J Cardiol 2006; 98(3):352–6.

35 Lee SW, Park SW, Hong MK, Kim YH, Lee BK, Song JM, Han KH, Lee CW, Kang DH, Song JK, Kim JJ, Park SJ. Triple versus dual antiplatelet therapy after coronary stenting: impact on stent thrombosis. J Am Coll Cardiol 2005;46(10):1833–7.

36 Tina L. Pinto Slottow RW. Overview of the 2006 Food and Drug Administration Circulatory System Devices Panel meeting on drug-eluting stent thrombosis. Catheterization Cardiovasc Interv 2007;69 (7):1064–74.

CHAPTER 7

Intravascular ultrasound and new imaging in bifurcation stenting

Seung-Jung Park, MD, PhD *and Soo-Jin Kang,* MD, PhD
University of Ulsan College of Medicine, Asan Medical Center, Seoul, Korea

Introduction

Although drug-eluting stents (DES) reduced the rate of restenosis and the need for repeat revascularization compared with bare metal stents (BMS), there is a concern that delayed arterial healing may be a mechanism for late "catch-up" and stent thrombosis [1–5]. Bifurcation stenting still remains technically challenging and is a major determinant of lower procedural success rates as well as adverse outcomes. Intravascular ultrasound (IVUS) provides unique insights into the extent and distribution of coronary atherosclerosis pre-intervention and plays a role in stent optimization by identifying underexpansion and edge problems that contribute to DES failure [6–10].

IVUS-guided PCI and predictors of restenosis and thrombosis

In the BMS era IVUS guidance during percutaneous coronary intervention (PCI) had a favorable impact on restenosis [11–14]. Although IVUS predictors for restenosis and stent thrombosis have been reported in the DES era, it is still uncertain that routine use of IVUS guidance with DES implantation can prevent stent thrombosis or restenosis. Roy *et al.* compared the clinical outcomes of 884 patients undergoing IVUS-guided DES implantation with a propensity-score matched population with angiographic guidance [15]. A higher rate

of definite stent thrombosis was observed in the angiographic-guidance group at 30 days (0.5% vs 1.4%; p = 0.046) and at 12 months (0.7% vs 2.0%; p = 0.014), respectively. IVUS guidance was an independent predictor of freedom from cumulative stent thrombosis at 12 months and also reduced thrombosis and repeat revascularization at 12 months.

The IVUS-measured minimum stent area (MSA) has been the best IVUS predictor for DES restenosis. Although operators routinely depend on manufacturer-supplied compliance charts based on stent size and inflation pressure to predict final stent dimensions, IVUS analyses report that manufacturer-supplied charts underestimated final stent dimensions. Cypher and Taxus achieved only $75 \pm 10\%$ of predicted minimal stent diameter and $66 \pm 17\%$ of predicted MSA. Thus, approximately 25% of Cypher and Taxus implanted into >3.0-mm vessels did not achieve an MSA >5.0 mm^2, a standard definition of adequate DES expansion [16]. Previous studies emphasized that the MSA and the degree of stent expansion were significantly smaller in the stent thrombosis group compared with matched controls [17,18]. Therefore, proper stent expansion is essential to prevent DES stent thrombosis as well as restenosis at follow-up. Serial IVUS analysis from the sirolimus-eluting stent (SES) in coronary lesions (SIRIUS) trial indicated that a MSA <5.0 mm^2 was responsible for the majority of restenosis [19]. Hong *et al.* also found that the

Bifurcation Stenting, First Edition. Edited by Ron Waksman and John A. Ormiston.
© 2012 Blackwell Publishing Ltd. Published 2012 by Blackwell Publishing Ltd.

MSA that best separated restenosis from no restenosis was 5.5 mm^2 in a large series of patients treated with the SES implantation. [20] Finally, data from the TAXUS trials identified 6.0 mm^2 as the MSA to reduce the risk of revascularization. Examination of sensitivity and specificity curves in these three analyses confirmed that the MSA that best separated DES restenosis from no restenosis was 5.0–6.0 mm^2. However, an MSA >5.0 mm^2 may not be achievable in small vessels where stent expansion represented as MSA/reference lumen area in smaller vessels may be the best predictor of an adequate lumen at follow-up [21].

Residual plaque burden is also a predictor of late stent thrombosis and edge restenosis. Fujii et al. reported that the presence of a significant residual reference segment stenosis (defined as edge lumen cross-sectional area <4 mm^2 and a plaque burden >70%) was more common in a stent thrombosis group compared with a matched control group (67% vs 9%, p < 0.001) [17]. Independent predictors of stent thrombosis were stent underexpansion (p = 0.03) and a significant residual reference segment stenosis (p = 0.02). Consistently, Okabe et al. suggested that DES patients who developed stent thrombosis showed a smaller MSA and more residual disease at the stent edges with a larger plaque burden [18]. According to the results of SIRIUS trial, a larger percentage plaque area at the reference segment was associated with edge restenosis, indicating that inadequate lesion coverage may contribute to edge stenosis and target lesion revascularization (TLR) [22]. To confirm full lesion coverage and a proper match between the stented and adjacent segments, use of IVUS may improve outcomes in patients receiving DES implantation.

The impact of the final MSA and stent length on restenosis were relatively reduced in the DES era because of the profound anti-restenosis effect of the eluted drug. However, an IVUS-measured stent length >40 mm predicted 6-month angiographic restenosis after SES implantation with a sensitivity 81% and a specificity 78% [20]. This study also demonstrated the interaction between stent length and final MSA. When implanting long or overlapping SES (total length >40 mm), it is incrementally important to achieve adequate stent expansion, suggesting that the role of IVUS in clinical practice to reduce angiographic restenosis may be greater in complex lesions (very long lesions in small vessels) than in the simple lesions.

Complete stent-vessel wall apposition appeared to be less important than adequate stent expansion. Most acute stent malapposition resolved over time and did not affect the incidence of stent thrombosis or in-stent restenosis. Hong et al. showed that post-procedure incomplete stent apposition occurred in 7.2% of DES-treated lesions and was not associated with major adverse cardiac events including TLR or even an increased amount of intimal hyperplasia [23]. In the TAXUS-II trial 8 of 13 acute stent malappositions in the slow-release group resolved, all acute stent malappositions in the moderate-release group resolved, and at 12 months acute stent malappositon was not associated with an increase in adverse clinical events [24]. Because of the lack of evidence of a relationship between acute incomplete stent apposition and DES failure, too aggressive additional inflations in order to eliminate malapposition seemed unwarranted.

Role of IVUS in PCI for bifurcating lesions

IVUS

There are only a few published data regarding the role of IVUS in bifurcation lesions. However, these data suggest that IVUS is useful to optimize stent placement and assess the risk and mechanism of stent failure. In the majority of bifurcation lesions treated with the crush technique, the smallest MSA appeared at the side branch ostium (68% of the lesions) [25]. For the side branch an MSA <4 mm^2 was found in 44%, and a MSA <5 mm^2 in 76%, typically at the ostium, this may contribute to a higher restenosis rate at the side branch ostium, the most common restenosis location. Furthermore, post-intervention imaging can determine whether the side branch has been compromised after provisional stenting or whether there is adequate stent expansion after stenting both branches. The use of IVUS demonstrated that incomplete crushing and ostial side branch stent underexpansion are common and often not suspected angiographically [26].

Hahn et al. suggested that inadequate post-procedural MSA with increased neointimal hyperplasia may cause the side branch ostium to be the most frequent site of restenosis after

T-stenting at bifurcation lesions [27]. The side branch ostium was the most frequent site of post-procedural MSA. The follow-up minimum lumen area correlated with post-procedural MSA (r = 0.81, p < 0.001) and the percentage of neointimal area was higher at the side branch ostium than other sites. The optimal threshold of post-procedural MSA to predict follow-up minimal lumen area ≥4 mm² at the side branch ostium was 4.83 mm² (area under the curve = 0.88, 95% confidence interval = 0.80 to 0.95).

In particular when using a one-stent cross-over technique, there are two suggested mechanisms of acute luminal loss at the ostium of the left circumflex: carina shift versus plaque shift [28–31] IVUS has been used to assess mechanisms and complications of stent implantation (Figure 7.1). Vassilev *et al.* reported that a smaller distal carina angle predicted higher side branch compromise and

major cardiovascular events at 1-year follow-up in patients with bifurcation lesions treated with single main vessel stent (cross-over technique) [28]. Although a negative correlation between the percentage stenosis and fractional flow reserve has been shown, there was a wide variation of functional significance, even among lesions with angiographically significant side branch stenosis [32]. Only 23% of the side branch lesions ≥75% diameter stenosis were functionally significant. Therefore, angiography is unreliable in the assessment of jailed side branch lesions and generally overestimates the functional severity, which may be explained by lesion eccentricity, stent strut artifacts, and relatively small myocardial territory of side branch. Moreover, the authors measured fractional flow reserve in the jailed side branch after main branch stenting [31,33] They suggested that preintervention percentage diameter stenosis of the side branch

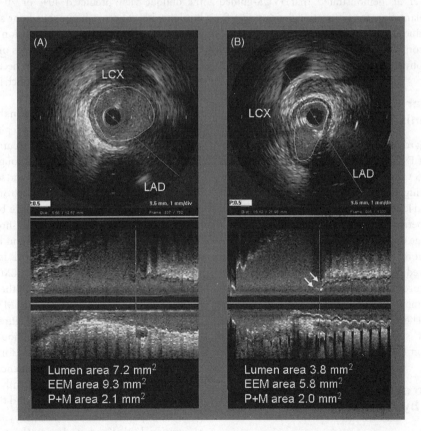

Figure 7.1 The LCX-pullback IVUS pre-stenting (a) and post-stenting (b). After cross-over stenting from the LAD to the LM, percentage change in the EEM area was −38% and percentage change in the lumen area was −47%. The longitudinal image reconstruction demonstrated carina shift into the LCX post-stenting (arrows).

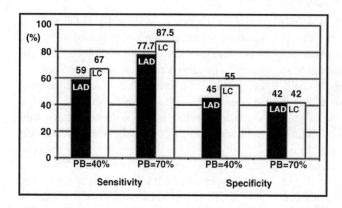

Figure 7.2 Accuracy of side branch plaque burden evaluation from main branch.

and minimum lumen diameter of main branch distal to the side branch were independent predictors of functionally significant side branch stenosis.

IVUS guidance of stent implantation might be even more beneficial in complex lesions such as bifurcation lesions. A current study conducted by Kim *et al.* demonstrated that IVUS-guided DES implantation for bifurcation lesions significantly reduced the 4-year mortality and very late stent thrombosis compared with conventional angiography-guided stenting [34].

Vascular responses and mechanisms of restenosis

With regard to OCT assessment of vascular response of DES-treated lesions [35], a sub-analysis of ODESSA demonstrated that at 6 months paclitaxel-eluting stents (PES) had the highest rate of uncovered lesions in side-branch ostium (60.1% of PES), whereas SES showed the highest rate of uncoverage opposite to the ostium (14.0% of SES). Furthermore, despite the use of a dedicated stent, malapposed struts were more frequent at the level of the bifurcation (33.3%) than in both the proximal segment (18.5%) and the distal segment (9.8%). The highest frequency and largest vessel wall-stent strut distance were observed in the bifurcation half toward the side branch [36].

How to evaluate bifurcating lesion by IVUS?

IVUS

Using a distal left main coronary artery (LMCA) stenosis as the model for a bifurcation lesion,

Oviedo *et al.* analyzed pullbacks from the left anterior descending artery (LAD) and the left circumflex artery (LCX) to evaluate whether IVUS assessment of the side branch ostium requires direct imaging or is accurate from the main vessel [37]. Using oblique versus direct comparisons, the oblique view predicted 40% or 70% plaque burden with good sensitivity, but poor specificity (Figure 7.2). Therefore, IVUS evaluation of a side branch ostium from the main vessel is only moderately reliable; and direct imaging is necessary for an accurate assessment of the side branch including its ostium.

Another study also by Oviedo *et al.* in the LMCA proposed an IVUS classification for bifurcation lesions illustrating longitudinal and circumferential spatial plaque distribution [38]. Although angiographic classifications of the location and severity of disease in the main vessel and side branch of left main coronary artery (LM) bifurcation have been proposed, they are rarely accurate. IVUS showed that bifurcation disease is mostly diffuse and not focal; and the carina (both sides of flow divider) is typically spared. Continuous plaque from the LM into the proximal LAD was seen in 90%, from the LM into the LCX artery in 66.4%, and from the LM into both the LAD and LCX arteries in 62% (Figure 7.3).

Ramcharitar *et al.* described a method for dedicated quantitative coronary analysis for bifurcations including the polygon of confluence (POC), the smallest region that behaves differently from the proximal and distal vessel segments and the region that encompasses the start and the end of the bifurcation [39]. Kang *et al.* recently studied the clinical impact of pre- and post-procedural IVUS findings in patients undergoing DES implantation

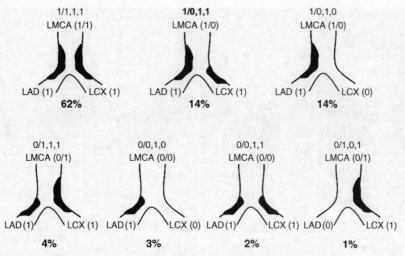

Figure 7.3 IVUS classification for LM bifurcation plaque distribution. Continuous involvement from the distal LMCA into the proximal LAD artery is present in 90%.

for unprotected LM bifurcation disease [40]. In parallel with the previous angiographic concepts, POC by IVUS was defined as a confluent zone of the LAD and LCX (Figure 7.4). The pre-procedural minimal lumen area within the LMCA was located within the POC in 41% of cases. Moreover, pre-procedural minimal lumen area within the POC reflecting the overall severity of LMCA bifurcation disease including the ostium of the LCX.

Beyond grayscale IVUS

Tissue characterization of atherosclerotic plaque using radiofrequency data analysis (virtual histology, VH) provides more detailed assessment of tissue composition than is possible with grayscale IVUS. Technologically, the main difference between grayscale IVUS and VH is that grayscale IVUS imaging is produced by the envelope (amplitude) of the ultrasound signal. However, the frequency and power of the signal commonly differ between tissues, regardless of similarities in amplitude. VH (Volcano Corp, Rancho Cordoba, USA) performs spectral analysis to construct tissue maps that classify plaques into four major components [41–43]. The accuracy of VH tissue characterization has been validated ex vivo by comparison with histology; the overall predictive accuracies were 93.5% for fibrous, 94.1% for fibro-fatty, 95.8% for necrotic core, and 96.7% for dense calcium, with sensitivities and specificities ranging from 72% to 99% [41–43].

Rodriguez-Granillo reported compositional characteristics of plaque located at distal LMCA bifurcating lesions [44]. A larger calcified and

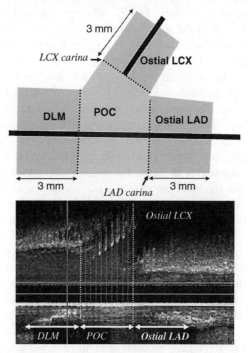

Figure 7.4 Four segments of LM bifurcation: POC (confluence zone of LAD and LCX on longitudinal IVUS image); distal LM (DLM) (3 mm-segment just proximal to the POC) assessed by LAD pullback; ostial LCX is separately assessed by LCX pullback.

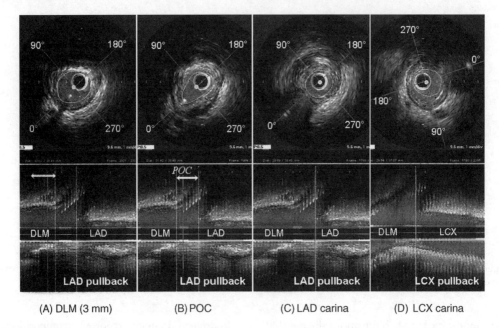

(A) DLM (3 mm)   (B) POC   (C) LAD carina   (D) LCX carina

Figure 7.4 (*Continued*)

necrotic core content was found distal to the circumflex take-off. Lesions were predominantly located in the outer wall of the carina, and this location was associated with larger necrotic core content. The pathophysiology of such phenomena can be explained briefly by the fact that the low endothelial shear stress induces a loss of the physiologic flow-oriented alignment of the endothelial cells, thus causing an enhancement of the expression of adhesion molecules and a weakening of cell junctions and ultimately leading to an increase in permeability to lipids and macrophages [45,46]. The results of the present study are in line with histopathologic data, showing higher concentrations of necrotic core and calcium in areas subject to low endothelial shear stress. However, irrespective of plaque size, plaques located in the LM stem contained minimal necrotic core. Thus, they mimic the distal but not the proximal tract of the LAD where plaque rupture or vessel occlusion occurs more frequently [47].

Optical coherence tomography (OCT) is a light-based imaging modality and its use has been increasingly in catherization laboratories. The ability to provide high spatial resolution (10–20 µm) images of the coronary artery in vivo has supported new possibilities for the precise plaque characterization pre-procedure and assessment of the immediate and long-term effects of the interaction between the stent and the vessel wall [36,48,49]. OCT tissue characterization includes lipid-rich plaque, fibrous plaque, calcium, red blood cell rich thrombus, platelet rich thrombus, and macrophages. OCT-derived TCFA is defined as fibrous cap thickness at the thinnest part ≤65 µm and an angle of lipidic tissue ≥180° [50–55]. In addition, OCT is capable of identifying the findings beyond the resolution IVUS, such as small-sized thrombus or tissue protrusion, intra-stent or edge dissections during PCI, and tissue coverage (especially small amounts of tissue coverage) and malapposition at follow-up. The major disadvantage of OCT is limited tissue penetration and, therefore, inability to image consistently the adventitia and assess the plaque burden. The original time-domain OCT technique requires continuous flushing with proximal balloon occlusion to displace the blood. The recent advance in new generation OCT system (Fourier-domain OCT, FD-OCT) allows rapid (15–30 mm/s) image acquisition of long segments with only a 3–5 second contrast or saline injection through the guiding catheter without the need for proximal balloon occlusion. Although OCT is currently used for long-term assessment of stent implantation, it is expected that OCT will be synergistically utilized with conventional IVUS to optimize the stent procedure.

OCT can provide new insights about the characteristics of the atherosclerotic plaque in bifurcations, another important factor that could potentially contribute to the higher risk of stent failure in these lesions. OCT can identify the extension and composition of the plaque along the main branch and in the ostium of the side branch. In vivo frequency and distribution of high-risk, necrotic core-rich plaques at bifurcations using a combined VH and OCT assessment was reported by Gonzalo *et al.* [48]. Fibroatheromas were identified in 26.2% and TCFAs in 17.4%. The percentage of necrotic core decreases from the proximal to the distal rim (16.8% vs 13.5%, p = 0.01), while the cap thickness had an inverse tendency. Overall, 44.1% of the TCFAs were located in the proximal rim, 41.2% within the bifurcation segment, and only 14.7% in the distal rim. The proximal rim of the ostium of the side branch was more likely to contain a thin fibrous cap and a greater proportion of necrotic core. More recent data showed that OCT-detected TCFAs were mostly distributed near side branches and opposite the side branch bifurcation [51]. Three-vessel OCT imaging in patients with acute myocardial infarction revealed that TCFAs tended to cluster in predictable spots within the proximal segment of the LAD, but developed relatively evenly in the LCX and right coronary artery.

OCT evaluation of bifurcation stenting

In vivo frequency and distribution of high-risk, necrotic core-rich plaques at bifurcations using a combined VH and OCT assessment was reported by Gonzalo *et al.* [44]. Fibroatheromas were identified in 26.2% and TCFAs in 17.4%. The percentage of necrotic core decreases from the proximal to the distal rim (16.8% vs 13.5%, p = 0.01), while the cap thickness had an inverse tendency. Overall, 44.1% of the TCFA were located in the proximal rim, and 41.2% in in-bifurcation segment and only 14.7% in the distal rim. The proximal rim of the ostium of the side branch was a region more likely to contain thin fibrous cap and a greater proportion

of necrotic core. More recent data showed that OCT-detected TCFAs were mostly distributed near side branches, mainly positioned opposite the side branch bifurcation [51]. Three-vessel OCT imaging in patients with acute myocardial infarction revealed that TCFAs tend to cluster in predictable spots within the proximal segment of the LAD, but develop relatively evenly in the LCX and right coronary artery.

With regard to the OCT follow-up study for vascular response of DES-treated lesions, there is strut-level analysis in human coronary bifurcations [35]. As a sub-analysis of ODESSA, 6-month follow-up OCT study demonstrate that paclitaxel-eluting stent (PES) had the highest rate of uncovered lesions in side-branch ostium (60.1% of PES), whereas SES showed the highest rate of uncoverage at opposite to the ostium (14.0% of SES), suggesting the variable patterns of strut coverage in the bifurcation according to the different stent technologies. Furthermore, despite the use of a dedicated stent, malapposed struts was more frequent at the level of the bifurcation (33.3%) than in both the proximal segment (18.5%) and the distal segment (9.8%). The highest frequency and largest vessel wall-stent strut distance are observed in the bifurcation half toward the side branch [47].

Conclusion

IVUS evaluation is useful to optimize the stent procedure and is the best way to identify and exclude causes of DES failure. The high resolution of OCT images gives us a new insight for the complex PCI for bifurcation lesions by supporting the precise information for lesion morphology and plaque composition.

References

1 Moses JW, Leon MB, Popma JJ, Fitzgerald PJ, Holmes DR, O'Shaughnessy C, Caputo RP, Kereiakes DJ, Williams DO, Teirstein PS, Jaeger JL, Kuntz RE; SIRIUS Investigators. Sirolimus-eluting stents versus standard stents in patients with stenosis in a native coronary artery. N Engl J Med 2003;349:1315–23.

2 Kastrati A, Dibra A, Mehilli J, Mayer S, Pinieck S, Pache J, Dirschinger J, Schomig A. Predictive factors of restenosis after coronary implantation of sirolimus- or paclitaxel-eluting stents. Circulation 2006;113:2293–100.

3　Park DW, Hong MK, Mintz GS, Lee CW, Song JM, Han KH, Kang DH, Cheong SS, Song JK, Kim JJ, Weissman NJ, Park SW, Park SJ. Two-year follow-up of the quantitative angiographic and volumetric intravascular ultrasound analysis after nonpolymeric paclitaxel-eluting stent implantation: late "catch-up" phenomenon from ASPECT Study. J Am Coll Cardiol 2006;48:2432–9.

4　Pfisterer M, Brunner-La Rocca H, Buser P, Rickenbacher P, Hunziker P, Mueller C, Jeger R, Bader F, Osswald S, Kaiser C; for the BASKET-LATE Investigators. Late clinical events after clopidogrel discontinuation may limit the benefit of drug-eluting stents an observational study of drug-eluting versus bare-metal stents. J Am Coll Cardiol 2006;48:2584–91.

5　Daemen J, Wenaweser P, Tsuchida K, Abrecht L, Vaina S, Morger C, Kukreja N, Juni P, Sianos G, Hellige G, van Domburg RT, Hess OM, Boersma E, Meier B, Windecker S, Serruys PW. Early and late coronary stent thrombosis of sirolimus-eluting and paclitaxel-eluting stents in routine clinical practice: data from a large two-institutional cohort study. Lancet 2007;369:667–78.

6　Hong MK, Mintz GS, Lee CW, Park DW, Choi BR, Park KH, Kim YH, Cheong SS, Song JK, Kim JJ, Park SW, Park SJ. Intravascular ultrasound predictors of angiographic restenosis after sirolimus-eluting stent implantation. Eur Heart J 2006;27:1305–10.

7　Takebayashi H, Kobayashi Y, Mintz GS, Carlier SG, Fujii K, Yasuda T, Moussa I, Mehran R, Dangas GD, Collins MB, Kreps E, Lansky AJ, Stone GW, Leon MB, Moses JW. Intravascular ultrasound assessment of lesions with target vessel failure after sirolimus-eluting stent implantation. Am J Cardiol 2005;95:498–502.

8　Fujii K, Mintz GS, Kobayashi Y, Carlier SG, Takebayashi H, Yasuda T, Moussa I, Dangas G, Mehran R, Lansky AJ, Reyes A, Kreps E, Collins M, Colombo A, Stone GW, Teirstein PS, Leon MB, Moses JW. Contribution of stent underexpansion to recurrence after sirolimus-eluting stent implantation for restenosis. Circulation 2004; 109:1085–8.

9　Fujii K, Carlier SG, Mintz GS, Yang YM, Moussa I, Weisz G, Dangas G, Mehran R, Lansky AJ, Kreps EM, Collins M, Stone GW, Moses JW, Leon MB. Stent underexpansion and residual reference segment stenosis are related to stent thrombosis after sirolimus-eluting stent implantation: an intravascular ultrasound study. J Am Coll Cardiol 2005;45:995–8.

10　Okabe T, Mintz GS, Buch AN, Roy P, Hong YJ, Smith KA, Torguson R, Gevorkian N, Xue Z, Satler LF, Kent KM, Pichard AD, Weissman NJ, Waksman R. Intravascular ultrasound parameters associated with stent thrombosis after drug-eluting stent deployment. Am J Cardiol 2007;100:615–20.

11　Fitzgerald PJ, Oshima A, Hayase M, Metz JA, Bailey SR, Baim DS, Cleman MW, Deutsch E, Diver DJ, Leon MB, Moses JW, Oesterle SN, Overlie PA, Pepine CJ, Safian RD, Shani J, Simonton CA, Smalling RW, Teirstein PS, Zidar JP, Yeung AC, Kuntz RE, Yock PG. Final results of the can routine ultrasound influence stent expansion (CRUISE) study. Circulation 2000;102:523–30.

12　Oemrawsingh PV, Mintz GS, Schalij MJ, Zwinderman AH, Jukema JW, van der Wall EE, TULIP Study. Thrombocyte activity evaluation and effects of ultrasound guidance in long intracoronary stent placement intravascular ultrasound guidance improves angiographic and clinical outcome of stent implantation for long coronary artery stenoses: final results of a randomized comparison with angiographic guidance (TULIP Study). Circulation 2003;107:62–7.

13　Moussa I, Di Mario C, Reimers B, Akiyama T, Tobis J, Colombo A. Subacute stent thrombosis in the era of intravascular ultrasound-guided coronary stenting without anticoagulation: frequency, predictors and clinical outcome. J Am Coll Cardiol 1997;29:6–12.

14　Cheneau E, Leborgne L, Mintz GS, Kotani J, Pichard AD, Satler LF, Canos D, Castagna M, Weissman NJ, Waksman R. Predictors of subacute stent thrombosis: results of a systematic intravascular ultrasound study. Circulation 2003;108:43–7.

15　Roy P, Steinberg DH, Sushinsky SJ, Okabe T, Pinto Slottow TL, Kaneshige K, Xue Z, Satler LF, Kent KM, Suddath WO, Pichard AD, Weissman NJ, Lindsay J, Waksman R. The potential clinical utility of intravascular ultrasound guidance in patients undergoing percutaneous coronary intervention with drug-eluting stents. Eur Heart J. 2008;29:1851–7.

16　de Ribamar Costa J Jr, Mintz GS, Carlier SG, Fujii K, Sano K, Kimura M, Tanaka K, Costa RA, Lui J, Na Y, Castellanos C, Biro S, Moussa I, Stone GW, Moses JW, Leon MB. Intravascular ultrasound assessment of drug-eluting stent expansion. Am Heart J. 2007;153:297–303.

17　Fujii K, Carlier SG, Mintz GS, Yang YM, Moussa I, Weisz G, Dangas G, Mehran R, Lansky AJ, Kreps EM, et al. Stent underexpansion and residual reference segment stenosis are related to stent thrombosis after sirolimus-eluting stent implantation. J Am Coll Cardiol 2005;945:995–8.

18　Okabe T, Mintz GS, Buch AN, Roy P, HongYJ, Smith KA, Torguson R, Gevorkian N, Xue Z, Satler LF, et al. Intravascular ultrasound parameters associated with stent thrombosis after drug-eluting stent deployment. Am J Cardiol 2007;100:615–20.

19　Sonoda S, Morino Y, Ako J, Terashima M, Hassan AH, Bonneau HN, Leon MB, Moses JW, Yock PG, Honda Y, Kuntz RE, Fitzgerald PJ, SIRIUS Investigators. Impact of final stent dimensions on long-term results following sirolimus-eluting stent implantation. J Am Coll Cardiol 2004;43:1959–63.

20 Hong MK, Mintz GS, Lee CW, Park DW, Choi BR, Park KH, Kim YH, Cheong SS, Song SS, Kim JJ, Park SW, Park SJ. Intravascular ultrasound predictors of angiographic restenosis after sirolimus-eluting stent implantation. Eur Heart J 2006;27:1305–10.

21 Shimada Y, Honda Y, Hongo Y, et al. Sirolimus-eluting stent implantation in small coronary arteries: predictors of long-term stent patency and neointimal hyperplasia (abstr). Circulation 2005;112:II736.

22 Sakurai R, Ako J, Morino Y, Sonoda S, Kaneda H, Terashima M, Hassan AH, Leon MB, Moses JW, Popma JJ, et al. and SIRIUS Trial Investigators, Predictors of edge stenosis following sirolimus-eluting stent deployment (a qualitative intravascular ultrasound analysis from the SIRIUS Trial. Am J Cardiol 2005;96:1251–3.

23 Hong M-K, Mintz GS, Lee CW, et al. Late stent malapposition after drug-eluting stent implantation: an intravascular ultrasound analysis with long-term follow-up. Circulation 2006;113:414–9.

24 Tanabe K, Serruys PW, and Degertekin M, et al. Incomplete stent apposition after implantation of paclitaxel-eluting stents or bare metal stents: insights from the randomized TAXUS-II trial. Circulation 2005;111:900–5.

25 Costa RA, Mintz GS, Carlier SG, et al. Bifurcation coronary lesions treated with the "crush" technique: an intravascular ultrasound analysis. J Am Coll Cardiol 2005;46:599–605.

26 Mintz GS, Weissman NJ. Intravascular ultrasound in the drug-eluting stent era. J Am Coll Cardiol 2006;48:421–9. [Review].

27 Hahn JY, Song YB, Lee SY, Choi JH, Choi SH, Kim DK, Lee SH, Gwon HC. Serial intravascular ultrasound analysis of the main and side branches in bifurcation lesions treated with the T-stenting technique. J Am Coll Cardiol 2009;54:110–7.

28 Gil RJ, Vassilev D, Formuszewicz R, Rusicka-Piekarz T, Doganov A. The carina angle-new geometrical parameter associated with periprocedural side branch compromise and the long-term results in coronary bifurcation lesions with main vessel stenting only. J Interv Cardiol 2009;22:E1–10.

29 Shimada Y, Courtney BK, Nakamura M, Hongo Y, Sonoda S, Hassan AH, Yock PG, Honda Y, Fitzgerald PJ. Intravascular ultrasonic analysis of atherosclerotic vessel remodeling and plaque distribution of stenotic left anterior descending coronary arterial bifurcation lesions upstream and downstream of the side branch. Am J Cardiol 2006;98:193–6.

30 Vassilev D, Gil R. Clinical verification of a theory for predicting side branch stenosis after main vessel stenting

in coronary bifurcation lesions. J Interv Cardiol 2008; 21:493–503.

31 Koo BK, Waseda K, Kang HJ, Kim HS, Nam CW, Hur SH, Kim JS, Choi D, Jang Y, Hahn JY, Gwon HC, Yoon MH, Tahk SJ, Chung WY, Cho YS, Choi DJ, Hasegawa T, Kataoka T, Oh SJ, Honda Y, Fitzgerald PJ, Fearon WF. Anatomic and functional evaluation of bifurcation lesions undergoing percutaneous coronary intervention. Circ Cardiovasc Interv 2010;3:113–9.

32 Koo BK, Kang HJ, Young TJ, et al. Physiologic assessment of jailed side branch lesions using fractional flow reserve. J Am Coll Cardiol 2005;46:633–7.

33 Koo BK, Park KW, Kang HJ, et al. Physiological evaluation of the provisional side-branch intervention strategy for bifurcation lesions using fractional flow reserve. Eur Heart J 2008;29:726–32.

34 Kim SH, Kim YH, Kang SJ, Park DW, Lee SW, Lee CW, Hong MK, Cheong SS, Kim JJ, Park SW, Park SJ. Long-term outcomes of intravascular ultrasound-guided stenting in coronary bifurcation lesions. Am J Cardiol 2010; 106:612–8.

35 Kyono H, Guagliumi G, Sirbu V, Rosenthal N, Tahara S, Musumeci G, Trivisonno A, Bezerra HG, Costa MA. Optical coherence tomography (OCT) strut-level analysis of drug-eluting stents (DES) in human coronary bifurcations. EuroIntervention 2010;6:69–77.

36 Tyczynski P, Ferrante G, Kukreja N, Moreno-Ambroj C, Barlis P, Ramasami N, De Silva R, Beatt K, Di Mario C. Optical coherence tomography assessment of a new dedicated bifurcation stent. EuroIntervention 2009;5: 544–51.

37 Oviedo C, Maehara A, Mintz GS, Tsujita K, Kubo T, Doi H, Castellanos C, Lansky AJ, Mehran R, Dangas G, Leon MB, Stone GW, Templin B, Araki H, Ochiai M, Moses JW. Is accurate intravascular ultrasound evaluation of the left circumflex ostium from a left anterior descending to left main pullback possible? Am J Cardiol 2010;105: 948–54.

38 Oviedo C, Maehara A, Mintz GS, Araki H, Choi SY, Tsujita K, Kubo T, Doi H, Templin B, Lansky AJ, Dangas G, Leon MB, Mehran R, Tahk SJ, Stone GW, Ochiai M, Moses JW. Intravascular ultrasound classification of plaque distribution in left main coronary artery bifurcations: where is the plaque really located? Circ Cardiovasc Interv 2010;3:105–12.

39 Ramcharitar S, Onuma Y, Aben JP, Serruys PW, et al. A novel dedicated quantitative coronary analysis methodology for bifurcation lesions. EuroIntervention 2008; 3:553–7.

40 Kang SJ, Mintz GS, Kim WJ, Lee JY, Park DW, Yun SC, Lee SW, Kim YH, Lee CW, Han KH, Kim JJ, Park SW, Park SJ. Effect of intravascular ultrasound findings on the long-term repeat revascularization in patients

undergoing drug-eluting stent implantation for severe unprotected left main bifurcation narrowing. Am J Cardiol 2011;107(3):367–73.

41 Nair A, Kuban BD, Tuzcu EM, Schoenhagen P, Nissen SE, Vince DG. Coronary plaque classification with intravascular ultrasound radiofrequency data analysis. Circulation 2002;106:2200–6.

42 Garcia-Garcia HM, Gonzalo N, Regar E, Serruys PW. Virtual histology and optical coherence tomography: from research to a broad clinical application. Heart 2009;95:1362–74.

43 Moore MP, Spencer T, Salter DM, et al. Characterization of coronary atherosclerotic morphology by spectral analysis of radiofrequency signal: in vitro intravascular ultrasound study with histological and radiological validation. Heart 1998;79:459–67.

44 Rodriguez-Granillo GA, García-García HM, Wentzel J, Valgimigli M, Tsuchida K, van der Giessen W, de Jaegere P, Regar E, de Feyter PJ, Serruys PW. Plaque composition and its relationship with acknowledged shear stress patterns in coronary arteries. J Am Coll Cardiol 2006;47: 884–5.

45 Slager CJ, Wentzel J, Gijsen FJH, Schuurbiers JCH, van der Wal AC, van der Steen AFW, Serruys PW. The role of shear stress in the generation of rupture-prone vulnerable plaques. Nat Clin Pract 2005;2:401–7.

46 Kornet L, Hoeks AP, Lambregts J, Reneman RS. In the femoral artery bifurcation, differences in mean wall shear stress within subjects are associated with different intima-media thicknesses. Arterioscler Thromb Vasc Biol 1999; 19:2933–9.

47 Valgimigli M, Rodriguez-Granillo GA, Garcia-Garcia HM, Vaina S, De Jaegere P, De Feyter P, Serruys PW. Plaque composition in the left main stem mimics the distal but not the proximal tract of the left coronary artery: influence of clinical presentation, length of the left main trunk, lipid profile, and systemic levels of C-reactive protein. J Am Coll Cardiol 2007;49:23–31.

48 Gonzalo N, Garcia-Garcia HM, Regar E, Barlis P, Wentzel J, Onuma Y, Ligthart J, Serruys PW. In vivo assessment of high-risk coronary plaques at bifurcations with combined intravascular ultrasound and optical coherence tomography. JACC Cardiovasc Imaging 2009;2:473–82.

49 Jang IK, Bouma BE, Kang DH, Park SJ, Park SW, Seung KB, Choi KB, Shishkov M, Schlendorf K, Pomerantsev E, Houser SL, Aretz HT, Tearney GJ. Visualization of coronary atherosclerotic plaques in patients using optical coherence tomography: comparison with intravascular ultrasound. J Am Coll Cardiol 2002;39:604–9.

50 Regar E, van Beusekom HMM, van der Gissen WJ, Serruys PW. Optical coherence tomography findings at 5-year follow-up after coronary stent implantation. Circulation 2005;112:e345–6.

51 Fujii K, Kawasaki D, Masutani M, Okumura T, Akagami T, Sakoda T, Tsujino T, Ohyanagi M, Masuyama T. OCT assessment of thin-cap fibroatheroma distribution in native coronary arteries. JACC Cardiovasc Imaging 2010;3:168–75.

52 Kume T, Akasaka T, Kawamoto T, Watanabe N, Toyota E, Neishi Y, Sukmawan R, Sadahira Y, Yoshida K. Assessment of coronary arterial plaque by optical coherence tomography. Am J Cardiol 2006;97:1172–5.

53 Kume T, Akasaka T, Kawamoto T, Ogasawara Y, Watanabe N, Toyota E, Neishi Y, Sukmawan R, Sadahira Y, Yoshida K. Assessment of coronary arterial thrombus by optical coherence tomography. Am J Cardiol 2006; 97:1713–7.

54 Kume T, Akasaka T, Kawamoto T, Okura H, Watanabe N, Toyota E, Neishi Y, Sukmawan R, Sadahira Y, Yoshida K. Measurement of the thickness of the fibrous cap by optical coherence tomography. Am Heart J 2006;152:755. e1–e4.

55 Yabushita H, Bouma BE, Houser SL, Aretz HT, Jang IK, Schlendorf KH, Kauffman CR, Shishkov M, Kang DH, Halpern EF, Tearney GJ. Characterization of human atherosclerosis by optical coherence tomography. Circulation 2002;106:1640–5.

8

CHAPTER 8

Drug-eluting balloons and bifurcations, a new future for treatment?

Pierfrancesco Agostoni, MD, PhD, *Anouar Belkacemi*, MD, *Michiel Voskuil*, MD, PhD *and Pieter R. Stella*, MD, PhD

University Medical Center Utrecht, Department of Interventional Cardiology, Utrecht, The Netherlands

Overview

Coronary bifurcation lesions remain hampered by procedural difficulties, post-procedural complications and suboptimal long-term results, even with the introduction of drug-eluting stents. In particular, side branch restenosis remains a drawback even with the provisional T-stenting technique. The introduction of drug-eluting balloons (DEB) creates a new hope for this technique by maintaining the relatively easy provisional T-stenting technique but promising better long-term outcomes for the SB treated with DEB. The DEB locally delivers a high concentration of an anti-restenotic drug, paclitaxel, thereby potentially reducing restenosis rate as compared to a regular balloon. However, little is still known on the optimal use and long-term outcome of DEB in bifurcations. The results of the "DEb in BIfUrcaTion trial (DEBIUT)" will help us to understand current achievements and future directions in the development of this new and promising device for this specific lesion subset.

Introduction

Coronary bifurcation lesions make up 15–20% of all percutaneous coronary interventions [1]. This subset of lesions is shown to be complex, with inferior angiographic and clinical results at follow-up compared with non-bifurcation lesions. In particular, the restenosis rate in the side branch (SB) remains the Achilles's heel of bifurcation lesions [2–5]. Besides, bifurcations are a known risk factor for increased late stent thrombosis particularly when using drug-eluting stents (DES) [6,7]. This warrants prolonged double antiplatelet therapy (DAPT) when compared with bare metal stents (BMS). Low compliance to DAPT has recently been shown to result in higher numbers of stent thrombosis in clinical practice [8].

Therefore, the search for alternative treatment strategies, with better outcomes than BMS, combined with a reduction of DAPT seems appropriate. A new device that potentially fulfills all these characteristics is the drug-eluting balloon (DEB).

Drug-Eluting balloons

Drug-eluting balloons are regular semi-compliant angioplasty balloons covered with an anti-restenotic drug, which is released into the vessel wall during inflation of the balloon, usually at nominal pressures with a specific minimal inflation time. The active substance on the DEB should be lipophilic enough to have a high absorption rate through the vessel wall [9], compensating for the short time of contact between the inflated balloon and the vessel wall itself, and to maintain a sustained effect once released [10]. The drug of choice at this moment is paclitaxel. Paclitaxel is a broad-spectrum anti-mitotic agent that inhibits cell division in the G2/M phase, stabilizing the polymerized microtubules, thus inhibiting cell replication of the smooth muscle cells, and by that reducing neo-intimal hyperplasia [11]. Paclitaxel was identified as the primary drug for DEB due to its right pharmacological characteristics such as high lipophilic property and ability to remain in the vessel wall for nearly a week [12]. Thus, a stent-driven sustained drug release may not be necessary in all cases [13].

Therefore, the potential advantages for the use of a DEB in bifurcations are: (1) homogeneous administration of the drug to the vessel wall (specifically at the ostium of the SB), whereas the DES only delivers the drug in the proximity of the struts; (2) delivery of high concentrations of drug into the vessel wall at the moment of highest injury; (3) no distortion of the original anatomy of the bifurcation; (4) minimization of strut deformation, of polymer crushing and of potential uncontrolled drug release (in case of multiple DES) and therefore; (5) potential decrease in dual anti-platelet therapy.

Technical aspects

A high degree of similarity exists among DEB manufacturers in terms of basic principles, however the Sequence Please (or its predecessor PACCO-CATH) and the DIOR have been investigated extensively in accessible studies, giving insight into certain important properties (e.g. delivery dose of paclitaxel in the vessel wall, and drug release properties).

Coating with matrix carrier

SeQuent Please (B. Braun Melsungen AG, Melsungen, Germany), Protégé (Blue Medical Devices BV, Helmond, Netherlands), Pantera Lux (Biotronik, Berlin, Germany), and In.Pact Falcon (Medtronic inc., Minnesota, *USA)* catheters are all coated with paclitaxel ($3\,\mu g/mm^2$). In general they are coated with a matrix composed of paclitaxel and a hydrophilic spacer (matrix carrier). This coating method

improves the solubility of paclitaxel and its transfer to the vessel wall [14]. The hydrophilic character of the matrix carrier and the lipophilic properties of paclitaxel support the release of the drug from the balloon surface and its delivery into the vascular wall by preventing paclitaxel to lump.

Different types of hydrophilic spacers have been introduced by the manufacturers (Table 8.1) [27], all relying on the same concept that has been firstly developed in the SeQuent Please DEB. Paclitaxel, in the beginning delivered intracoronary by dilution in hydrophilic contrast medium (iopromide) [15] and later directly loaded on a balloon catheter [14], resulted in concentrations of the drug in vascular tissue that were high enough to have anti-proliferative effects. The SeQuent Please DEB currently used is coated with paclitaxel and a small amount of iopromide as spacer, using acetone as the main solvent [14,16].

Protégé, Pantera Lux, and In.Pact Falcon have been introduced using the same coating principle, these three DEB are the latest introduced devices. Next to the matrix carrier technology, both Protégé and Pantera Lux use a shielding technique. This is a dedicated folding of the balloon in its non-inflated status in order to prevent paclitaxel release from an early wash-off effect. The clinical value of the shielding technique is still not proven. It has been shown on the contrary that, while using the SeQuent Please, which is manufactured without a shielding technique, at least 6% of the paclitaxel is released into the systemic circulation [14]. Most likely this amount has no harmful effect as during chemotherapy much higher doses of paclitaxel are reached (50–1000 times higher).

Coating without matrix carrier

The DIOR (Eurocor GmbH, Bonn, Germany) catheter is coated with paclitaxel ($3\,\mu g/mm^2$). The first generation DIOR-I (which is no longer produced) was manufactured with a roughened balloon surface, containing a crystalline coating. The currently available DIOR-II has a coating consisting of a 1:1 mixture of paclitaxel with shellac applied to the balloon by a micro-pipetting procedure. Shellac is a natural coating layer derived from a resin secreted by the female lac bug and it is approved as a coating for food. In the DIOR-II the hydrophilic shellac-network, once in contact with body tissues, swells

Table 8.1 Overview of CE approved drug-eluting balloons

DEB	Drug dose	Coating with matrix carrier (hydrophilic spacer)	Hydrophilic spacer	Coating without matrix carrier (hydrophilic spacer)	Shielding technique	Release from balloon surface 30 s	Release from balloon surface 60 s	Vessel wall paclitaxel concentration after DEB treatment: concentration (µg) – time of inflation (s) – time after measuring vessel wall paclitaxel concentration (min)
Sequent please	3 µg/mm²	+	PACCOCATH + Paclitaxel	–	–	NA	93%	~45–95 µg – 60 s – 40–60 min
Protégé	3 µg/mm²	+		–	+ (3-fold)	NA	NA	NA
Pantera Lux	3 µg/mm²	+	BTHC + Paclitaxel	–	+	NA	NA	165 µg – 30 s – 30 min
In.Pact Falcon	3 µg/mm²	+	FREEPAC + Paclitaxel	–	–	NA	NA	NA
First-generation DIOR	3 µg/mm²	–	–	Rough balloon surface; Crystalline + paclitaxel	+ (3-fold)	20 %	25 %	~1.5 – 6 µg – 60 s – 90 min
Second-generation DIOR	3 µg/mm²	–	–	Shellac + paclitaxel	+ (3-fold)	75 %	85 %	167 µg – 30 s – 45 min

NA = not available; BTHC = Butyryl-tri-hexyl citrate; – = No; + = Yes and opens its structure for the pressure-induced fast release of paclitaxel on the inflated balloon. The advised inflation time in order to deliver the adequate amount of drug to the vessel tissue is 30–45 seconds.

The DIOR was the first DEB adopting the already mentioned shielding technique, by which the non-inflated DEB is 3-folded and protects the loaded drug from an early wash-off effect during insertion into the vasculature and tracking to the lesions (Table 8.1). In contrast with SeQuent Please, no plasma concentrations of paclitaxel can be detected after DIOR inflation, indicating no systemic release in the circulation with the use of a DIOR [10].

One of the drawbacks of DIOR-I was the low delivery dose of paclitaxel into the vessel wall (25% of the dose loaded on the balloon), the DIOR-II has a higher delivery dose (up to 85% of the dose loaded on the balloon), comparable with the delivery dose of the Pantera Lux. The DIOR-II showed significant better distribution properties into the vessel wall with a 5–20-fold higher tissue drug concentration with respect to DIOR-I, resulting in shorter inflation times [17].

Animal studies

Neo-intimal hyperplasia (i.e. proliferation of smooth muscle cells) is a patho-physiologic cause of restenosis after stent placement. Already in the late 1990s it was shown that paclitaxel is a potent inhibitor of this process [13]. Consequently, studies delivering paclitaxel locally to the coronary arteries were performed. The first preclinical study compared a combination of paclitaxel solved in a contrast agent (iopromide) with a control group with iopromide only, after stent placement. The study showed that the combination of paclitaxel solved in iopromide inhibited the neo-intimal hyperplasia process better than the control group [18]. Sequentially, the same authors compared the delivery mode of paclitaxel and iopromide after stent placement. Intracoronary injection of paclitaxel and iopromide inhibited the neo-intimal hyperplasia process more profoundly than intravenous injection [15]. Hence, a local delivery platform was developed. An angioplasty balloon was coated with the combination of paclitaxel and iopromide to generate a DEB. After stent placement, DEB

inflations (with an inflation time of 60 seconds to allow paclitaxel to "impregnate" the vessel wall) were performed, showing a reduction of neo-intimal hyperplasia as compared with inflations with normal balloons [14].

Still there was some uncertainty about the warranted inflation times and distribution rates of paclitaxel into the vessel wall. Cremers et al. showed that even with shorter inflation times, 10 seconds instead of 60 seconds in the previous studies, sufficient paclitaxel was absorbed by the vessel wall. Moreover, they found no increased safety risk after two overlapping DEB inflations (2 times $5 \mu g/mm^2$) in the same vascular segment [16].

Clinical studies with DEB

Several randomized clinical studies have shown promising results; however these trials have been performed in small numbers of patients. While most studies have focused on in-stent restenotic lesions (PACOCATH ISR I and II, and PEPCAD II), only recently new data have been published on de novo coronary lesions (PEPCAD I and III, PICCO-LETO and the Spanish multicenter registry), and just one on bifurcation lesions (DEBIUT trial).

In-stent restenosis

The PACOCATH ISR I and II [19,20] trials were the first benchmark studies that showed clinical superiority of SeQuent Please DEB in comparison with a regular balloon in the treatment of BMS or DES restenosis, with sustained results up to 24 months. Furthermore, 6-month angiographic follow-up demonstrated significant reductions in late lumen loss and binary restenosis with DEB.

Similar positive results were found in the PEPCAD II trial, comparing the SeQuent Please DEB with paclitaxel eluting stent (PES) to treat BMS restenosis. Superior angiographic results were found for the DEB at 12-month follow-up. In addition, not significant trends towards reduced major adverse cardiac events (mainly driven by target lesion revascularization) were found for the DEB group [21].

De novo lesions

Inconsistent data were found for de novo lesions. The PEPCAD I [22], a prospective registry on the treatment of de novo small coronary arteries with a SeQuent Please DEB (and provisional bare metal stenting), demonstrated that DEB possibly yields the potential as treatment alternative for these types of lesions. In the PICCOLETO [23] randomized trial, the DIOR-I DEB (with provisional stenting) was compared with PES in de novo lesions in small vessels. The trial was interrupted after enrolment of two–thirds of patients due to clear superiority of the PES group over the DEB group. It should be noticed, however, that both groups had significant differences at index procedure: (1) in the DEB arm only 25% pre-dilatation with conventional balloons was performed; (2) considerably lower inflation pressures were used (on average, maximal inflation pressure of 7.7 atmospheres in the DEB group versus 13.4 atmospheres in the PES group). Clinical and angiographic results in the DEB group were considerably worse than in the PEPCAD I study. One explanation could be that the PICCOLETO study was performed with DIOR-I where the SeQuent Please as used in PEPCAD I can probably be considered as superior to the DIOR-I in terms of tissue dosage [24]. A second explanation could be the occurrence of so-called "geographical miss", which lead to restenosis in stented lesion sites that were not adequately pre-treated with DEB.

The PEPCAD III trial (Hamm C, unpublished data, presented at the American Heart Association meeting 2009 in Orlando, Florida) investigated a new hybrid DEB/stent system (Coroflex DEBlue) as an alternative to DES. This study failed to show non-inferiority, angiographically and clinically at 9 months, for the DEB group in comparison with the DES group (Cypher sirolimus-eluting stent). Although the study failed to show non-inferiority, outcome measures for DEB were very reasonable, with a late luminal loss of 0.41 mm and a target lesion revascularization rate of 10.5% at 9 months if compared to historically known BMS data.

The Spanish, prospective non-randomized, registry (Vaquerizo B, unpublished data, presented at the American Heart Association meeting 2009 in Orlando, Florida) assessed the value of DIOR-I DEB in; (1) in stent restenosis (BMS and DES); (2) de novo small vessels (including also bifurcation lesions); and (3) patients with contraindication to DAPT. Only a 3.4% MACE rate in all three groups was found at 3-months follow-up. Results

seem to be good, however cautious interpretation of these results is warranted since all limitations of a nonrandomized registry apply. Data on de novo small vessel lesions remain therefore inconclusive; larger randomized trials comparing latest DEB versus latest DES are warranted to define the value of DEB in this subgroup of patients.

Bifurcation lesions

Currently two pilot studies and one randomized trial have been performed with DEB in bifurcation lesions. In the first pilot study performed [25], DIOR DEB was used and among the 20 patients enrolled, no major adverse cardiac events at 4-month clinical follow-up were reported.

The second, PEPCAD V, enrolled 28 patients with bifurcation lesions in two centres. Both main and side branch were ballooned with a Sequent Please DEB, with BMS deployment in the MB. The primary endpoint, procedural success, was met in all cases. At 9-month follow-up one target lesion revascularization was needed, next to two significant restenosis (7.1%) of the side branch without a target lesion revascularization. At 9-month angiographic follow-up late luminal loss was 0.38 mm in the MB and 0.21 mm in the SB. Comparing these results with historical data of DES treatment, restenosis percentages are seemingly not higher in this pilot study.

The third, an international multicenter randomized trial was initiated, aimed at comparing a provisional T-stenting technique for coronary bifurcation lesions with pre-dilatation using DEB followed by BMS implantation (group A), versus standard BMS implantation (group B) versus standard DES implantation (group C). The main inclusion criteria were stable or unstable angina pectoris or silent ischemia, due to de novo coronary artery lesions (stenosis >50% and <100%) at the level of a bifurcation. Eligible patients were assigned to one of the three treatment groups with all three groups using a stent with the same design in order to exclude this confounding factor. A BMS stent was implanted in the main branch (MB) in groups A and B, after predilatation of both MB and SB with respectively DIOR DEB or regular balloon. In group C, a paclitaxel DES was implanted after dilatation with a regular balloon of both MB and SB. Final kissing balloon dilatation with regular balloons was mandated in all groups. After the procedure, patients were treated with 3 months of DAPT in groups A and B, or 12 months of DAPT in group C. A control coronary angiography was performed at 6-month follow-up. Major adverse cardiac events (death, myocardial infarction, target vessel revascularization) were recorded up to 12 months. The primary endpoint was 6-month angiographic late luminal loss and the power analysis was based on the angiographic superiority of group A (DEB) over group B (BMS).

Overall, 117 patients (group A: 40, group B: 37, group C: 40) with suitable bifurcation lesions were treated according to the protocol. A total of eight (6.8%) peri-procedural non-Q wave myocardial infarctions occurred during the initial hospitalization without differences between groups. No further in-hospital MACE occurred. Considering the primary endpoint, group A showed a numerically similar late luminal loss as group B. The values of late luminal loss in group C were numerically and statistically better than the other groups. Binary restenosis rates per bifurcation and 12-month MACE rates were 24.2%, 28.6%, and 15% ($p = 0.45$) and 20%, 29.7%, and 17.5% ($p = 0.40$) in groups A, B and C, respectively.

Future perspective

The recently introduced DEB potentially can overcome some of the limitations of bifurcation PCI with stent delivery in the main vessel and normal balloon angioplasty of the side branch. By means of releasing an anti-proliferative drug combined with a BMS, not only vessel recoil can be tackled but potentially also restenosis rates can be reduced. Besides, a potential reduction of the added risk of stent thrombosis, as accounted for DES, may be realized. Eventually this may result in a shorter prescription of DAPT.

However, results of the DEBIUT study showed comparable results for the DEB group and the BMS group, while the DES group showed superior angiographic results with respect to the other two groups, indicating no benefit for DEB with respect to current treatment strategies.

Nevertheless, as summarized in Table 8.1, the technical and pharmacological aspects of DEB have to be still clarified. With drug dose and release kinetics being the only variables among the three treatment groups in the DEBIUT study, these findings suggest that the pharmacokinetics of paclitaxel with DIOR-I may have been insufficient to provide comparable benefits, in terms of late luminal loss, to those observed in the DES arm. Hence, the use of a second generation, higher tissue delivery dose, DIOR-II DEB in combination with a BMS, might lead to better angiographic and clinical outcomes when used in bifurcation lesions.

Apart from these technical improvements (i.e. release kinetics), it will be interesting to see whether other drug-based DEB will provide further improvements. Two preclinical studies using the delivery of sirolimus and zotarolimus have shown encouraging results so far. In the first study, local administration of sirolimus during angioplasty showed inhibition of both smooth muscle cells as well as the expression of extracellular matrix components [26]. In the second study, a porcine animal study, a zotarolimus eluting balloon showed a marked reduction in neo-intimal proliferation with respect to normal balloon angioplasty. Interestingly even better angiographic results for the zotarolimus eluting balloon were found when compared to the established zotarolimus eluting stent [28].

Next to efficacy assessment, most important is the safety profile of DEB. Although, the DEBIUT study did not show an increased safety hazard, the study size was not aimed at drawing conclusions on any clinical hazards of DEB. Also other DEB studies were not powered to detect increased clinical risks. Considering both efficacy and clinical aspects so far, a new large randomized study with a latest generation high-concentration DEB combined with a DES in the MB is warranted.

At this point of development of DEB it is still difficult to understand if this new technique will remain a promise or become a real asset. Different technical and safety aspects have to be clarified yet, in studies large enough to address these aspects.

Thus, as accounted for DES, a thorough validation of various DEB has to be performed in order to exploit their full potential, and determine the different values of each individual DEB. Because, baseline conceptual characteristics of the different DEB appear to be the same, however, the technical and pharmacologic aspects of the various DEB remain under-evaluated. Especially actual tissue delivery dosages as achieved and measured in animal testing should be reported, in order to provide more insights into the technical properties of the different DEB. At present, in-stent restenosis treatment is the only clear indication for DEB use. Until new data are forthcoming, DEB remains a promising future treatment option for coronary bifurcation lesions.

References

1 Meier B, Gruentzig AR, King SB, 3rd, Douglas JS, Jr., Hollman J, Ischinger T, *et al.* Risk of side branch occlusion during coronary angioplasty. Am J Cardiol 1984;53:10–4.

2 Iakovou I, Schmidt T, Bonizzoni E, Ge L, Sangiorgi GM, Stankovic G, *et al.* Incidence, predictors, and outcome of thrombosis after successful implantation of drug-eluting stents. JAMA 2005;293:2126–30.

3 Galassi AR, Tomasello SD, Capodanno D, Barrano G, Ussia GP, Tamburino C. Mini-crush versus T-provisional techniques in bifurcation lesions: clinical and angiographic long-term outcome after implantation of drug-eluting stents. JACC Cardiovasc Interv 2009;2:185–94.

4 Ge L, Iakovou I, Cosgrave J, Agostoni P, Airoldi F, Sangiorgi GM, *et al.* Treatment of bifurcation lesions with two stents: one year angiographic and clinical follow up of crush versus T stenting. Heart 2006;92:371–6.

5 Palmerini T, Marzocchi A, Tamburino C, Sheiban I, Margheri M, Vecchi G, *et al.* Impact of bifurcation technique on 2-year clinical outcomes in 773 patients with distal unprotected left main coronary artery stenosis treated with drug-eluting stents. Circ Cardiovasc Interv 2008;1:185–92.

6 Nakazawa G, Vorpahl M, Finn AV, Narula J, Virmani R. One step forward and two steps back with drug-eluting-stents: from preventing restenosis to causing late thrombosis and nouveau atherosclerosis. JACC Cardiovasc Imaging 2009;2:625–8.

7 Ong AT, McFadden EP, Regar E, de Jaegere PP, van Domburg RT, Serruys PW. Late angiographic stent thrombosis (LAST) events with drug-eluting stents. J Am Coll Cardiol 2005;45:2088–92.

8 Jarvie JL, Foody JM. Predictors of early discontinuation of dual-antiplatelet therapy: room for improvement. Circulation 2010;122:946–8.

9 Rowinsky EK, Donehower RC. Paclitaxel (taxol). N Engl J Med 1995;332:1004–14.

10 Posa A, Hemetsberger R, Petnehazy O, Petrasi Z, Testor M, Glogar D, *et al.* Attainment of local drug delivery with paclitaxel-eluting balloon in porcine coronary arteries. Coron Artery Dis 2008;19:243–7.

11 Finn AV, Nakazawa G, Joner M, Kolodgie FD, Mont EK, Gold HK, *et al.* Vascular responses to drug eluting stents: importance of delayed healing. Arterioscler Thromb Vasc Biol 2007;27:1500–10.

12 Mori T, Kinoshita Y, Watanabe A, Yamaguchi T, Hosokawa K, Honjo H. Retention of paclitaxel in cancer cells for 1 week in vivo and in vitro. Cancer Chemother Pharmacol 2006;58:665–72.

13 Axel DI, Kunert W, Goggelmann C, Oberhoff M, Herdeg C, Kuttner A, *et al.* Paclitaxel inhibits arterial smooth muscle cell proliferation and migration in vitro and in vivo using local drug delivery. Circulation 1997;96:636–45.

14 Scheller B, Speck U, Abramjuk C, Bernhardt U, Bohm M, Nickenig G. Paclitaxel balloon coating, a novel method for prevention and therapy of restenosis. Circulation 2004;110:810–4.

15 Scheller B, Speck U, Schmitt A, Bohm M, Nickenig G. Addition of paclitaxel to contrast media prevents restenosis after coronary stent implantation. J Am Coll Cardiol 2003;42:1415–20.

16 Cremers B, Speck U, Kaufels N, Mahnkopf D, Kuhler M, Bohm M, *et al.* Drug-eluting balloon: very short-term exposure and overlapping. Thromb Haemost 2009;101:201–6.

17 Posa A, Nyolczas N, Hemetsberger R, Pavo N, Petnehazy O, Petrasi Z, *et al.* Optimization of drug-eluting balloon use for safety and efficacy: evaluation of the 2nd generation paclitaxel-eluting DIOR-balloon in porcine coronary arteries. Catheter Cardiovasc Interv 2010;76:395–403.

18 Scheller B, Speck U, Romeike B, Schmitt A, Sovak M, Bohm M, *et al.* Contrast media as carriers for local drug delivery. Successful inhibition of neointimal proliferation in the porcine coronary stent model. Eur Heart J 2003;24:1462–7.

19 Scheller B, Hehrlein C, Bocksch W, Rutsch W, Haghi D, Dietz U, *et al.* Treatment of coronary in-stent restenosis with a paclitaxel-coated balloon catheter. N Engl J Med 2006;355:2113–24.

20 Scheller B, Hehrlein C, Bocksch W, Rutsch W, Haghi D, Dietz U, *et al.* Two year follow-up after treatment of coronary in-stent restenosis with a paclitaxel-coated balloon catheter. Clin Res Cardiol 2008;97:773–81.

21 Unverdorben M, Vallbracht C, Cremers B, Heuer H, Hengstenberg C, Maikowski C, *et al.* Paclitaxel-coated balloon catheter versus paclitaxel-coated stent for the treatment of coronary in-stent restenosis. Circulation 2009;119:2986–94.

22 Unverdorben M, Kleber FX, Heuer H, Figulla HR, Vallbracht C, Leschke M, *et al.* Treatment of small coronary arteries with a paclitaxel-coated balloon catheter. Clin Res Cardiol 2010;99:165–74.

23 Cortese B, Micheli A, Picchi A, Coppolaro A, Bandinelli L, Severi S, *et al.* Paclitaxel-coated balloon versus drug-eluting stent during PCI of small coronary vessels, a prospective randomised clinical trial. The PICCOLETO study. Heart 96: 1291–6.

24 Cremers B, Biedermann M, Mahnkopf D, Bohm M, Scheller B. Comparison of two different paclitaxel-coated balloon catheters in the porcine coronary restenosis model. Clin Res Cardiol 2009;98:325–30.

25 Fanggiday JC, Stella PR, Guyomi SH, Doevendans PA. Safety and efficacy of drug-eluting balloons in percutaneous treatment of bifurcation lesions: the DEBIUT (drug-eluting balloon in bifurcation Utrecht) registry. Catheter Cardiovasc Interv 2008;71: 629–35.

26 Buerke M, Guckenbiehl M, Schwertz H, Buerke U, Hilker M, Platsch H, *et al.* Intramural delivery of Sirolimus prevents vascular remodeling following balloon injury. Biochim Biophys Acta 2007;1774:5–15.

27 Stella PR, Belkacemi A, Agostoni P. Drug-eluting balloons and Bifurcations, a new future for treatment? EuroIntervention 2010;6(Supplement J): J161–J164.

28 Cremers B, Toner J, Schwartz LB, *et al.* Inhibition of coronary neointimal hyperplasia in swine using a novel zotarolimus-eluting balloon catheter. Eur Heart J. 2009;30(abstract supplement): 532.

CHAPTER 9

Percutaneous coronary intervention for bifurcation lesions: Bench testing and the real world

John A. Ormiston, MBChB, *Mark Webster,* MBChB
and Bruce Webber, MHSc
Mercy Angiography, Auckland, New Zealand

Introduction

The first dedicated bifurcation coronary stent, the Y-shaped Carina Bard, was first implanted in a patient by Patrick Serruys at the Rotterdam Live Course in 1997 [1]. A subsequent case report [2] described another implantation of the stent, and highlighted some its limitations including the large crossing profile and propensity for wire twisting (wrap) that limited delivery. Since then, no dedicated bifurcation stents have been approved by the United States Food and Drug Administration (FDA), or are in widespread clinical use in the rest of the world. Greater attention to insights from bench-top testing might have avoided some of the pitfalls encountered over the past decade or so in developing a clinically useful bifurcation stent.

The FDA stipulates in its guidance for industry that non-clinical testing should support the safety and effectiveness of intracoronary stents and their delivery systems (dsmica@fda.hhs.gov). Such testing helps determine the limits to which a device can be pushed, such as evaluating the device at extreme dimensions, and to assess performance at the outer limits of physiologic variables such as blood pressure, vascular compliance, and anatomic types.

At least as importantly, bench testing can provide crucial information on stenting techniques, how a device works, and whether there are any concerns about or limitations of device function. Bench testing may predict stent behaviour, technical results and, in some cases, clinical outcomes thereby reducing the need for preclinical in vivo and human clinical testing. Various device iterations can be evaluated and compared in a cost effective way, before preclinical testing. The ultimate aim of bench testing is to improve human outcomes.

Bench testing has provided useful insights into the mechanical properties of stents such as flexibility and profile[3] technical challenges to stent delivery (Figure 9.1), optimization of stent deployment especially in bifurcations [4,5], and damage to stent polymer coatings (http://www.tctmd.com/show.aspx?id=57090) This chapter outlines the bench testing methods, including phantom (mock artery) evolution, deployment recording, and various imaging modalities.

Testing of mechanical properties

Stent mechanical properties determine stent performance in different coronary artery anatomies. Testing of mechanical properties can provide

---

Bifurcation Stenting, First Edition. Edited by Ron Waksman and John A. Ormiston.
© 2012 Blackwell Publishing Ltd. Published 2012 by Blackwell Publishing Ltd.

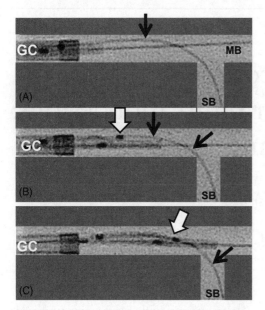

Figure 9.1 A bench deployment shows that wire bias directs the side-branch component of a two wire dedicated bifurcation stent away from the side-branch (SB) ostium preventing rotation and alignment. (a) The black arrow shows the SB wire curving away from the SB before it enters the SB; (b) The dedicated device is advanced from the guide catheter (GC) and the SB component (white arrow) is directed away from the SB; (c) With further advancement of the device, the SB component (white arrow) has not rotated so that alignment and delivery were not possible. This problem is most marked with steep SB angles and with proximal SBs.

GC = guide catheter, MB = main branch, SB = side-branch

the interventional cardiologist with independent objective data on which to base rational stent selection. The ease with which a stent can be delivered to a lesion is, at least in part, dependent on measurable characteristics including stent delivery system flexibility and diameter [3,6]. The ideal stent delivery system should be highly flexible and have a very low crossing profile. The low profile is important in direct stenting without predilatation, crossing tight stenoses and when smaller calibre guide catheters are employed [7]. When assessing characteristics associated with stent deliverability, the stent must be evaluated on its delivery balloon as the balloon has a greater influence than the stent on the deliverability current systems as a whole [6]. The expanded stent should retain flexibility and have desirable characteristics

such as adequate radial strength and lesion coverage. The expanded flexibility is important to allow the stent to conform to vessel contours and to minimize distortion at the stent-vessel junction when stents are deployed on bends. The radial strength of the expanded stent determines resistance to compressive forces such as those found in some calcified, fibrotic and ostial lesions [6]. Subjective assessments of stent characteristics can differ substantially from objective measurements.

Testing of device delivery

To understand better the clinical challenges of deploying both dedicated bifurcation stents and conventional stents deployed in bifurcations, stent delivery is evaluated through a guiding catheter into a bifurcation phantom submerged in a water bath. Cine angiographic recording, including contrast injection, documents each step in delivery and deployment to understand better delivery challenges and the adequacy of deployment. This bench model predicted the difficulties of passive delivery system rotation experienced in the first-in-human trials [8,9] with the Petal (Boston Scientific, Natick, MA) and the Branch (Medtronic, Santa Rosa, CA) dedicated bifurcation stents. Some were initially sceptical of the findings, attributing the delivery problems to limitations of the phantoms (Figure 9.1). Bench testing predicted that the major restriction to passive rotational alignment was guide wire bias, with the wire curving from the upstream main branch into the side branch directing the side branch component of the stent to the opposite vessel wall immediately upstream from the bifurcation (Figure 9.1). In addition, guide wire wrap or twisting frequently prevented device advancement and delivery. If wire wrap was observed, withdrawing and readvancing either the main or side branch wires could overcome the problem, albeit with potential loss of guide wire position. Passive rotational alignment was also limited by the oval cross-sectional nature of the device. This oval cross-section is likely to limit rotation in clinical situations where there is eccentric plaque or calcification. Bench testing predicts that a delivery system shaft that can be actively rotated under fluoroscopic control may overcome these problems, even in tortuous vessel phantoms.

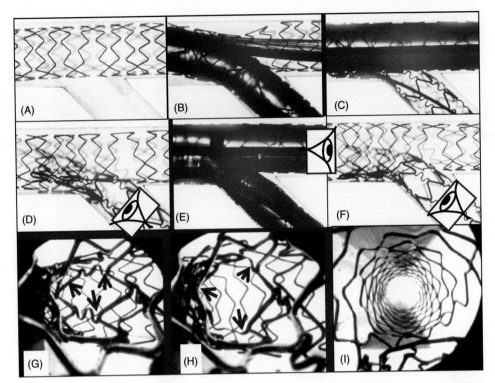

Plate 1 Bench deployment with the "internal crush" technique of provisional side-branch (SB) stenting using a ring design stent in the main branch (MB) and a slotted tube design stent in the SB. Use of different stent designs in bench testing assists in differentiating between struts from the different stents enhancing understanding of deployments. In (a), the ring design stent is deployed in the MB. In (b), the second stent is deployed into the SB then an inflated MB balloon crushes that component of the SB that lies in the MB (c). The diagram of an eye symbolizes the direction of an endoscopic view. (d) and (g) demonstrate endoscopy of the SB before kissing post-dilatation with a single layer of struts between the MB and SB (arrows). This is in contrast to conventional external crush where there are two layers of struts (ref crush papers). After kissing post-dilatation (e), endoscopy (f and h) shows that the struts covering the SB ostium are partially removed from the SB ostium (arrows). Endoscopy of the MB after kissing (i) shows that the MB stent is widely patent without protruding struts.

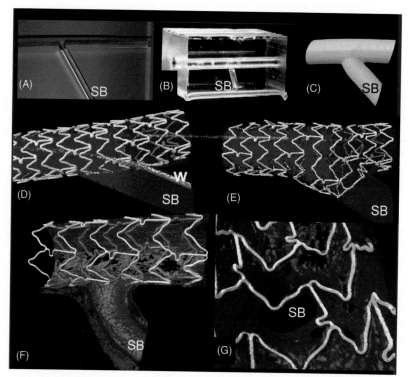

Plate 2 Progression of phantom development (a–d), phantom lumen identification (d, e) and phantom wall identification (f, g); (a) Our first phantom was a square-sided trough cut in a perspex sheet; (b) A silicone phantom constructed by casting silicone over rods; (c) A phantom constructed by stereolithography; (d, e) The phantom lumen is identified by exploiting the difference in Housfield number between the metallic stent and the air in the lumen (d) The guide wire (w) has crossed to the SB close to the carina distally in relation to SB so that after kissing post-dilatation (e) optimal protrusion of stent struts into the SB ostium has occurred; (f, g) The lumen of a phantom has been painted with metallic paint so that the stent can be differentiated on CT from the phantom vessel wall. The phantom in (f) has been cut electronically to show the relationship of struts covering the SB ostium; (g) is an image from a "fly-though" display showing the stent struts overlying the SB ostium and "jailing" the SB.

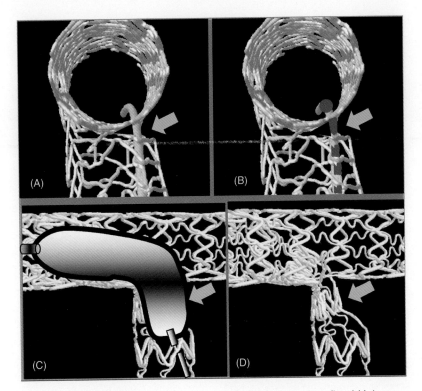

Plate 3 The mechanism for the development of gaps in strut coverage that may occur with crush stenting. (a) The wire has passed from the MB lumen above, traversed the "V" shaped gap between the two stents and re-entered the SB stent below; (b) When a balloon (blue) follows the wire and is inflated (c), it can cause a gap (yellow arrow in d) that may result in a suboptimal acute ostial lumen or lead to ostial restenosis because of lack of scaffolding and drug application.

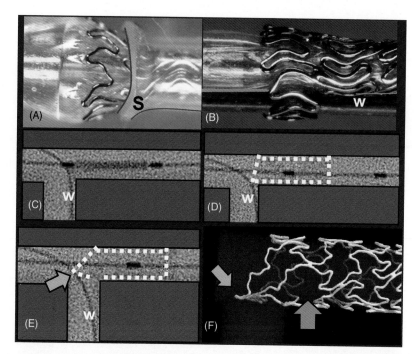

Plate 4 Unexpected stent distortion with the Szarbo technique for ostial deployment. (a) The balloon is inflated to 2 atmospheres with a sheath (S) restricting the expansion of all but the proximal ring of struts that become elevated from the balloon; (b) A wire (w) has been passed under the proximal strut that is then manually re-crimped onto the balloon; (c) This wire (w) prevents the proximal end of the stent advancing beyond the ostium. After stent deployment (broken line in d and e), retraction of the wire has caused stent distortion with displacement of struts proximal to the ostium (yellow arrow) and enlargement of spaces between struts at the ostium; (f) These gaps may reduce uniformity of scaffolding (blue arrow), reduce stent radial strength where maximum support is needed and reduce drug application to the site were restenosis is most common.

Polymeric stents such as the Bioresorbable Vascular Scaffold (BVS, Abbott Vascular, Santa Clara, CA) used in the Absorb Trial [10] need to be tested in a fluid bath at body temperature as testing in air or at room temperature where the polymer is much less flexible profoundly affects stent and coating integrity. If polymeric coatings are of interest, deployment of stents should be under similar conditions to limit non-physiologic polymer damage.

Evolution of imaging modalities and phantom construction

Conventional photography

Conventional photography, used when we began imaging stents, enabled us to identify that dilatation through the side of a stent improved SB access, protruded struts into the SB but distorted the stent[11]. This distortion could be repaired by kissing balloon post-dilatation while retaining the SB ostial diameter and desirable strut protrusion into the SB [11]. Conventional photography after crush deployment clearly revealed for the first time the three layers of crushed struts upstream from the side-branch ostium and the two layers separating the main branch from the side-branch [4]. Images were of high resolution but limitations included the concealment of the inside of the stent by the struts, and the need for a phantom that was an unroofed trough to enable high-quality images without degradation by overlying plastic.

Pediatric endoscope

Limited imaging of the inside of stents was made possible for the first time by photography through a pediatric endoscope (See Colour Plate 1). Kissing balloon post-dilatation after crush stenting improved SB ostial patency by partially removing the two layers of struts separating the SB from the MB [4] (See Colour Plate 1). The implication that kissing balloon post-dilatation after crush stenting might improve clinical outcomes has been confirmed in studies whose authors stipulate that kissing post-dilatation is mandatory after crush stenting [12,13].

Phantom development

Our first phantoms were troughs (See Colour Plate 2) cut in a perspex plate [11]. Because there was no phantom material between the camera and stent, there was no light image distortion and high resolution images could be obtained. However these phantoms were rigid, non-circumferential and very unlike a flexible, distensible tubular coronary artery. Securing the stent during deployment and post-dilatation was suboptimal.

MicroCT has allowed development of more complex and more anatomically correct phantoms. In contrast to images using light, images constructed from X-ray photons are not distorted by common phantom materials such as silicone. For microCT imaging, we initially deployed stents in silicone block phantoms made by casting silicone over a metallic model of a bifurcation. While these had radial flexibility compared with perspex, they did not have the longitudinal flexibility of a coronary artery. In addition it was difficult to build anatomically true phantoms by this method.

As knowledge of bifurcation anatomy improves, potentially more anatomically accurate phantoms can be constructed. Stereolithography [14,15] is a powerful tool that can be computer directed to construct antomically true phantoms using an appropriate material (See Colour Plate 2, C, F and G). The manufacturing process involves progressive, layer by layer, alternate deposition and curing of a light curable polymer to create a 3-dimensional structure from a predefined design. Technical specifications were derived from a human necropsy bifurcation study [16], input into an Eden 500V 3-dimensional printing system (Objet, Rehovot, Israel) creating mock vessels from an acrylic-based photopolymer (TriReme Medical Inc, Pleasantville, CA). Any shape can be generated. These models are tubular and of similar compliance to human coronary arteries.

In order to understand stent deployment better, ways to differentiate stent struts from the phantom arterial wall and from the lumen are being developed. The relationship of stent to lumen can be determined by exploiting the difference in radiodensity between the metallic stent and air (See Colour Plate 2, D and E). Assessing the relationship between the phantom vessel wall and the stent is more challenging. Increasing the radiodensity of the vessel by adding radioopaque material to the phantom material or painting the luminal surface of the phantom with metallic paint (See Colour Plate 2, F and G) has been met with only partially success.

Micro-computed tomography

The development of micro computed tomographic (microCT) imaging of stents (SkyScan 1172, SkyScan, Belgium) particularly in bifurcations has been a further advance [5]. The 3D images can be cut electronically and opened out, rotated, tumbled, and magnified. A "fly through" presentation is possible so that unprecedented complete examination of the adequacy of the stent deployment is achieved (See Colour Plate 2).

MicroCT has led to further insights into the potential importance of seemingly modest changes in stent deployment technique. One example was a study of 116 stents deployed using the "crush" technique [5], SB ostial stenosis was common after conventional kissing post-dilatation (Figure 9.2). This could be minimized by "two step" kissing post-dilatation, which involved high-pressure SB post-dilatation with a non-compliant balloon followed by lower pressure kissing post-dilatation [5] to correct the distortion caused by SB dilatation. A subsequent clinical study using IVUS to evaluate patients undergoing crush stenting for bifurcation lesions suggested that ostial SB stent underexpansion may be the commonest underlying cause of drug-eluting stent restenosis [17]. Optimizing stent deployment by two-step kissing post-dilatation should reduce clinical stent restenosis and thrombosis after crush stenting; this remains to be confirmed clinically.

Unexpected stent behavior can be found on bench testing. In this study of crush stenting it was surprising to find on occasion regardless of stent design that gaps in stent strut support and thus drug application could occur [5]. Sometimes a guide wire may pass for a short distance outside the stents in the "V" shaped junction between the crushed stents (See Colour Plate 3). The post-dilating balloon follows the wire and when inflated pushes struts aside to cause the gap in strut coverage [5] (See Colour Plate 3). This may be an important unpredictable limitation to crush stenting.

Bench testing has provided other surprises. The "Szabo" technique [18] was designed to facilitate correct placement of a stent at a vessel ostium (See Colour Plate 4). The concept is that a wire is placed under a proximal strut to limit advancement of the proximal stent beyond the ostium. Unfortunately, and surprisingly, after ostial deployment, wire removal from under the strut caused stent distortion with retraction of stent struts proximal to the ostium. There was distortion and enlargement of the unsupported area between struts at the ostium, where restenosis is highest. Whether this translates

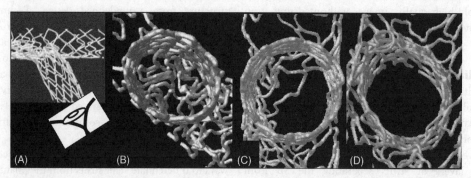

(A)   (B)   (C)   (D)

Figure 9.2 Frames from microCT imaging of crush stent deployments showing post-dilatation strategies. (a) The eye symbol depicts the direction from which crush deployments are viewed in (b–d). Note that the side of the stent opposite the SB has been removed electronically so that the struts across the SB ostium can be clearly seen; (b) Following deployment using the crush technique there are two layers of struts separating the MB from the SB; (c) Conventional kissing post-dilatation partially clears these struts from the SB ostium; (d) After two-step post-dilatation (very high pressure SB dilatation with a non-compliant balloon followed by low pressure kissing post-dilatation), there is full expansion of struts at the SB ostium.

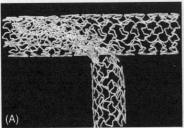
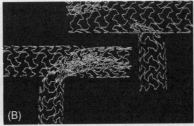
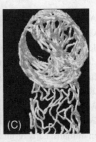

Figure 9.3 MicroCT imaging of the simultaneous kissing stent (SKS) technique for coronary bifurcation stenting [19]. The two stents deployed using the SKS technique (a) have, been electronically cut longitudinally and laid open; (b) to show the considerable intracoronary metal; (c) Looking "down the barrel" of the MB stent showing the spiralling metallic "septum" dividing the lumen of the phantom artery asymmetrically.

into suboptimal clinical outcomes is yet to be determined.

While the simultaneous kissing stent (SKS) technique [19] for bifurcation stenting, where two stents side by side are deployed simultaneously, is quick and easy, there are a number of microCT findings that raise concerns about this strategy. If there is long stent overlap, microCT imaging (Figure 9.3) shows a long metallic "septum" composed of two layers of struts so that there may be a predisposition to stent thrombosis especially in smaller calibre coronary arteries or if there is reduced flow. In addition, microCT shows that the two stents may spiral around each other dividing the artery asymmetrically. Reewiring may be a challenge if repeat treatment is necessary.

Summary

Bench testing has provided considerable insight into stent deployment and how different techniques might impact on clinical outcomes. Bench testing of stents is essential to support the safety and effectiveness of coronary stents and their delivery systems. It can provide critical information on stenting techniques, how a device works, whether there are likely to be concerns about device function, and may predict clinical outcomes. Evaluation of device iterations is possible, speeding up device development and limiting the need for preclinical and clinical testing at each stage. Greater attention to bench results would certainly have avoided some of the mistakes of the past.

In the future, progress in phantom development and bench testing techniques will better replicate the clinical environment. A missing component in current testing is the effect of different techniques on flow and shear stress. Coronary blood flow impacts restenosis, atheroma development and thrombosis. There is potential to explore how flow changes in different coronary anatomies, and to explore how stent designs and deployment techniques may optimize flow and clinical outcomes.

References

1 Carlier S, Van der Giessen W, Foley D, Kutryk M, Rensing B, Carleton M, Serruys PW. Stenting with a true bifurcated stent: acute and mid-term follow-up results. Cathet Cardiovasc Interv 1999;47:361–96.

2 Colombo A, Airoldi F, Sheiban I, Di Mario C. Successful treatment of a bifurcation lesion with the Carina Bard stent: A case report. Cathet Cardiovasc Interv 1999;48: 89–92.

3 Ormiston J, Dixon S, Webster M, Ruygrok P, Stewart J, Minchington I, West T. Stent longitudinal flexibility: A comparison of 13 stent designs before and after expansion. Cathet Cardiovasc Interv 2000;50:120–4.

4 Ormiston J, Currie E, Webster M, Kay I, Ruygrok P, Stewart J, Padgett R, Panther M. Drug-eluting stents for coronary bifurcations: insights into the crush technique. Cathet Cardiovasc Interv 2004;63:332–6.

5 Ormiston J, Webster M, Webber B, Stewart J, Ruygrok P, Hatrick R. The "crush" technique for coronary bifurcation stenting: Insights from micro-computed tomographic imaging of bench deployments. J Am Coll Cardiol Interv 2008;1:351–7.

6 Ormiston J, Blake J, Peebles C, Webster M, Stewart J, Ruygrok P, O'Shaughnessy B. Expanded stent radial strength and flexibility: Benchtop testing of 10 stents. Am J Cardiol 2002;90(Suppl 6A): 76H.

7 Ormiston J, Dixon S, Webster M, Ruygrok P. 5 French guide catheters for percutaneous coronary intervention:

A feasibility study in 100 consecutive patients. Cathet Cardiovasc Interv 2001;52:45–8.

8 Johnson T, Kay I, Ormiston J. A novel paclitaxel-eluting dedicated bifurcation stent: A case report from the first human use Taxus Petal Trial. Cathet Cardiovasc Interv 2009;73:637–40.

9 Meredith I, Whitbourn R, Ormiston J, Worthley S. Feasibilty study evaluating a bare metal bifurcation stent in humans: Early results from the BRANCH clinical trial. Am J Cardiol 2009;104:98D.

10 Ormiston J, Webster M, Armstrong G. First-in-human implantation of a fully bioabsorbable drug-eluting stent: The BVS poly-L-lactic acid everolimus-eluting coronary stent. Cathet Cardiovasc Interv 2007;69:128–31.

11 Ormiston J, Webster M, Ruygrok P, Stewart J, White H, Scott D. Stent deformation following simulated side-branch dilatation: A comparison of five stent designs. Cathet Cardiovasc Interv 1999;47:258–63.

12 Ge L, Airoldi F, Iakovou I, Cosgrove J, Michev I, Sangiorgi G, Montorfano M, Chieffo A, Carlino M, Corvaja M, Colombo A. Clinical and angiographic outcome after implantation of drug-eluting stents in bifurcation lesions with the crush technique. J Am Coll Cardiol 2005; 46:613–20.

13 Hoye A, Iakovou I, Ge L, von Mieghem C, Ong A, Cosgrave J, Sangiorgi G, Airoldi F, Montorfano M, Michev I, Chieffo A, Carlino M, Corvaja M, Aoki J, Granillo G, Valgimigli M, Sianos G, van der Giessen W, de Feyter PJ, van Domburg R, Serruys PW. Long-term outcomes after stenting of bifurcation lesions with the "crush" technique. J Am Coll Cardiol 2006;47: 1949–58.

14 Wetzel S, Ohta M, Handa A, Auer J-M, Lylyk P, Lovblad K-O, Babic D, Rufenacht D. From patient to model: Stereolithographic modeling of cerebral vasculature based on rotational angiography. Am M Neuroradiol 2005;26:1425–7.

15 Knoxa K, Kerber C, Singel S, Bailey M, Imbesi S. Stereo-lithographic vascular replicas from CT scans: Choosing treatment strategies, teaching, and research from live patient scan data. Am M Neuroradiol 2005;26:1428–31.

16 Russell M, Binyamin G, Konstantino E. Ex vivo analysis of human coronary bifurcation anatomy: defining the main vessel-to-side-branch transition zone. Eurointerv 2009; 5:96–103.

17 Costa R, Mintz G, Carlier S, Lansky A, Moussa I, Fujii K, Takebayashi H, Yasuda T, Costa J, Tsuchiya Y, Jensen L, Cristea E, Mehran R, Dangas G, Iyer S, Collins M, Kreps E, Colombo A, Stone G, Leon M, Moses J. Bifurcation Coronary Lesions treated with the "crush" technique. J Am Coll Cardiol 2005;46:599–605.

18 Szabo S, Abrahamowitz B, Vaitkus P. Am J Cardiol 2005;96:212H.

19 Shama S, Choudhury A, Lee J, Kim M, Kataoka T, Fisher E, Steinheimer A, Kini A. Simultaneous kissing stents (SKS) technique for treating bifurcation lesions in medium-to-large size coronary arteries. Am J Cardiol 2004;94:913–17.

CHAPTER 10

Coronary bifurcation stenting and stent thrombosis

Michael Mahmoudi, MD, PhD *and Ron Waksman,* MD

Division of Cardiology, Washington Hospital Center, Washington, DC, USA

Introduction

Coronary bifurcation lesions are encountered in approximately 15% of percutaneous coronary interventions (PCI) [1]. Early experience using balloon angioplasty was discouraging due to complications such as acute closure and restenosis in both the main branch (MB) and the side branch (SB) [2]. Although the introduction of bare metal stents (BMS) in the treatment of bifurcation lesions provided some improvement over balloon angioplasty, results continued to be disappointing with a 38% rate of target lesion revascularization (TLR) at 6 months and a 32% rate of major adverse cardiac events (MACE) at 1 year [3,4]. The beneficial effects of drug-eluting stents (DES) in reducing restenosis in both simple and complex coronary lesions appear to extend to bifurcation lesions regardless of whether a one-stent or two-stent strategy is deployed [5–12]. However, despite advances in both stent technology and techniques, the treatment of bifurcation lesions continues to pose a challenge due to a combination of technical complexity and associated morbidity and mortality.

Pathophysiology

The development of atherosclerotic plaque is orchestrated by a dynamic combination of endothelial dysfunction, increased permeability of lipoproteins, up-regulation of adhesion molecules and transmigration of monocytes, T-lymphocytes and vascular smooth muscle cells [13]. More specifically, atherosclerotic lesions exhibit a predilection for bifurcation points as evidenced by a greater prevalence of both plaque and necrotic core formations along the lateral wall of bifurcation points. Plaque formation in native coronary bifurcations and neointimal growth after DES implantation was significantly less at the flow divider versus the lateral wall. A higher prevalence of late stent thrombosis in DES compared with BMS was associated with greater uncovered struts at flow divider sites, which is likely to be due to flow disturbances [14]. In addition, the contribution of low-shear stress and changes in oscillatory flow, along with variations in the bifurcation angle, are being increasingly recognized as fundamental to both the development and the progression of atherosclerosis at these sites. Indeed, a number of studies have demonstrated an association between areas of low-shear stress and the up-regulation of intracellular and vascular adhesion molecules, as well as increases in the turbulent flow as the angle of bifurcation increases thus making coronary bifurcations a primary target in both the development and the progression of atherosclerotic lesions [15–17].

Stent thrombosis

A persisting challenge in the treatment of coronary bifurcation lesions remains the issue of stent

Bifurcation Stenting, First Edition. Edited by Ron Waksman and John A. Ormiston.

thrombosis even in the current era of DES. A variety of risk factors have been implicated for the development of stent thrombosis. These include factors related to the procedure itself, such as stent malapposition and/or under-expansion; patient characteristics, particularly diabetes mellitus; lesion characteristics such as ST-elevation and non ST-elevation MI; the thrombus burden of a given lesion; and factors related to the stent itself, such as delayed healing and persistent inflammation, as well as premature discontinuation of dual antiplatelet therapy [18–22].

Bifurcation lesions themselves have indeed been shown to be independent predictors of stent thrombosis, with several studies showing stenting in such lesions to be an independent factor for stent thrombosis with a risk ratio of 3–10x that associated with stenting of a non-bifurcation lesion [18,23–25]. Pathological analysis of 40 stented bifurcation lesions (21 with BMS and 19 with DES) obtained from the CVPath Sudden Death Registry has also shown that the use of DES at these sites was associated with a greater delay in arterial healing, particularly at flow divider sites where thrombi

could be seen to originate at the sites of uncovered struts [14]. Although this study was limited by sample size and selection bias, it does provide some mechanistic insight as to how bifurcation stenting may lead to a greater risk for stent thrombosis.

Stent thrombosis at the bifurcation can occur with BMS, DES, or in combination of the two. Doubling the metallic surface is a predisposition for increased acute and subacute stent thrombosis and can occur even in the presence of adequate expansion of the stents at the bifurcation (Figure 10.1) However, the impact of double stenting as an independent predictor of stent thrombosis remains controversial. An analysis of the major randomized studies and clinical registries comparing a single versus two-stent strategy (Tables 10.1 and 10.2, Figure 10.2) has confirmed both the safety and efficacy of the two-stent strategy with acceptable rates of stent thrombosis. The 3.5% rate of stent thrombosis observed in the study by Colombo *et al.* remains the highest rate reported in the randomized literature to date [5,11,26–28]. This study was indeed the first randomized study to compare a two-stent strategy via the crush technique against

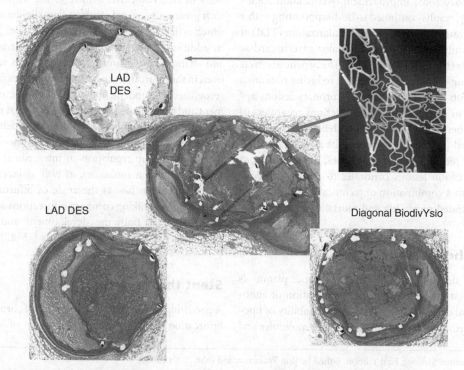

Figure 10.1 Stent thrombosis at the bifurcation of a DES in the LAD and BMS at the diagonal.

Table 10.1 Summary of randomized clinical trials addressing the treatment of coronary bifurcation lesions

Study	Number of patients	Techniques	Primary end point	Outcome	Stent thrombosis
Colombo	85	Crush, Culotte, T	Angiographic restenosis	18.7 vs. 28% (p = NS)	3.5%
Pan	91	T	Angiographic restenosis	7% vs. 25% (p = NS)	
NORDIC	413	Crush, Culotte, T	Death, MI, TVR or stent thrombosis	2.9% vs. 3.4% (p = NS)	0% vs. 0.5% (p = NS)
BBK	202	T	Angiographic restenosis	23% vs. 27.7% (p = NS)	2% vs. 1% (p = NS)
CACTUS	350	Crush	Death, MI, TVR	15% vs. 15.8% (p = NS)	1.7% vs. 1.1% (p = NS)
BBC ONE	500	Crush, Culotte	Death, MI, TVF	8% vs. 15.2% (p = NS)	2% vs. 0.4% (p = NS)

MI, myocardial infarction; TVR, target vessel revascularization; TVF, target vessel failure; NS, not significant

Table 10.2 Summary of the large clinical registries addressing the treatment of coronary bifurcation stenting

Author	Number of patients	Technique	End point	Outcome	Stent thrombosis
Sharma	200	SKS	In-hospital and 30-day MACE and 9-month TLR	3%, 5%, 4%	1%
Ge	181	Culotte	In-hospital and 9-month MACE	8.8%; 26.5%	2.8%
Hoye	231	Crush	In-hospital MACE; Survival free MACE at 9 months	4.8%; 83.5%	4.3%
Moussa	120	Crush	6-month MACE	13%	1.7%
Ge	182	Crush vs T	12-month MACE	26.4% vs 36.1%; p = 0.23	1.7% vs 0.0%; p = 0.8

SKS, simultaneous kissing stents; MACE, major adverse cardiovascular events

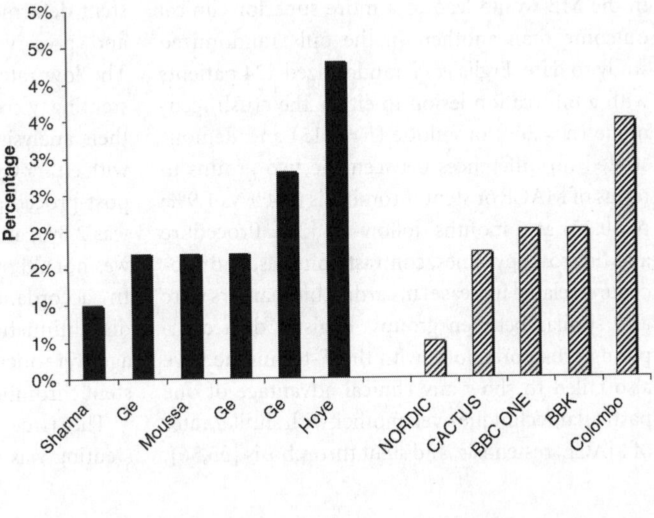

Figure 10.2 Stent thrombosis rates in the major studies of coronary bifurcation stenting in the DES era.

a strategy of stenting the MB and provisional stenting of the SB. However, a number of subsequent studies by the same group have suggested that the addition of a two-step final kissing balloon dilatation (FKBD) to the crush technique can lead to lower rates of restenosis in the SB, lower rates of MACE and the need for subsequent TLR [29]. Furthermore, in a sub-analysis of the data from the coronary bifurcations: application of the crushing technique using sirolimus-eluting stents (CACTUS) study, the performance of FKBD in both the crush and provisional groups was associated with lower incidences of in-hospital and follow-up MI, target vessel revascularization (TVR), stent thrombosis and angiographic restenosis in both the MB and SB. The rationale for this benefit may be explained by a more complete apposition of the crushed stent struts against the main vessel wall as inadequate apposition has been postulated to be a contributing mechanism for the development of stent thrombosis in bifurcation lesions treated with the crush technique [30]. Classic crush stenting may also predispose to stent thrombosis as a consequence of multiple layering of stent struts, which has been associated with reduced endothelialization and reduced tissue coverage [31,32]. Although not assessed in the context of a randomized clinical study, mini-crush variations of classic crush have been suggested to reduce multiple layering of DES struts and lead to a more complete endothelialization, thus minimizing the risk of stent thrombosis [33].

There is currently limited data to suggest whether a bifurcation technique entailing less metal in the MB would lead to a more superior clinical outcome than another. In the only randomized study to date, Erglis et al. randomized 424 patients with a bifurcation lesion to either the crush technique (n = 209) or culotte (n = 215) and demonstrated no differences between the two groups in terms of MACE or stent thrombosis (1.4% vs 1.9%; p = 0.73) at 6 months' follow-up [34]. Procedure and fluoroscopy times, contrast volumes, and procedure-related increases in cardiac biomarkers were also similar between groups. Registry data comparing crush or culotte with the T-technique have also failed to show any clinical advantage of one particular technique over another with similar rates of MACE, restenosis, and stent thrombosis [35,36].

Although the rates of stent thrombosis observed in the randomized studies have been reassuringly low and not significantly different from the single stent strategy arm, such results must be interpreted with caution. Firstly, none of the randomized studies so far has been adequately powered to assess stent thrombosis. Secondly, with the exception of the British bifurcation coronary study (BBC ONE) and bifurcations Bad Krozingen (BBK) studies, the duration of follow-up has been limited to less than 12 months, a period that may not be sufficiently long enough to adequately assess the rates of stent thrombosis. Finally, the patient population enrolled into these studies represents a heterogeneous population with differing clinical characteristics, differing anatomical classification of bifurcation disease, as well as differing rates of cross-over from one arm of the study to another, as exemplified by the study by Colombo et al. where the rate of cross-over from the double to single stent strategy was 51.2%.

Clinical registries have served as excellent complements to randomized clinical studies on bifurcation techniques. Such registries for the most part have confirmed the relatively low rates of stent thrombosis associated with bifurcation techniques (Table 10.2). Using the simultaneous kissing stent (SKS) technique in 200 consecutive patients undergoing bifurcation stenting with the Cypher stent, Sharma reported a stent thrombosis rate of 1% at an average follow-up of 9 months [37]. The rate of stent thrombosis compared favorably with those of randomized studies utilizing the crush and culotte techniques, perhaps as a consequence of less stent deformation, full coverage of the SB ostium and preservation of the bifurcation geometry. The low rates of stent thrombosis in bifurcation stenting were further confirmed by Ge et al. in their analysis of 181 consecutive patients treated with either Cypher or Taxus stents [29]. The rate of post-procedural stent thrombosis in this registry was 2.8%, and, in contrast to the CACTUS study, was not altered by FKBD (2.6% vs 3.1%; p = 0.78). In accordance with other reports, premature discontinuation of dual antiplatelet therapy and age were identified as the strongest predictors of stent thrombosis [38,39].

The issue of stent thrombosis in bifurcation stenting was once again brought into sharp focus by Hoye *et al.* who evaluated the clinical and angiographic outcomes of 231 consecutive patients with coronary bifurcation lesions treated with either Cypher or Taxus stents[40]. The rate of stent thrombosis was as high as 4.3% with a trend toward a higher rate in patients who had received the Taxus stent (6.9% vs 2.2%; p = 0.08). However, it is noteworthy that of the 10 patients who had stent thrombosis, only two were documented angiographically and four patients had discontinued dual antiplatelet therapy within 7 months of their procedure, a factor that has been established beyond doubt as one of the most important predictors of stent thrombosis. Furthermore, such high rates of stent thrombosis have not been replicated in either randomized studies or clinical registries.

Conclusion

Stent thrombosis is a potentially catastrophic consequence of PCI and remains the Achilles's heel of modern interventional cardiology. Although there is currently no convincing evidence that the use of DES in bifurcation lesions is associated with a greater risk of stent thrombosis, the treatment of bifurcation lesions must aim to achieve the optimal result in both the main and side braches.

References

1 Meier B, Gruentzig AR, King SB, 3rd, Douglas JS, Jr., Hollman J, Ischinger T, Aueron F, Galan K. Risk of side branch occlusion during coronary angioplasty. Am J Cardiol 1984;53:10–4.

2 Pinkerton CA, Slack JD, Van Tassel JW, Orr CM. Angioplasty for dilatation of complex coronary artery bifurcation stenoses. Am J Cardiol 1985;55:1626–8.

3 Yamashita T, Nishida T, Adamian MG, Briguori C, Vaghetti M, Corvaja N, Albiero R, Finci L, Di Mario C, Tobis JM, Colombo A. Bifurcation lesions: two stents versus one stent – immediate and follow-up results. J Am Coll Cardiol 2000;35:1145–51.

4 Al Suwaidi J, Yeh W, Cohen HA, Detre KM, Williams DO, Holmes DR, Jr., Immediate and one-year outcome in patients with coronary bifurcation lesions in the modern era (NHLBI dynamic registry). Am J Cardiol 2001;87:1139–44.

5 Colombo A, Moses JW, Morice MC, Ludwig J, Holmes DR, Jr., Spanos V, Louvard Y, Desmedt B, Di Mario C, Leon MB. Randomized study to evaluate sirolimus-eluting stents implanted at coronary bifurcation lesions. Circulation 2004;109:1244–9.

6 Kelbaek H, Thuesen L, Helqvist S, Klovgaard L, Jorgensen E, Aljabbari S, Saunamaki K, Krusell LR, Jensen GV, Botker HE, Lassen JF, Andersen HR, Thayssen P, Galloe A, van Weert A. The stenting coronary arteries in non-stress/benestent disease (SCANDSTENT) trial. J Am Coll Cardiol 2006;47:449–55.

7 Morice MC, Serruys PW, Sousa JE, Fajadet J, Ban Hayashi E, Perin M, Colombo A, Schuler G, Barragan P, Guagliumi G, Molnar F, Falotico R. A randomized comparison of a sirolimus-eluting stent with a standard stent for coronary revascularization. N Engl J Med 2002;346:1773–80.

8 Moses JW, Leon MB, Popma JJ, Fitzgerald PJ, Holmes DR, O'Shaughnessy C, Caputo RP, Kereiakes DJ, Williams DO, Teirstein PS, Jaeger JL, Kuntz RE. Sirolimus-eluting stents versus standard stents in patients with stenosis in a native coronary artery. N Engl J Med 2003;349:1315–23.

9 Pan M, de Lezo JS, Medina A, Romero M, Segura J, Pavlovic D, Delgado A, Ojeda S, Melian F, Herrador J, Urena I, Burgos L. Rapamycin-eluting stents for the treatment of bifurcated coronary lesions: a randomized comparison of a simple versus complex strategy. Am Heart J 2004;148:857–64.

10 Schofer J, Schluter M, Gershlick AH, Wijns W, Garcia E, Schampaert E, Breithardt G. Sirolimus-eluting stents for treatment of patients with long atherosclerotic lesions in small coronary arteries: double-blind, randomised controlled trial (E-SIRIUS). Lancet 2003;362:1093–9.

11 Steigen TK, Maeng M, Wiseth R, Erglis A, Kumsars I, Narbute I, Gunnes P, Mannsverk J, Meyerdierks O, Rotevatn S, Niemela M, Kervinen K, Jensen JS, Galloe A, Nikus K, Vikman S, Ravkilde J, James S, Aaroe J, Ylitalo A, Helqvist S, Sjogren I, Thayssen P, Virtanen K, Puhakka M, Airaksinen J, Lassen JF, Thuesen L. Randomized study on simple versus complex stenting of coronary artery bifurcation lesions: the Nordic bifurcation study. Circulation 2006;114:1955–61.

12 Thuesen L, Kelbaek H, Klovgaard L, Helqvist S, Jorgensen E, Aljabbari S, Krusell LR, Jensen GV, Botker HE, Saunamaki K, Lassen JF, van Weert A. Comparison of sirolimus-eluting and bare metal stents in coronary bifurcation lesions: subgroup analysis of the stenting coronary arteries in non-stress/benestent disease trial (SCANDSTENT). Am Heart J 2006;152:1140–5.

13 Hansson GK. Inflammation, atherosclerosis, and coronary artery disease. N Engl J Med 2005;352:1685–95.

14 Nakazawa G, Yazdani SK, Finn AV, Vorpahl M, Kolodgie FD, Virmani R. Pathological findings at bifurcation lesions: the impact of flow distribution on atherosclerosis

and arterial healing after stent implantation. J Am Coll Cardiol 2010;55:1679–87.

15 Cheng C, van Haperen R, de Waard M, van Damme LC, Tempel D, Hanemaaijer L, van Cappellen GW, Bos J, Slager CJ, Duncker DJ, van der Steen AF, de Crom R, Krams R. Shear stress affects the intracellular distribution of eNOS: direct demonstration by a novel in vivo technique. Blood 2005;106:3691–8.

16 Cheng C, Tempel D, van Haperen R, van der Baan A, Grosveld F, Daemen MJ, Krams R, de Crom R. Atherosclerotic lesion size and vulnerability are determined by patterns of fluid shear stress. Circulation 2006;113:2744–53.

17 Perktold K, Peter RO, Resch M, Langs G. Pulsatile non-Newtonian blood flow in three-dimensional carotid bifurcation models: a numerical study of flow phenomena under different bifurcation angles. J Biomed Eng 1991;13:507–15.

18 Daemen J, Wenaweser P, Tsuchida K, Abrecht L, Vaina S, Morger C, Kukreja N, Juni P, Sianos G, Hellige G, van Domburg RT, Hess OM, Boersma E, Meier B, Windecker S, Serruys PW. Early and late coronary stent thrombosis of sirolimus-eluting and paclitaxel-eluting stents in routine clinical practice: data from a large two-institutional cohort study. Lancet 2007;369:667–78.

19 Farb A, Burke AP, Kolodgie FD, Virmani R. Pathological mechanisms of fatal late coronary stent thrombosis in humans. Circulation 2003;108:1701–6.

20 Finn AV, Joner M, Nakazawa G, Kolodgie F, Newell J, John MC, Gold HK, Virmani R. Pathological correlates of late drug-eluting stent thrombosis: strut coverage as a marker of endothelialization. Circulation 2007; 115:2435–41.

21 Chen BX, Ma FY, Luo W, Ruan JH, Xie WL, Zhao XZ, Sun SH, Guo XM, Wang F, Tian T, Chu XW. Neointimal coverage of bare-metal and sirolimus-eluting stents evaluated with optical coherence tomography. Heart 2008;94:566–70.

22 Alfonso F, Suarez A, Perez-Vizcayno MJ, Moreno R, Escaned J, Banuelos C, Jimenez P, Bernardo E, Angiolillo DJ, Hernandez R, Macaya C. Intravascular ultrasound findings during episodes of drug-eluting stent thrombosis. J Am Coll Cardiol 2007;50:2095–7.

23 Iakovou I, Schmidt T, Bonizzoni E, Ge L, Sangiorgi GM, Stankovic G, Airoldi F, Chieffo A, Montorfano M, Carlino M, Michev I, Corvaja N, Briguori C, Gerckens U, Grube E, Colombo A. Incidence, predictors, and outcome of thrombosis after successful implantation of drug-eluting stents. JAMA 2005;293:2126–30.

24 Ong AT, McFadden EP, Regar E, de Jaegere PP, van Domburg RT, Serruys PW. Late angiographic stent thrombosis (LAST) events with drug-eluting stents. J Am Coll Cardiol 2005;45:2088–92.

25 Kuchulakanti PK, Chu WW, Torguson R, Ohlmann P, Rha SW, Clavijo LC, Kim SW, Bui A, Gevorkian N, Xue Z, Smith K, Fournadjieva J, Suddath WO, Satler LF, Pichard AD, Kent KM, Waksman R. Correlates and long-term outcomes of angiographically proven stent thrombosis with sirolimus- and paclitaxel-eluting stents. Circulation 2006;113:1108–13.

26 Ferenc M, Gick M, Kienzle RP, Bestehorn HP, Werner KD, Comberg T, Kuebler P, Buttner HJ, Neumann FJ. Randomized trial on routine vs. provisional T-stenting in the treatment of de novo coronary bifurcation lesions. Eur Heart J 2008;29:2859–67.

27 Colombo A, Bramucci E, Sacca S, Violini R, Lettieri C, Zanini R, Sheiban I, Paloscia L, Grube E, Schofer J, Bolognese L, Orlandi M, Niccoli G, Latib A, Airoldi F. Randomized study of the crush technique versus provisional side-branch stenting in true coronary bifurcations: the CACTUS (Coronary Bifurcations: Application of the Crushing Technique Using Sirolimus-Eluting Stents) Study. Circulation 2009;119:71–8.

28 Hildick-Smith D, de Belder AJ, Cooter N, Curzen NP, Clayton TC, Oldroyd KG, Bennett L, Holmberg S, Cotton JM, Glennon PE, Thomas MR, Maccarthy PA, Baumbach A, Mulvihill NT, Henderson RA, Redwood SR, Starkey IR, Stables RH. Randomized trial of simple versus complex drug-eluting stenting for bifurcation lesions: the British bifurcation coronary study: old, new, and evolving strategies. Circulation 2010;121:1235–43.

29 Ge L, Airoldi F, Iakovou I, Cosgrave J, Michev I, Sangiorgi GM, Montorfano M, Chieffo A, Carlino M, Corvaja N, Colombo A. Clinical and angiographic outcome after implantation of drug-eluting stents in bifurcation lesions with the crush stent technique: importance of final kissing balloon post-dilation. J Am Coll Cardiol 2005;46:613–20.

30 Costa RA, Mintz GS, Carlier SG, Lansky AJ, Moussa I, Fujii K, Takebayashi H, Yasuda T, Costa JR, Jr., Tsuchiya Y, Jensen LO, Cristea E, Mehran R, Dangas GD, Iyer S, Collins M, Kreps EM, Colombo A, Stone GW, Leon MB, Moses JW. Bifurcation coronary lesions treated with the "crush" technique: an intravascular ultrasound analysis. J Am Coll Cardiol 2005;46:599–605.

31 Finn AV, Kolodgie FD, Harnek J, Guerrero LJ, Acampado E, Tefera K, Skorija K, Weber DK, Gold HK, Virmani R. Differential response of delayed healing and persistent inflammation at sites of overlapping sirolimus-or paclitaxel-eluting stents. Circulation 2005;112:270–8.

32 Awata M, Kotani J, Uematsu M, Morozumi T, Watanabe T, Onishi T, Iida O, Sera F, Nanto S, Hori M, Nagata S. Serial angioscopic evidence of incomplete neointimal coverage after sirolimus-eluting stent

implantation: comparison with bare-metal stents. Circulation 2007;116:910–6.

33 Ormiston JA, Currie E, Webster MW, Kay P, Ruygrok PN, Stewart JT, Padgett RC, Panther MJ. Drug-eluting stents for coronary bifurcations: insights into the crush technique. Catheter Cardiovasc Interv 2004;63:332–6.

34 Erglis A, Kumsars I, Niemela M, Kervinen K, Maeng M, Lassen JF, Gunnes P, Stavnes S, Jensen JS, Galloe A, Narbute I, Sondore D, Makikallio T, Ylitalo K, Christiansen EH, Ravkilde J, Steigen TK, Mannsverk J, Thayssen P, Hansen KN, Syvanne M, Helqvist S, Kjell N, Wiseth R, Aaroe J, Puhakka M, Thuesen L. Randomized comparison of coronary bifurcation stenting with the crush versus the culotte technique using sirolimus eluting stents: the Nordic stent technique study. Circ Cardiovasc Interv 2009;2:27–34.

35 Ge L, Iakovou I, Cosgrave J, Agostoni P, Airoldi F, Sangiorgi GM, Michev I, Chieffo A, Montorfano M, Carlino M, Corvaja N, Colombo A. Treatment of bifurcation lesions with two stents: one year angiographic and clinical follow up of crush versus T stenting. Heart 2006;92:371–6.

36 Kaplan S, Barlis P, Dimopoulos K, La Manna A, Goktekin O, Galassi A, Tanigawa J, Di Mario C. Culotte versus T-stenting in bifurcation lesions: immediate clinical and angiographic results and midterm clinical follow-up. Am Heart J 2007;154:336–43.

37 Sharma SK. Simultaneous kissing drug-eluting stent technique for percutaneous treatment of bifurcation lesions in large-size vessels. Catheter Cardiovasc Interv 2005;65:10–16.

38 Jeremias A, Sylvia B, Bridges J, Kirtane AJ, Bigelow B, Pinto DS, Ho KK, Cohen DJ, Garcia LA, Cutlip DE, Carrozza JP, Jr., Stent thrombosis after successful sirolimus-eluting stent implantation. Circulation 2004; 109:1930–2.

39 Schuhlen H, Kastrati A, Dirschinger J, Hausleiter J, Elezi S, Wehinger A, Pache J, Hadamitzky M, Schomig A. Intracoronary stenting and risk for major adverse cardiac events during the first month. Circulation 1998;98:104–11.

40 Hoye A, Iakovou I, Ge L, van Mieghem CA, Ong AT, Cosgrave J, Sangiorgi GM, Airoldi F, Montorfano M, Michev I, Chieffo A, Carlino M, Corvaja N, Aoki J, Rodriguez Granillo GA, Valgimigli M, Sianos G, van der Giessen WJ, de Feyter PJ, van Domburg RT, Serruys PW, Colombo A. Long-term outcomes after stenting of bifurcation lesions with the "crush" technique: predictors of an adverse outcome. J Am Coll Cardiol 2006;47:1949–58.

CHAPTER 11

Bifurcation angles during the cardiac cycle

Satoko Tahara, MD, PhD[1], *Hiram G. Bezerra,* MD, PhD[1],
Pieter H. Kitslaar, Msc[2], *Johan HC Reiber,* PhD[2]
and Marco A. Costa, MD, PhD, FACC, FSCAI[1]

[1]Harrington-McLaughlin Heart and Vascular Institute, University Hospitals, Case Western Reserve University, Cleveland, OH, USA
[2]Department of Radiology, Leiden University Medical Center, Leiden, The Netherlands

Introduction

Bifurcations of coronary arteries are predilection sites for atherosclerosis and expansive remodeling associated with plaque vulnerability. Clinical outcomes remain unsatisfactory despite multiple percutaneous approaches toward them, as the continuous dynamic variation in the three-dimensional (3D) anatomical configurations exists in coronary bifurcations. Although interventional procedures in a coronary system use two-dimensional X-ray-based imaging as the major imaging modality for procedure guidance and quantification of key parameters, specific coronary vascular curvilinearity delineated in bifurcations is considered one of the key parameters that requires a four-dimensional (4D) format or 3D anatomical representations that change during the cardiac cycle. A 4D imaging modality would likely have an impact on furthering our understanding of the unique intricacies of bifurcation disease. Recently, new methods have been developed for reconstruction and analysis of patient-specific 4D datasets utilizing routine diagnostic tools in cardiac imaging.

In the field of cardiac CT, multidetector-row acquisition provides improved spatial resolution for multidetector CT angiography (MDCTA) of the coronary arteries and makes 3D imaging of the coronary vasculature possible. A novel method to acquire images in multiple phases of the cardiac cycle, which allowed for the evaluation of the 3D anatomical changes that occur at coronary artery bifurcations over time, has recently been developed. In this chapter, the necessity of 4D imaging for bifurcations, the present status of 3D bifurcation imaging preceding 4D imaging and this novel method of 4D multidetector computed tomography (MDCT) imaging are described.

Bifurcation as the "Achilles' heel" of PCI

Bifurcation coronary artery disease occurs in 15–20% of all patients undergoing percutaneous coronary interventions. Treatment of bifurcation lesions has been suboptimal and dissatisfying [1–5]. Balloon angioplasty results were suboptimal and led to a high frequency of restenosis [6,7]. Use of bare metal stents (BMS) in either the main branch or in both the main branch and side branch produced similarly disappointing results [8–13].

Bifurcation Stenting, First Edition. Edited by Ron Waksman and John A. Ormiston.
© 2012 Blackwell Publishing Ltd. Published 2012 by Blackwell Publishing Ltd.

Despite the introduction of drug-eluting stents (DES), different stent technique implantations involving DES still yielded suboptimal results for bifurcation lesions [2,14]. Moreover, restenosis rates of the side branch with either BMS or DES have remained unacceptable, as high as 22% [15]. The side branch ostium remains one of the few scenarios where BMS or DES is not superior to balloon angioplasty. The reason for this phenomenon seems to be multifactorial, and the failure of ostium coverage by the stent may only partially explain the poor outcome. However, even using the technique for full coverage, bifurcation ostium is still susceptible to higher rate of major adverse outcome compared with non-bifurcation lesions.

Importance of 4D imaging for bifurcation

Bifurcation lesions have specific features related with cardiac movements. First, specific arteries follow the underlying wall motion. The LAD follows the anterior wall, while the LCX follows the lateral wall, and then the maximal attrition is considered to likely occur at the carina [16]. Second, there is a difference in the timing of activation and contraction of different regions of the entire heart. This dynamic variation in the 3D anatomical configurations of coronary bifurcations during the cardiac cycle is suggested to be a potential cause of bifurcation coronary device failure. The placement of rigid metallic prostheses at these areas of constant motion has a susceptibility to fracture, recoil or impart excess injury to the underlying vessel after long-lasting stress. Thus, to demonstrate and quantify the dynamic changes in coronary bifurcation anatomy, the use of 4D imaging seems to be essential.

Development of coronary bifurcation 3D imaging preceding 4D imaging

Although specific anatomical assessment of bifurcations was supposed to be useful in achieving better outcomes, insufficient investigational approaches toward bifurcation imaging had been done because of difficulties in the evaluation of

their structural diversity (angulation, position) and dynamic conformational change affected by cardiac contraction [17]. However, following unsatisfactory results of DES in bifurcation stenting and the overwhelming improvement in MDCT [18,19], bifurcation imaging studies using cardiac CT have emerged since 2006. Pflederer *et al.* performed bifurcation angle measurements by contrast-enhanced CT in comparison with invasive angiography by examining the average angles of four main coronary bifurcations: left anterior descending artery (LAD)-left circumflex artery (LCX); LAD-first diagonal branch (D1); LCX-oblique marginal branch (OM1); and posterior descending coronary artery (PDA)-right posterolateral branch (RPLD) [20]. Interobserver variability was also determined in 15 patients, both in 16-row MDCT data sets and invasive coronary angiograms, by two independent observers. In their results, MDCT allowed assessment of coronary bifurcation angles with a higher accuracy with lower interobserver variability ($r = 0.91$) than invasive angiography ($r = 0.62$). Additionally, analysis of the natural distribution of bifurcation angles by MDCT revealed average values of 80 ± 27 degrees (LAD-LCX), 46 ± 19 degrees (LAD-D1), 48 ± 24 degrees (LCX-OM1), and 53 ± 27 degrees (PDA-RPLD), respectively. Kawasaki *et al.* [21] measured the coronary bifurcation angles of 209 patients suspected of having angina pectoris using 64-row MSCT. In their study, the average left main coronary artery (LM) bifurcation angles (LM-LAD, LM-LCX, and LAD-LCX) were 143 ± 13 degrees, 121 ± 21 degrees, and 72 ± 22 degrees, respectively. The average LAD-D1 was 138 ± 19 degrees, the average LCX-OM was 134 ± 23 degrees, the average distal RCA bifurcation angles (RCA-4AV, RCA-4PD, and 4AV-4PD) were 152 ± 15 degrees, 137 ± 20 degrees, and 61 ± 21 degrees, respectively. In addition, a percentage of steep angled bifurcations (<110 degrees) was higher in the LM (26%) than in other bifurcations ($p < 0.05$). Rodriguez-Granillo *et al.* determined using a 40-row MDCTA the differences in plaque burdens at different segments of the left main bifurcation and their relationship with the bifurcation angle [22]. Seventeen (34%) patients presented with at least wall irregularities in the LM and in the ostial LCX, whereas the ostial LAD was affected in 32 (64%) patients. More than 90% of plaques were located opposite to the flow divider. In their study, the median LMCA bifurcation angle was 88.5 degrees (IQR 68.8 degrees, 101.4 degrees). Interestingly, of the 18 patients with a normal ostial LAD, 13 (72%) had a bifurcation angle < 88.5 degrees, whereas the 63% of the patients with any LAD disease had an angle ≥88.5 degrees (p = 0.018), which led to the conclusion that the angle of the left main bifurcation and the presence of plaques within the bifurcation were closely related. In bifurcation stent analysis, Murasato *et al.* performed three different double-stentings: crush, kissing, and modified T stentings using a silicon model of the LM bifurcation and 3D reconstruction images created with micro-focus X-ray computed tomography (MFCT) with a minimal resolution of 0.06 mm [23]. Close apposition of the stent to the vessel at the ostium of the LCX was difficult to achieve at the LM bifurcation, regardless of which double-stent technique was employed. This presented a possible relation between the wider angle of LM bifurcation and restenosis in the double-stent technique. 3D imaging has been credited with a lot of findings of bifurcations and provided partial explanations for higher incidences of bifurcation restenosis. However, without considering a cardiac cycle, dramatic improvements don't seem to be accomplished.

Novel methodology of 4D multidetector computed tomography (MDCT) imaging

Image acquisition
The target bifurcations of our study were the LM-LAD, LM-LCX and LCX-LAD artery bifurcations. Anonymous five image datasets with good quality were selected for analysis.

4D post-processing and bifurcation angle determination
The optimal phase was found to be around the 70% R-R interval value. The high-quality phases were used as an aid during the processing of the lesser quality phases. Center lines for the vessels were obtained at the bifurcation point, as well as the two vessels (Figure 11.1). The technique used to obtain

the vessel centerlines consisted of two phases. First, an initial segmentation of the arterial lumen volume of the bifurcation was obtained using a threshold-based region growing scheme with occasional manual correction. Second, a 3D tracking algorithm was used to define paths through the segmentation running from the distal end points of the bifurcation to the proximal start point in the common branch. A third path was next derived that was located in the middle of these two initial paths. This third path followed the main direction of the common branch, and at a certain point, intersected the carina to leave the segmented bifurcation volume. The bifurcation point was next defined at a fixed distance proximal from this intersection point along the defined third path. The position of the bifurcation point was chosen such that the distance to the carina equaled half of the diameter of the common vessel segment at that distance. Using this definition, the bifurcation point could be reproducibly defined in all the phases of the cardiac cycle. Once this bifurcation point was obtained, two new paths from the distal end points to the bifurcation point were calculated using the tracking algorithm [24]. Once these steps were completed, it was possible to make additional corrections to the centerlines. The manual corrections did not influence the location of the bifurcation point.

Using this representation, the relative angle between two branches, which was calculated by virtually projecting the 3D direction vectors of the different branches onto the defined planes and by measuring the 2D angle that were made by these projected vectors, was measured within the 3 planes that they spanned, 3D angles. Adding temporal information, the 4D dataset of the three pairs of branches (LM-LAD, LM-LCX, and LAD-LCX) could be obtained. Geometrically, there was no definition for the angle between the two curved lines. Therefore the obtained centerlines were approximated as a straight line between the bifurcation point and a point at a fixed distance along the curved centerline. The obtained angles for a chosen distance (10 mm, 15 mm, 20 mm, 25 mm, 30 mm, etc) could be calculated for each phase in the cardiac cycle. The values related with 10 mm distance values for angle comparisons are reported.

Figure 11.1 Coronary segmentation and angle determination. Coronary segmentation was performed removing the surrounding tissue. A vessel center line was placed and manually corrected (Figure 11.1a). This procedure was repeated for each phase (eight phases), generating a dynamic data set. Angles, defined as **(1)** LAD-LCX, **(2)** LCX-LM, and **(3)** LAD-LM, were assessed. Each angle was automatically determined in 3D (x, y and z planes) (Figure 11.1b).

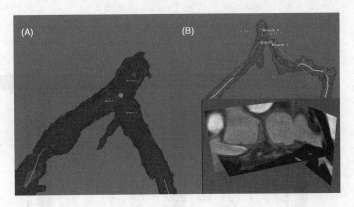

Results

Mean angle and variability

Figure 11.2 shows the variability of mean angles of the three bifurcations during the cardiac cycle. There were large variations in all three measured angles (LM-LAD, LM-LCX, and LAD-LCX) throughout the cardiac cycle. Furthermore, angle variations were not uniform between the LM-LAD, LM-LCX and LAD-LCX, and the widest variation occurred in different cardiac planes for each of the bifurcations. In the LAD-LCX carina, the widest range of variation was observed in the axial plane (16.2% coefficient of variance (CV) and 38.2 °Δ). For the main-LAD carina, the highest variability was located in the sagittal plane (21.6% CV and 73.6 °Δ). The main-LCX carina had high variability in both the axial and sagittal planes (22% CV and 43 °Δ; 17% CV and 55.4 °Δ, respectively).

Correlation between mean angle and the range of variability along the cardiac cycle

There was no correlation between the mean bifurcation angle and the absolute variation range of the bifurcation during phases, except for a trend towards an inverse correlation between the LM-LCX carina mean angle and range of variation, resulting in that a smaller LM-LCX angle predicted a higher range of variability throughout the cardiac cycle.

Correlation between the anatomic planes

A correlation between the changes on angulation of the LM-LAD bifurcation was observed between the axial and sagittal planes (r = 0.68, p < 0.001), but no correlation was observed between the other planes. On the LM-LCX bifurcation, none of the angulations correlated between the different cardiac planes. For the LAD-LCX bifurcation, a weak correlation among the axial and sagittal planes (r = 0.32, p = 0.047), a moderate correlation between the axial and coronal planes (r = 0.47, p = 0.003), and a strong correlation between the sagittal and coronal plane angulations were observed (r = 0.821, p < 0.0001).

The 4D assessment of cardiac MDCT images revealed a marked 3D variance of coronary bifurcations over the cardiac cycle. Such constant changes in anatomical coronary configurations pose a significant challenge to current devices and therapeutic strategies. It was previously proposed that the dynamic changes that occur in coronary artery bifurcations during the cardiac cycle represent a potential explanation for the marginal results with current percutaneous therapeutic approaches [17]. The motion of the heart produces movement of the coronary arteries in various directions throughout the cardiac cycle. Unfortunately, the continuous dynamic variation in the 3D anatomical configurations of coronary bifurcations has been largely overlooked. The repeated failure of double stent techniques for bifurcations may be explained, among other factors, by the constant complex movement of the MB and SB during the cardiac cycle. A number of new devices and techniques have been developed; unfortunately, most of them were developed based on a 2D static anatomical concept. The lack of a 4D imaging modality of coronary circulation likely limited the understanding of the unique intricacies of bifurcation disease.

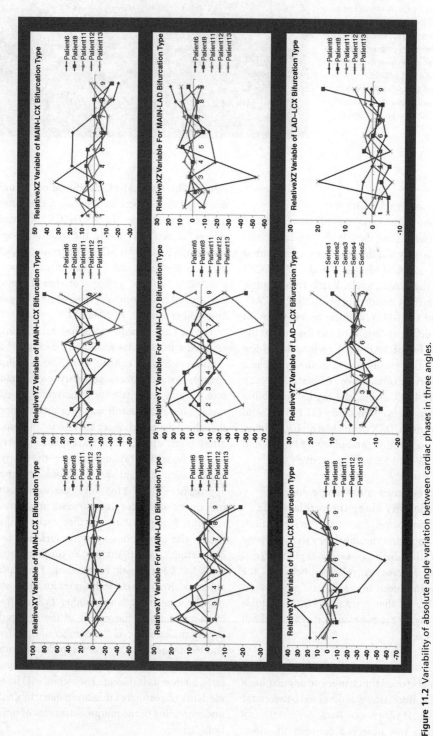

Figure 11.2 Variability of absolute angle variation between cardiac phases in three angles.
The baseline angle was calculated as the mean of the angles along eight phases; all angles minus this baseline angle were used as y, and phases were used as x.

The 4D assessment also demonstrated that the average bifurcation angle could not predict the variation range along the cardiac cycle. An average acute or obtuse angle will not predict on how much variation the bifurcation will face during the cardiac cycle. One exception to this rule is the LM-LCX bifurcation that demonstrates an inverse correlation between average bifurcation angulation and the range of variability; acute angles correlate with high variability in the cardiac cycle. Interestingly, the correlation between the different cardiac planes is dependent on the bifurcation type. In the LM-LCX bifurcation, the angle varied independently on each of the anatomic planes. On the other hand, a good correlation was observed between the sagittal and coronal planes on the LAD-LCX bifurcation.

This study has limitations because the sample size was small and clinical data on patients was not considered. It is necessary to perform further studies to determine if similarities in particular populations exist that could be classified into specific types of angle variations by adjusting cardiac phases.

Conclusion

These seminal findings on the dynamics of bifurcations in the cardiac cycle are critical for future developments of percutaneous strategies and technologies to treat bifurcation disease or other segments of the coronary tree subject to motion. After establishing a standardized methodology, it would be applied to define the different patterns of dynamic angle variations between pre-stenting and post-stenting. Getting this particular information on the dynamics of bifurcations might provide an important clue for preventing restenosis in bifurcation stenting. Furthermore, novel devices, such as biodegradable stents or composite hybrid stents, might incorporate such concepts and be capable of sustaining dynamic morphologic changes. Bench testing of these devices should be performed in 4D models, instead of static, planar bench systems. Beyond technological developments, 4D models provide important clues for daily practices and in our understanding of device failures in coronary bifurcations. Although the true clinical impact of such a prognostic tool rests in its ability to improve

outcomes, it is clear that the 4D assessment of bifurcation coronary artery disease provides the clinician, the investigator and the engineer with a formal tool to quantitatively assess the dynamic nature of coronary anatomy.

References

1 Ong AT, Hoye A, Aoki J, van Mieghem CA, Rodriguez Granillo GA, Sonnenschein K, Regar E, McFadden EP, Sianos G, van der Giessen WJ, de Jaegere PP, de Feyter P, van Domburg RT, Serruys PW. Thirty-day incidence and six-month clinical outcome of thrombotic stent occlusion after bare-metal, sirolimus, or paclitaxel stent implantation. J Am Coll Cardiol 2005;45:947–53.

2 Tanabe K, Hoye A, Lemos PA, Aoki J, Arampatzis CA, Saia F, Lee CH, Degertekin M, Hofma SH, Sianos G, McFadden E, Smits PC, van der Giessen WJ, de Feyter P, van Domburg RT, Serruys PW. Restenosis rates following bifurcation stenting with sirolimus-eluting stents for de novo narrowings. Am J Cardiol 2004;94:115–18.

3 Pan M, de Lezo JS, Medina A, Romero M, Segura J, Pavlovic D, Delgado A, Ojeda S, Melian F, Herrador J, Urena I, Burgos L. Rapamycin-eluting stents for the treatment of bifurcated coronary lesions: a randomized comparison of a simple versus complex strategy. Am Heart J 2004;148(5):857–64.

4 Colombo A, Stankovic G, Orlic D, Corvaja N, Liistro F, Airoldi F, Chieffo A, Spanos V, Montorfano M, Di Mario C. Modified T-stenting technique with crushing for bifurcation lesions: immediate results and 30-day outcome. Catheter Cardiovasc Interv 2003;60:145–51.

5 Ge L, Airoldi F, Iakovou I, Cosgrave J, Michev I, Sangiorgi GM, Montorfano M, Chieffo A, Carlino M, Corvaja N, Colombo A. Clinical and angiographic outcome after implantation of drug-eluting stents in bifurcation lesions with the crush stent technique: importance of final kissing balloon post-dilation. J Am Coll Cardiol 2005;46:613–20.

6 Weinstein JS, Baim DS, Sipperly ME, McCabe CH, Lorell BH. Salvage of branch vessels during bifurcation lesion angioplasty: acute and long-term follow-up. Cathet Cardiovasc Diagn 1991;22:1–6.

7 Mathias DW, Mooney JF, Lange HW, Goldenberg IF, Gobel FL, Mooney MR. Frequency of success and complications of coronary angioplasty of a stenosis at the ostium of a branch vessel. Am J Cardiol 1991;67:491–5.

8 Al Suwaidi J, Berger PB, Rihal CS, Garratt KN, Bell MR, Ting HH, Bresnahan JF, Grill DE, Holme DR, Jr. Immediate and long-term outcome of intracoronary stent implantation for true bifurcation lesions. J Am Coll Cardiol 2000;35:929–36.

9 Chevalier B, Glatt B, Royer T, Guyon P. Placement of coronary stents in bifurcation lesions by the "culotte" technique. Am J Cardiol 1998;82:943–9.

10 Yamashita T, Nishida T, Adamian MG, Briguori C, Vaghetti M, Corvaja N, Albiero R, Finci L, Di Mario C, Tobis JM, Colombo A. Bifurcation lesions: two stents versus one stent--immediate and follow-up results. J Am Coll Cardiol 2000;35:1145–51.

11 Pan M, Suarez de Lezo J, Medina A, Romero M, Hernandez E, Segura J, Castroviejo JR, Pavlovic D, Melian F, Ramirez A, Castillo JC. Simple and complex stent strategies for bifurcated coronary arterial stenosis involving the side branch origin. Am J Cardio. 1999; 83:1320–25.

12 Anzuini A, Briguori C, Rosanio S, Tocchi M, Pagnotta P, Bonnier H, Gimelli G, Airoldi F, Margonato A, Legrand V, Colombo A. Immediate and long-term clinical and angiographic results from Wiktor stent treatment for true bifurcation narrowings. Am J Cardiol. 2001;88:1246–50.

13 Al Suwaidi J, Yeh W, Cohen HA, Detre KM, Williams DO, Holmes DR, Jr. Immediate and one-year outcome in patients with coronary bifurcation lesions in the modern era (NHLBI dynamic registry). Am J Cardiol. 2001; 87:1139–44.

14 Colombo A, Moses JW, Morice MC, Ludwig J, Holmes DR, Jr., Spanos V, Louvard Y, Desmedt B, Di Mario C, Leon MB. Randomized study to evaluate sirolimus-eluting stents implanted at coronary bifurcation lesions. Circulation 2004;109:1244–9.

15 Pan M, Suarez de Lezo J, Medina A, Romero M, Hernandez E, Segura J, Castroviejo JR, Pavlovic D, Melian F, Ramirez A, Castillo JC. Simple and complex stent strategies for bifurcated coronary arterial stenosis involving the side branch origin. Am J Cardiol 1999;83:1320–5.

16 Pao YC, Lu JT, Ritman EL. Bending and twisting of an in vivo coronary artery at a bifurcation. J Biomech 1992; 25:287–95.

17 Suzuki N, Angiolillo DJ, Kawaguchi, et al. Percutaneous coronary intervention of the bifurcation coronary disease. Minerva Cardiology 2007;55:57–71.

18 Achenbach S, Moshage W, Daniel WG, et al. Value of electronbeam computed tomography for the noninvasive detection of high-grade coronary artery stenoses and occlusions. N Engl J Med 1998;339:1964–71.

19 Kopp AF, Schroeder S, Claussen CD, et al. Non-invasive coronary angiography with high resolution multidetector-row computed tomography. Results in 102 patients. Eur Heart J 2002;23:1714–25.

20 Pflederer T, Ludwig J, Achenbach S, et al. Measurement of coronary bifurcation angles by multidetector computed tomography. Invest Radiol 2006;41:793–8.

21 Kawasaki T, Koga H, Koga N, et al. The bifurcation study using 64 multislice computed tomography. Catheter Cardiovasc Interv 2009;73:653–8.

22 Rodriguez-Granillo GA, Rosales MA, Rodriguez AE, et al. Multislice CT coronary angiography for the detection of burden, morphology and distribution of atherosclerotic plaques in the left main bifurcation. Int J Cardiovasc Imaging 2007;23:389–92.

23 Murasato Y, Horiuchi M, Otsuji Y. Three-dimensional modeling of double –stent techniques at the left main coronary artery bifurcation using micro-focus X-ray computed tomography. Catheter Cardiovasc Interv 2007;70:211–20.

24 Kitslaar PH, Marquering HA, Jukema WJ, Koning G, Nieber M, Vossepoel AM, Bax JJ, Reiber JHC. Automated determination of optimal angiographic viewing angles for coronary artery bifurcations from CTA data. Proc SPIE 2008;6918: 69181J–10.

CHAPTER 12

OCT in coronary bifurcations

Juan Luis Gutiérrez-Chico, MD, PhD, FESC, *Robert Jan van Geuns,* MD, PhD, FESC, *Patrick Serruys,* MD, PhD, FESC, FACC *and Evelyn Regar,* MD, PhD, FESC

Erasmus Medisch Centrum, Thoraxcentrum, Rotterdam, The Netherlands

Introduction

Optical coherence tomography (OCT) is currently the most accurate intracoronay invasive imaging technology. It provides with the highest axial resolution (10–15 microns), thus enabling a precise quantitative in-vivo evaluation of stents, such as apposition or coverage [1–4]. These parameters influence the quality of the result immediately after the procedure or at follow-up respectively, and may potentially impact clinical outcome [5–10]. The interest in OCT has grown since the advent of drug-eluting stents (DES). In the bare metal stent (BMS) era, the main concern after a percutaneous coronary intervention (PCI) was restenosis [11], which was the result of an excessive neointimal proliferation after the vascular injury induced by PCI [12–19]. Restenosis could be reliably quantified with quantitative coronary angiography (QCA) [20–37] or with intravascular ultrasound (IVUS) [38–41]. DES have successfully addressed the problem of restenosis [42–44]; however, some reports have also suggested higher incidence of stent thrombosis [45–50]. Delayed neointimal healing with incomplete endothelialization is a common substrate in cases of late stent thrombosis when assessed by pathology [8,9]. While the axial resolution of conventional IVUS (around 100 μm) yields an accurate assessment of restenosis, the thin neointimal layer covering DES struts is normally below this range, and therefore cannot be reliably measured by IVUS. OCT has arisen as the golden standard for the in-vivo assessment of struts coverage after stenting. OCT tissue coverage shows good correlation with histological neointimal coverage in animal studies [51–53], with superior accuracy compared with IVUS [(51], and higher reproducibility [1,54]. The ability of OCT to implement this hitherto unmet need of evaluating the tissue coverage after stenting has been the main driving force for the growing interest toward this technology applied to coronary heart disease [55,56].

Nevertheless, OCT is an extraordinary research tool with multiple applications in coronary heart disease, other than tissue coverage and apposition after stenting [57]. Bifurcations are clearly one of the fields where OCT could contribute the most. In spite of some progress achieved during the past years, bifurcations are still a topic resisting to a scientific quantitative study. Problems such as strut apposition, overlap, non-apposed side-branch (NASB) struts, scaffolding or the access to the side branch, that are still today a pending issue for the investigators, could be efficiently evaluated and quantified by OCT. However, the intrinsic geometric, anatomic and methodologic complexity of bifurcations also represents a challenge that has not been satisfactorily solved yet even by OCT. This chapter illustrates the potential of OCT to shed "light" on the scope of bifurcations.

Bifurcation Stenting, First Edition. Edited by Ron Waksman and John A. Ormiston.
© 2012 Blackwell Publishing Ltd. Published 2012 by Blackwell Publishing Ltd.

Methodological problems in the study of bifurcations

Complex geometry

The first challenge in the study of bifurcations is finding a suitable model for its peculiar geometry. Initially, all the quantitative parameters to assess stenosis severity or the result of an intervention have been conceived for a cylindrical geometry. In these cylindrical models the proximal and distal reference segments will provide directly with the reference parameters required for the quantitative assessment. Thus, for calculation of percentage area stenosis in a cylindrical model, the reference area can be reliably estimated from the average of mean area in the proximal and in the distal lumen areas, for example, and the percentage area stenosis will be hence defined as the quotient between minimal lumen area and the reference area, times 100.

In case of vessel tapering, the above approach is no longer valid, because the reference area (or diameter) will vary depending on the location of the minimal lumen area (or diameter), and hence it is not possible to calculate an average reference area valid for any location along the diseased or stented segment. The challenge of tapering is efficiently solved by means of interpolation, using an iterative regression method.

In bifurcations, neither the cylindrical nor the tapering models are valid. Bifurcations follow a model of fractal geometry [58,59] with morphologic self-similarity. From a physiologic point of view, this geometry is efficient to preserve the hydrodynamic energy in the vascular system [60]. A fractal object is defined by a pattern that is similar at whatever level of observation: this is known as self-similarity or homothetic invariance [61]. There have been several attempts to model the pattern of self-similarity in the coronary arteries [(62], but the most popular ones among cardiologists are Murray's law [60] and Finet's law [59]. Both define the relation in size between the parental vessel or proximal main vessel (PMV) and the two filial ramifications, namely the distal main vessel (DMV) and the side branch (SB), according to their corresponding diameters. In Murray's law the cube of the diameter in the PMV equals the sum of the cubes of the diameters of DMV and SB.

Murray's law: $D_{PMV}^3 = D_{DMV}^3 + D_{SB}^3$

Finet's law is a linearization of Murray's law to simplify the calculations.

Finet's law: $D_{PMV} = 0.678(D_{DMV} + D_{SB})$

According to this geometry, the change in diameter/area between the proximal and the distal segments of a bifurcation is not gradual, like, typically, in vessel tapering, but abrupt at the point of bifurcation. This is known as the step-down phenomenon (Figure 12.1), and must be taken into account for defining valid reference values. As a consequence, neither averaging nor interpolation will calculate valid reference parameters, and the best methodological alternative seems to analyze separately each segment of the bifurcation: PMV, DMV and SB.

As an additional turn of the screw, there is a fourth segment whose geometry is totally irregular and cannot be assimilated by any means to a cylindrical model: the segment around the take-off of the side branch. This segment has received diverse denominations by the different bifurcation- dedicated QCA softwares: "polygon of confluence" or "bifurcation core" [63]. For invasive imaging "bifurcation core" is preferable, because the definition of the polygon of confluence makes sense only for QCA but is conceptually inappropriate for technologies rendering cross-sectional views. In order to overcome the intrinsic geometric complexity of coronary bifurcations, the separate analysis is suggested of four different portions:

1 PMV
2 Bifurcation core
3 DMV
4 SB

Complex anatomy

Beyond the geometric complexity there exist multiple anatomic variations diversifying the problem to the limit and sometimes jeopardizing the required homogeneity in definitions for a systematic approach. Below are some considerations about some of these anatomic issues.

Relevance of the side branch

The relevance of the side branch is important even for the definition of bifurcation itself. The coronary

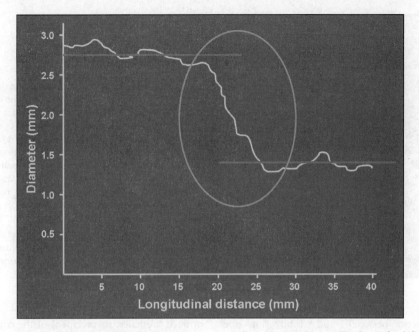

Figure 12.1 Step-down phenomenon. The change in diameter/area between the proximal and the distal segments of a bifurcation is not gradual, like in tapering, but abrupt at the point of bifurcation. This is known as the step-down phenomenon, and is relevant for defining valid reference values for quantitative analysis in bifurcations. Modified from Lansky et al. [95].

tree is rich in ramifications, but not all of them gather the minimal magnitude required to be considered a bifurcation: only those giving a "relevant" side branch are considered as such. However, it is very difficult to define what a "relevant" side branch is. In the past, an objective threshold (>2mm diameter) was proposed, but in practice it proved too rigid and often did not meet other functional considerations. The current consensus is rather flexible, and defines a relevant side branch as a side branch that an operator does not want to loose. This definition implies that the decision about its relevance is fully left to the operator's discretion.

The designation of the filial vessels deserves also some considerations: which is the DMV and which is the SB? There are two possible approaches: the nosological, which follows the anatomic hierarchy (LAD or LCX will be always the main vessel in relation to the diagonals or the OM, respectively), or the QCA approach, which considers DMV the filial branch with the largest diameter. Thus, in a bifurcation LCX-OM such as the one showed in Figure 12.2, the OM could be considered either DMV or SB depending on the adherence to one approach or to the other. The QCA criterion seems to fit better to the usual practice in interventional

cardiology of deploying the stent from the PMV to the vessel of larger calibre, across the vessel of smaller calibre. Nevertheless, a too strict application of this rule could often disregard relevant functional factors. Again, the current consensus leaves the decision of the designation of the filial vessels up to the operator, provided that it is taken upfront, before initiation of the procedure.

Angulation

The angulation determined by the take-off of the SB needs three angles to be properly defined: the angle PMV-SB, the angle DMV-SB and the angle PMV-DMV. Each angle is relevant for specific issues that fall out of the scope of this chapter. In bifurcation-dedicated QCA software, the angulation plays a major role, and in some cases it had led to the definition of "T-bifurcations" and "Y-bifurcations". OCT, however, cannot estimate any of the angles of the bifurcations, and it is uncertain if they could affect significantly the measurements or the quality of the image. The angulation could influence the eccentricity of the guide wire, or the disalignment between the longitudinal axis of the vessel and the OCT imaging catheter, but its overall impact on the OCT analysis seems rather moderate.

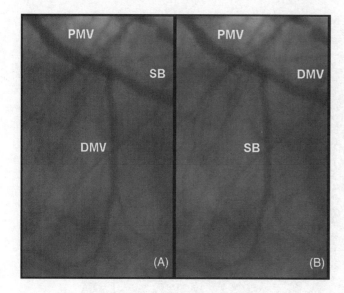

(A) (B)

Figure 12.2 Designation of the filial vessels. Bifurcation LCX-OM, illustrating how the designation of the filial vessels can change depending on the adherence to a nosological; (a) or a QCA criterion (b). In the nosological approach (a) the anatomical hierarchy is strictly followed, and thus the distal LCX is considered the DMV. In the QCA approach (b), conversely, the OM is considered the DMV, because its diameter is larger than that of the distal LCX.

DMV: distal main vessel; LCX: left circumflex; OM: obtuse marginal; PMV: proximal main vessel; QCA: quantitative coronary angiography; SB: side branch.

The distinction between T and Y bifurcations does not seem to make sense for OCT, although T-bifurcations will present in-vivo some methodological advantages that we will address properly later, namely they will improve the reproducibility of the delimitation of the bifurcation core.

Varied atherosclerotic affectation

On top of the geometrical and intrinsic anatomical complexity of non-diseased bifurcations, we must add the multiple ways how atherosclerosis can affect its structure, increasing the complexity of the problem even more. After several classification attempts that demanded memoristic efforts, angiography-based Medina classification [64] has been accepted in consensus [65], with the aim of promoting methodological homogeneity and simplifying the problem as far as possible. Nonetheless, Medina classification is currently receiving a lot of criticism, because its appealing simplicity might eventually not cover a rich spectrum of relevant details, and hence not be predictive of procedural or clinical outcomes.

The role of OCT

OCT analysis pre-stenting

OCT can provide insights of the lesion prior to the intervention, thus being potentially helpful to guide the procedure [66,67]. The severity of the stenosis in both branches, involvement of the ostia or the carina, extension of the plaque, calcification, etc, are important issues that can be accurately studied by OCT, whose assessment could have a relevant impact in planning the procedure, and that are often not correctly visualized by angiography, mainly due to foreshortening of vessels overlap. The operator may need to know the real extent of the atherosclerotic plaque and the size of the reference lumen, in order to choose a stent of the appropriate length and diameter, respectively. Likewise, the extent of the plaque around the carina region [68] or the minimal lumen in the side branch access are relevant parameters to estimate the likelihood of some intra-procedural complications, like the snow-plough phenomenon or the transient occlusion. OCT can provide this information on a direct, clear and quick fashion after a minimal training of the interventional cardiologist, without need for complex interpretation [69]. The pre-intervention OCT study is essentially qualitative, with minimal lumen measurements [70,71], and not as methodologically challenging as the quantitative post-stenting analysis, but still requires a minimum of two pullbacks (in the main vessel and in the side branch) for a systematic and reliable assessment of the above mentioned parameters, that could let the operator tailor the intervention to meet the specific requirements of each single case.

OCT analysis post-stenting

OCT is also useful to estimate the success of our intervention immediately after stenting [72] and at follow-up [73]. An immediate and direct qualitative assessment will allow the evaluation as to whether the stent covers the whole length of the plaque, or if there are remaining areas of uncovered necrotic core at the stent edges. Likewise, the analysis of apposition will confirm if the choice for the stent size was correct [74], and how the device has conformed to the complex geometry of the bifurcation. In techniques where it is attempted to keep a patent access to the side branch, OCT is the best tool to assess the final result in this regard, showing whether the intervention has modified the structure of the bifurcation core or if the patency might be jeopardized by suboptimal scaffolding or by massive plaque displacement, for instance. Finally, OCT is sensitive enough to detect small structural damage of the vessel wall, such as intimal dissections and micro-dissections, which are often seen after stenting, and ballooning at the edges of the stent [75,76]. Nevertheless, it should be emphasized that the presence of these micro-dissections, otherwise unnoticed by angiography, should not be advocated to justify any additional intervention aimed at "optimizing" the result. The evaluation of edge dissections after stenting is a very interesting estimator of the vessel damage, but its clinical meaning has not yet been established.

Minimal methodological requirements

The quantitative analysis of OCT studies is time-consuming, and therefore the issue of optimizing the methodological approach is not trivial. An efficient method should be as simple and fast as possible, but still should not jeopardize the accuracy of OCT measurements. Some generic guidelines are proposed based on experience of bench-testing models. Further efforts in this kind of research are warranted.

Two pullbacks

The OCT study of any bifurcation requires the recording of **two different pullbacks**: one starting in the DMV, and another starting distally in the side branch. Studies recording a single pullback per bifurcation will be limited and cannot provide a comprehensive analysis. In some interventional techniques for bifurcations it is not possible to record two OCT pullbacks: for example, in a provisional stenting-across-SB where final kissing was not necessary, the pullback from the side branch cannot be obtained. This is an important limitation for the comparability of techniques and devices that must be taken into account in the studies involving OCT parameters.

Two landmarks

It is necessary to identify two landmarks in each pullback: the **carina** and the **countercarina**. These landmarks will be used to delineate the take-off of the side branch and further regions of interest. The carina frame is usually clearly identified in both pullbacks as the most distal frame of the pullback where a tissue structure separates completely both branches of the bifurcation, without any point of connection. Somewhat more problematic is the identification of the countercarina. In a precedent study with IVUS, it was proposed to define the countercarina frame as the one where the main vessel "assumed again a circular shape" [77], that is, the most distal frame where the main vessel assumed again a circular shape, proximal to the bifurcation core. Although the definition is conceptually correct, its reproducibility in in-vivo studies is very poor, because the transition between an oval to a circular lumen shape is usually very gradual, and often influenced by many other factors, as for instance the performance of a final kissing-balloon. The systematic use of the longitudinal pullback reconstruction could be helpful and improve the reproducibility. In T-bifurcations, the identification of the countercarina is easier and more reproducible than in Y-bifurcations, because the transition is usually sharper.

4 segments

Once we have identified the carina and countercarina frames in each pullback, we are in disposition to define the four segments of interest (Figure 12.3).

1 Distal main vessel (DMV)
   It is imaged only in the main vessel pullback, and extends from the most distal frame where struts

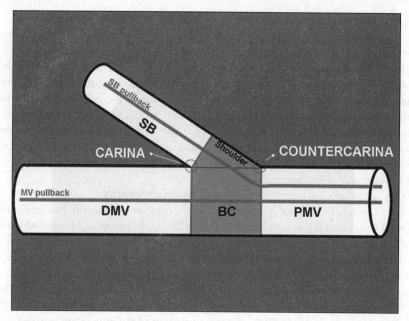

Figure 12.3 The four segments in the OCT study of a bifurcation. DMV: distal main vessel; it is imaged only from the main vessel pullback (MV pullback). SB: Side branch; imaged only from the side branch pullback (SB pullback). PMV: Proximal Main Vessel; imaged both from the MV and SB pullbacks, but analyzed only in the MV pullback. BC: Bifurcation core; one part is imaged in the MV pullback, and another part (the shoulder of the bifurcation) is imaged in the SB pullback. BC starts and ends in each pullback in the carina and countercarina frames, respectively.

are identified in a 360° circular shape till the carina frame.

2 Side branch (SB)

It is imaged only in the side branch pullback. In case the side branch has been stented, it will extend from the most distal frame where struts can be identified in a 360° circular shape up to the carina frame. In case the side branch has not been stented, it will extend from the most distal frame where any strut can be identified up to the carina frame.

o Proximal main vessel (PMV)

It is imaged both in the main vessel and the side branch pullbacks, and extends from the countercarina frame up to the most proximal frame where struts are identified in a 360° circular shape. Until the issues of how much wire eccentricity and vessel-catheter axial disalignment are further clarified, it is advised to consider only the measurements of the main vessel pullback, where these potential confounding factors are expected to be lower than in the side branch pullback.

o Bifurcation core (BC)

It is imaged partially in the main vessel pullback and partially in the side branch pullback. In both pullbacks it extends from the carina frame up to the contercarina frame. In order to avoid duplicity of measurements, it is advised to restrict the analysis to the branch where the optic catheter is placed in each case, disregarding the other branch and interpolating the lumen/stent contours whenever possible (Figure 12.4). If this method is followed, the BC in the main vessel pullback will represent the portion of MV where the take-off of the SB takes place; whilst the BC in the side branch pullback represents the shoulder of the bifurcation, which is a region of high interest, half way between the main vessel and the side branch, hot spot for malapposition and whose scaffolding or the lack of it is believed to be relevant for the outcome of the intervention [78,79].

3 Parameters of interest

The cornerstone of the OCT study of a bifurcation is defining the parameters of potential

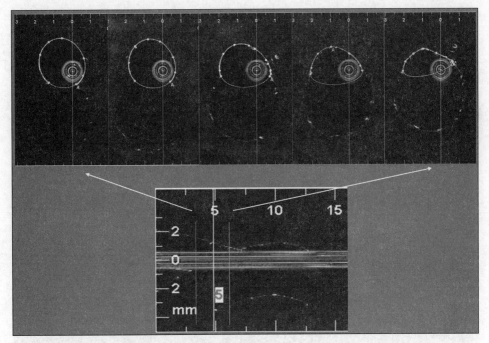

Figure 12.4 Interpolation of the lumen contours at the side branch pullback in the analysis of a silicon phantom.

interest that can be assessed. Below is a list of them, although their clinical relevance has not been properly tested yet in most of the cases.

a Apposition of the struts.

b Existence of overlap segments or regions with multiple layers of stent.

c Non-apposed side-branch (NASB) struts: struts suspended in the middle of the blood flow, without apparent connection with the rest of the stent structure and with no clear relation to the vessel walls.

d Scaffolding of the carina and the shoulder.

e Access to the side branch.

f Tissue coverage of the struts.

4 Location

Apposition, overlap and coverage are maybe the parameters where additional topographic specifications would be most interesting. The first obvious step is reporting the results per segment, but also some indications about the distribution within the cross-section would be very interesting, although methodologically challenging [80].

5 Defining the most efficient longitudinal interval between cross-sections for the analysis

In a conventional OCT analysis, stented segment cross-sections are analyzed at 1 mm longitudinal intervals. In bifurcations, however, this distance could be too large for the detection of subtle parameters, like the NASB, or the scaffolding. Little protrusions of struts into the lumen or small gaps in the scaffolding will be often of lower magnitude, thus the sensitivity of a method at 1mm intervals is not likely to be high. It seems principally reasonable to make an analysis at shorter intervals [81,82], at least in the bifurcation core, however, the most efficient analysis interval has not been established yet.

Apposition

Incomplete stent apposition (ISA) is associated with worse outcomes after stenting [5,6]. Although the mechanism explaining this association is still not clear, ISA struts could represent a handicap per se for a proper neointimal healing [83]. Bifurcations are particularly sensitive to malapposition, because stenting techniques using conventional cylindrical stents or bifurcation-dedicated devices

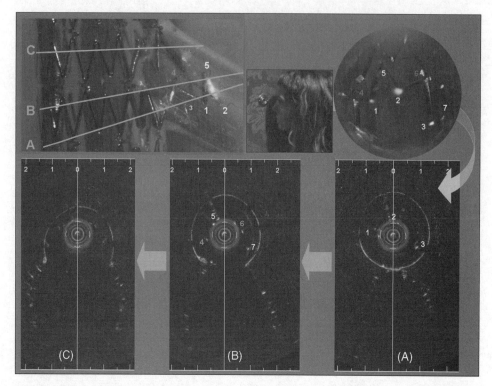

Figure 12.5 Malapposition at the shoulder of the bifurcation: micro-photography and OCT view in the bench-testing with silicon phantoms. Preclinical bench-testing of bifurcation-dedicated prototypes of stent. In the case illustrated, the prototype could not conform to the geometry of the bifurcation. To ease the understanding of the correspondence between the different images, the most distal struts in the side branch have been numbered. Struts with a connector appear in red: the connector can be preserved (6) or dislodged (4). The use of OCT during the bench testing permits a precise quantification and detection of subtle degrees of malapposition that are often unadverted by the micro-photography.

cannot always conform to their peculiar geometry and anatomy (Figure 12.5). Moreover, sequential balloon inflations or kissing-balloon techniques may distort the stent structure and induce some degree of malapposition [84].

OCT can assess ISA accurately. Since the light cannot penetrate the metallic structure of the stent, it is necessary to measure the distance from the leading edge of the strut reflection to the lumen contour. If this distance is higher than the strut thickness, then the strut is malapposed [85]. Therefore, precise knowledge of the type of stent implanted and the thickness of its struts is mandatory. The apposition will be quantified as a proportion of malapposed struts with respect to the total number of analyzed struts, or as ISA areas and volumes. In bifurcations it can be also inter-esting to report the localization of the ISA struts, because this information might help to improve the techniques or the devices. Some techniques or devices present typical ISA patterns at specific segments (Figure 12.6).

Strut overlap segments and multilayer segments

There is increasing evidence that strut overlap is associated with worse clinical and angiographic outcomes [86,87]. Most two-stent techniques in bifurcations entail some degree of overlap between the different stents implanted in order to avoid areas of incomplete scaffolding that are believed to be associated with worse outcomes [78,79]. In some cases, like the culotte or the crush techniques, there

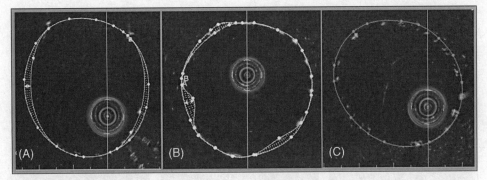

Figure 12.6 Typical malapposition patterns in the proximal main vessel (PMV) segment of some bifurcation dedicated stents: bench-testing with silicon phantoms.

Nile-Croco (Minvasys©) (a) is a modular stent whose deployment ends with simultaneous kissing-balloon inflation. Notice the typical oval pattern of the malapposition in the PMV, due to the 8-shaped disposition of the balloons. Tryton (Tryton Medical©) (b) is a side-branch stent, with a specifically-designed transition zone between the side branch and the main vessel, prolonged into the PMV through a minimal scaffold consisting of 3 legs. Notice how the presence of these 3 legs induces some degree of malapposition in the regions of overlap with the stent in the main vessel. Stentys (Stentys©) (c) is a self-expandable stent, with minimal malapposition in the main vessel.

will be regions where a double or even triple layer of stent has been implanted (Figure 12.7). OCT is able to visualize clearly these regions of multiple stent layers with the individual struts. The extension of these areas should be reported, and a methodical analysis should be performed.

NASB (non-apposed side-branch struts)

The struts corresponding to the portion of a stent across a side-branch deserve a separate category. Here they are designated as non-apposed side-branch (NASB) struts; but they have also been dubbed "floating" struts in the literature. They appear as "suspended" struts in the middle of the side branch ostium, with no apparent connection with the rest of the stent structure, and with no vessel wall behind in cross-sectional OCT images (Figure 12.8). Commonly these struts are reported as ISA struts, but it is not completely correct, because apposition was never pursued by the operator and cannot be assessed due to anatomical reasons. Their clinical implications might be also be different than for ISA struts: whilst ISA has been consistently associated with worse outcomes in intravascular ultrasound studies [5,6], the implications of NASB are still a matter of debate. Initial pathological studies suggested a higher risk of incomplete neointimal healing and stent thrombosis [9,88]; however, a recent randomized trial comparing stenting-across versus other bifurcation techniques or versus systematic kissing-balloon, did not confirm clinical disadvantage of the technique producing NASB [89,90].

In the stenting techniques that can be studied by OCT, small protrusions of struts at the level of the carina are frequently found: the NASB struts. Usually they will be visualized from both the main vessel and the side branch pullbacks, at the bifurcation core segment. Nonetheless, it is recommended that they are counted and measured only in the main vessel pullback, where they are best observed [91], in order to avoid duplication of measurements. As a result of the high spatial resolution of OCT, several NASB struts will be detected in non-bifurcation segments, due to the take-off of tiny side branches. They must be categorized as NASB, despite the fact of not being at the bifurcation under study.

Scaffolding of the carina and the shoulder

Incomplete scaffolding has been advocated to explain the worse results of stenting in bifurcations

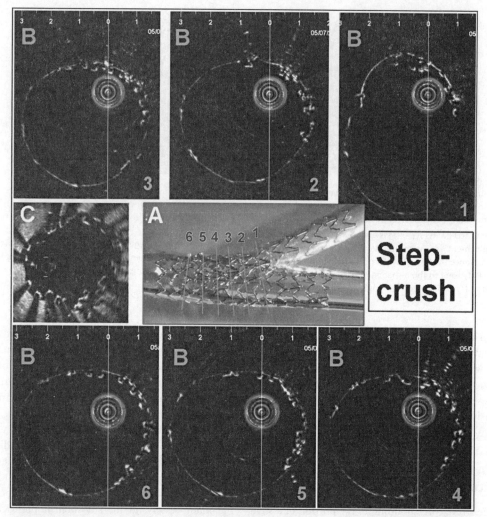

Figure 12.7

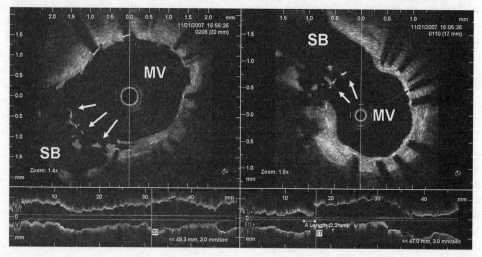

Figure 12.8

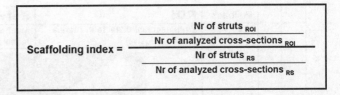

$$\text{Scaffolding index} = \dfrac{\dfrac{\text{Nr of struts}_{ROI}}{\text{Nr of analyzed cross-sections}_{ROI}}}{\dfrac{\text{Nr of struts}_{RS}}{\text{Nr of analyzed cross-sections}_{RS}}}$$

Figure 12.9

compared with straight vessels [78,79]. Assessing the scaffolding by OCT, despite its apparent simplicity, is complex. A systematic approach should include the assessment of scaffolding at three different levels:

1 Carina
   a Main vessel surface   Main vessel pullback
   b Side-branch surface   Side-branch pullback
2 Shoulder   Side-branch pullback

According to preliminary experience on bench-testing models, a scaffolding index is proposed. Averaging the number of struts per cross-section in the shoulder and in the region 2 mm distal to the carina frame could be a good estimator. By dividing this number by the average number of struts per cross-section in a 2 mm reference segment, it would result in a *scaffolding index* for each region (Figure 12.9). The corresponding reference segments for each region must be defined depending on the stenting technique, being in general 2 mm of a monolayer segment outside the bifurcation core (Figure 12.10).

Notice that the scaffolding index of the shoulder is based on the analysis of a narrower sector and therefore will score systematically lower than the carina indexes. Thus, it cannot be used for comparing the scaffolding of the shoulder versus that of the carina in a same bifurcation, but it is valid for comparison of the shoulder scaffolding between different patients or different devices.

Access to the side branch

Although there is no evidence to support this practice, preserving the access to the side branch is actively pursued by many operators in many procedures, particularly if the bifurcation involves vessels of large calibre, such as the left main-LAD-LCX. There are many clinical arguments that may

be advocated for this preference. Many bifurcation-dedicated devices concede importance to keeping a good access to the side branch, as well.

Conceptually, OCT analysis could define the access to the side branch as the smallest metal-free area that the blood traverses on its way to the SB (Figure 12.11). In practice, however, the variations in the take-off angle of the SB, or the different location of this minimal metal-free area depending on the technique and the devices employed (Figure 12.12) can make the assessment of SB access complex. Based on preliminary experiences on phantoms, we seem to have found a solid estimator, whose definition will change depending on the moment of assessment (acutely post-implantation versus follow-up) and on the stenting of the SB with a second stent (Figure 12.13). In all the cases, it will be defined in the side branch pull-back. This way, methodological problems due to SB take-off angle or to location variants can be overcome. The proposed definitions would not be valid for provisional stenting without final kissing, where the minimal metal-free area would be located in the main vessel (stent cells), but this technique is currently not suitable for OCT assessment, because the OCT catheter cannot be placed in the SB.

Coverage

The accuracy of OCT for the assessment of tissue coverage after stenting has been solidly addressed in the literature. OCT is currently the only technology able to assess in vivo the tissue coverage after stenting, due to its high axial resolution (14 μm). The OCT-derived tissue coverage seems to be a good surrogate for histological neointimal healing, according to several animal studies [51–53]. This gives OCT a paramount role in the evaluation of intracoronary devices, since delayed neointimal healing has been

		Pullback	**ROI**	**Reference segment**
carina	MV face	**MV**	2mm segment distal to the carina frame (inclusive)	Most proximal 2mm segment of a stented monolayer, distal to the ROI
	SB face *	**SB**	2mm segment distal to the carina frame (inclusive)	Most proximal 2mm segment of a stented monolayer, distal to the ROI
Shoulder		**SB**	Segment between the carina frame and the countercarina frame.	Most distal 2mm segment of a stented monolayer, proximal to the ROI

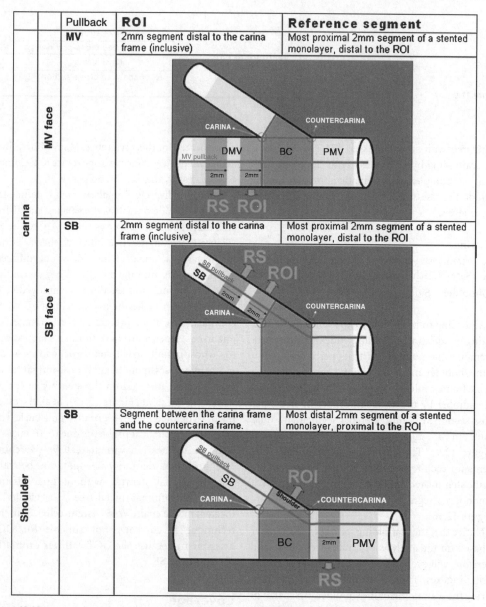

Figure 12.10

associated with stent thrombosis in several pathological studies [8,9]. Coverage can be assessed by OCT through different parameters, such as the proportion of non-covered struts, the mean thickness or the coverage areas/volumes [92]. In bifurcations, coverage can be repoted topographically considering the four segments separately. ISA areas and NASB struts deserve especial attention [83].

Advantages of fourier-domain versus time-domain OCT

Bifurcations are one of the fields where Fourier-domain OCT (FD OCT) systems are clearly preferable to time-domain systems, since the quality of the images is sensibly superior. The reason for this is that bifurcations often have relatively large diameters at the bifurcation core. Time domain OCT

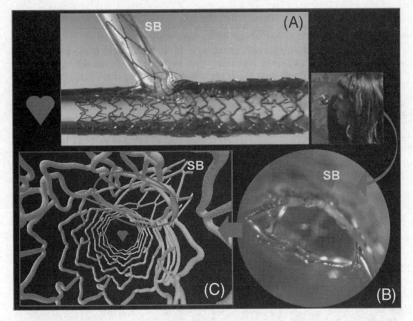

Figure 12.11

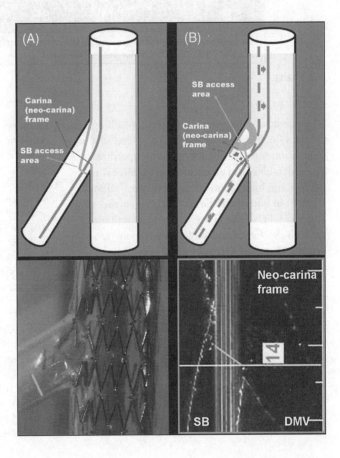

Figure 12.12

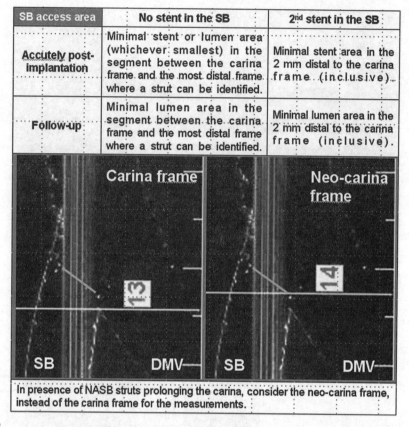

SB access area	No stent in the SB	2nd stent in the SB
Accutely post-implantation	Minimal stent or lumen area (whichever smallest) in the segment between the carina frame and the most distal frame where a strut can be identified.	Minimal stent area in the 2 mm distal to the carina frame (inclusive).
Follow-up	Minimal lumen area in the segment between the carina frame and the most distal frame where a strut can be identified.	Minimal lumen area in the 2 mm distal to the carina frame (inclusive).

In presence of NASB struts prolonging the carina, consider the neo-carina frame, instead of the carina frame for the measurements.

Figure 12.13

is hampered by poor penetration depth, resulting in frequent "out of view" artifacts at the level of the bifurcation core [93]. This limitation jeopardizes to a considerable extent the accuracy of the OCT study, because the bifurcation core is the most relevant segment in both pullbacks, as has been extensively addressed. FD OCT can overcome these limitations as it allows for considerably greater penetration depth and stable OCT catheter position, minimizing the "out of view" problem, and warranting a more accurate quantitative analysis [94].

References

1 Gonzalo N, Garcia-Garcia HM, Serruys PW, Commissaris KH, Bezerra H, Gobbens P, et al. Reproducibility of quantitative optical coherence tomography for stent analysis. EuroIntervention 2009 Jun; 5(2):224–32.

2 Barlis P, van SG, Serruys PW, Regar E. Intracoronary optical coherence tomography and the evaluation of stents. Expert Rev Med Devices 2009 Mar; 6(2):157–67.

3 Tanimoto S, Aoki J, Serruys PW, Regar E. Paclitaxel-eluting stent restenosis shows three-layer appearance by optical coherence tomography. EuroIntervention 2006 Feb; 1 (4):484.

4 Regar E, Schaar J, Serruys PW. Images in cardiology. Acute recoil in sirolimus eluting stent: real time, in vivo assessment with optical coherence tomography. Heart 2006 Jan; 92(1):123.

5 Cook S, Wenaweser P, Togni M, Billinger M, Morger C, Seiler C, et al. Incomplete Stent Apposition and Very Late Stent Thrombosis After Drug-Eluting Stent Implantation. Circulation 2007 May 8; 115(18): 2426–34.

6 Hassan AK, Bergheanu SC, Stijnen T, van der Hoeven BL, Snoep JD, Plevier JW, et al. Late stent malapposition risk is higher after drug-eluting stent compared with bare-metal stent implantation and associates with late stent thrombosis. Eur Heart J 2009 Jan 21.

7 Farb A, Heller PF, Shroff S, Cheng L, Kolodgie FD, Carter AJ, et al. Pathological analysis of local delivery of paclitaxel via a polymer-coated stent. Circulation 2001 Jul 24; 104(4):473–9.

8 Finn AV, Joner M, Nakazawa G, Kolodgie F, Newell J, John MC, *et al.* Pathological correlates of late drug-eluting stent thrombosis: Strut coverage as a marker of endothelialization. Circulation 2007 May 8; 115(18): 2435–41.

9 Farb AM, Burke APM, Kolodgie FDP, Virmani RM. Pathological mechanisms of fatal late coronary stent thrombosis in humans. Circulation 2003 Oct 7; 108(14): 1701–6.

10 Farb AM, Sangiorgi GM, Carter AJD, Walley VMM, Edwards WDM, Schwartz RSM, *et al.* Pathology of acute and chronic coronary stenting in humans. Circulation 1999 Jan 5; 99(1):44–52.

11 Kastrati A, Mehilli J, Dirschinger J, Pache J, Ulm K, Schuhlen H, *et al.* Restenosis after coronary placement of various stent types. Am J Cardiol 2001 Jan 1; 87(1): 34–9.

12 Liu MW, Roubin GS, King SB, III., Restenosis after coronary angioplasty. Potential biologic determinants and role of intimal hyperplasia. Circulation 1989 Jun 1; 79(6):1374–87.

13 Essed CE, van den BM, Becker AE. Transluminal coronary angioplasty and early restenosis. Fibrocellular occlusion after wall laceration. Br Heart J 1983 Apr; 49(4):393–6.

14 Giraldo AA, Esposo OM, Meis JM. Intimal hyperplasia as a cause of restenosis after percutaneous transluminal coronary angioplasty. Arch Pathol Lab Med 1985 Feb; 109(2):173–5.

15 Austin GE, Ratliff NB, Hollman J, Tabei S, Phillips DF. Intimal proliferation of smooth muscle cells as an explanation for recurrent coronary artery stenosis after percutaneous transluminal coronary angioplasty. J Am Coll Cardiol 1985 Aug; 6(2):369–75.

16 Bjorkerud S, Bondjers G. Arterial repair and atherosclerosis after mechanical injury. 5. Tissue response after induction of a large superficial transverse injury. Atherosclerosis 1973 Sep; 18(2):235–55.

17 Clowes AW, Clowes MM, Reidy MA. Kinetics of cellular proliferation after arterial injury. III. Endothelial and smooth muscle growth in chronically denuded vessels. Lab Invest 1986 Mar; 54(3):295–303.

18 Clowes AW, Schwartz SM. Significance of quiescent smooth muscle migration in the injured rat carotid artery. Circ Res 1985 Jan; 56(1):139–45.

19 Clowes AW, Reidy MA, Clowes MM. Mechanisms of stenosis after arterial injury. Lab Invest 1983 Aug; 49(2): 208–15.

20 Baim DS, Cutlip DE, O'Shaughnessy CD, Hermiller JB, Kereiakes DJ, Giambartolomei A, *et al.* Final results of a randomized trial comparing the NIR stent to the Palmaz-Schatz stent for narrowings in native coronary arteries. Am J Cardiol 2001 Jan 15; 87(2):152–6.

21 Serruys PW, de JP, Kiemeneij F, Macaya C, Rutsch W, Heyndrickx G, *et al.* A comparison of balloon-expandable-stent implantation with balloon angioplasty in patients with coronary artery disease. Benestent Study Group. N Engl J Med 1994 Aug 25; 331(8):489–95.

22 Serruys PW, van HB, Bonnier H, Legrand V, Garcia E, Macaya C, *et al.* Randomised comparison of implantation of heparin-coated stents with balloon angioplasty in selected patients with coronary artery disease (Benestent II). Lancet 1998 Aug 29; 352(9129):673–81.

23 Lansky AJ, Roubin GS, O'Shaughnessy CD, Moore PB, Dean LS, Raizner AE, *et al.* Randomized comparison of GR-II stent and Palmaz-Schatz stent for elective treatment of coronary stenoses. Circulation 2000 Sep 19; 102 (12):1364–8.

24 Schofer J, Schluter M, Gershlick AH, Wijns W, Garcia E, Schampaert E, *et al.* Sirolimus-eluting stents for treatment of patients with long atherosclerotic lesions in small coronary arteries: double-blind, randomised controlled trial (E-SIRIUS). Lancet 2003 Oct 4; 362 (9390):1093–9.

25 Kastrati A, Schomig A, Dirschinger J, Mehilli J, Dotzer F, von WN, *et al.* A randomized trial comparing stenting with balloon angioplasty in small vessels in patients with symptomatic coronary artery disease. ISAR-SMART Study Investigators. Intracoronary stenting or angioplasty for restenosis reduction in small arteries. Circulation 2000 Nov 21; 102(21):2593–8.

26 Park SW, Lee CW, Hong MK, Kim JJ, Cho GY, Nah DY, *et al.* Randomized comparison of coronary stenting with optimal balloon angioplasty for treatment of lesions in small coronary arteries. Eur Heart J 2000 Nov; 21(21): 1785–9.

27 Koning R, Eltchaninoff H, Commeau P, Khalife K, Gilard M, Lipiecki J, *et al.* Stent placement compared with balloon angioplasty for small coronary arteries: in-hospital and 6-month clinical and angiographic results. Circulation 2001 Oct 2; 104(14):1604–8.

28 Doucet S, Schalij MJ, Vrolix MC, Hilton D, Chenu P, de BB, *et al.* Stent placement to prevent restenosis after angioplasty in small coronary arteries. Circulation 2001 Oct 23; 104(17):2029–33.

29 Moer R, Myreng Y, Molstad P, Albertsson P, Gunnes P, Lindvall B, *et al.* Stenting in small coronary arteries (SISCA) trial. A randomized comparison between balloon angioplasty and the heparin-coated beStent. J Am Coll Cardiol 2001 Nov 15; 38(6):1598–603.

30 Morice MC, Serruys PW, Sousa JE, Fajadet J, Ban HE, Perin M, *et al.* A randomized comparison of a sirolimus-eluting stent with a standard stent for coronary revascularization. N Engl J Med 2002 Jun 6; 346(23):1773–80.

31 Fischman DL, Leon MB, Baim DS, Schatz RA, Savage MP, Penn I, *et al.* A randomized comparison of

coronary-stent placement and balloon angioplasty in the treatment of coronary artery disease. Stent Restenosis Study Investigators. N Engl J Med 1994 Aug 25; 331(8): 496–501.

32 Kereiakes DJ, Cox DA, Hermiller JB, Midei MG, Bachinsky WB, Nukta ED, et al. Usefulness of a cobalt chromium coronary stent alloy. Am J Cardiol 2003 Aug 15; 92(4):463–6.

33 Kastrati A, Mehilli J, Dirschinger J, Dotzer F, Schuhlen H, Neumann FJ, et al. Intracoronary stenting and angiographic results: strut thickness effect on restenosis outcome (ISAR-STEREO) trial. Circulation 2001 Jun 12; 103(23):2816–21.

34 Grube E, Sonoda S, Ikeno F, Honda Y, Kar S, Chan C, et al. Six- and twelve-month results from first human experience using everolimus-eluting stents with bioabsorbable polymer. Circulation 2004 May 11; 109(18):2168–71.

35 Gershlick A, De S, I, Chevalier B, Stephens-Lloyd A, Camenzind E, Vrints C, et al. Inhibition of restenosis with a paclitaxel-eluting, polymer-free coronary stent: the European evaLUation of pacliTaxel Eluting Stent (ELUTES) trial. Circulation 2004 Feb 3; 109(4):487–93.

36 Schampaert E, Cohen EA, Schluter M, Reeves F, Traboulsi M, Title LM, et al. The Canadian study of the sirolimus-eluting stent in the treatment of patients with long de novo lesions in small native coronary arteries (C-SIRIUS). J Am Coll Cardiol 2004 Mar 17; 43(6):1110–5.

37 Lansky AJ, Costa RA, Mintz GS, Tsuchiya Y, Midei M, Cox DA, et al. Non-polymer-based paclitaxel-coated coronary stents for the treatment of patients with de novo coronary lesions: angiographic follow-up of the DELIVER clinical trial. Circulation 2004 Apr 27; 109 (16):1948–54.

38 Serruys PW, Degertekin M, Tanabe K, Abizaid A, Sousa JE, Colombo A, et al. Intravascular ultrasound findings in the multicenter, randomized, double-blind RAVEL (RAndomized study with the sirolimus-eluting VElocity balloon-expandable stent in the treatment of patients with de novo native coronary artery Lesions) trial. Circulation 2002 Aug 13; 106(7):798–803.

39 Degertekin M, Serruys PW, Foley DP, Tanabe K, Regar E, Vos J, et al. Persistent inhibition of neointimal hyperplasia after sirolimus-eluting stent implantation: long-term (up to 2 years) clinical, angiographic, and intravascular ultrasound follow-up. Circulation 2002 Sep 24; 106(13): 1610–3.

40 Park SJ, Shim WH, Ho DS, Raizner AE, Park SW, Hong MK, et al. A paclitaxel-eluting stent for the prevention of coronary restenosis. N Engl J Med 2003 Apr 17; 348(16):1537–45.

41 Sonoda S, Morino Y, Ako J, Terashima M, Hassan AH, Bonneau HN, et al. Impact of final stent dimensions on

long-term results following sirolimus-eluting stent implantation: serial intravascular ultrasound analysis from the sirius trial. J Am Coll Cardiol 2004 Jun 2; 43(11): 1959–63.

42 Morice MC, Serruys PW, Sousa JE, Fajadet J, Ban Hayashi E, Perin M, et al. A randomized comparison of a sirolimus-eluting stent with a standard stent for coronary revascularization. N Engl J Med 2002 Jun 6; 346(23):1773–80.

43 Moses JW, Leon MB, Popma JJ, Fitzgerald PJ, Holmes DR, O'Shaughnessy C, et al. Sirolimus-Eluting Stents versus Standard Stents in Patients with Stenosis in a Native Coronary Artery. N Engl J Med 2003 Oct 2; 349 (14):1315–23.

44 Stone GW, Ellis SG, Cox DA, Hermiller J, O'Shaughnessy C, Mann JT, et al. A polymer-based, paclitaxel-eluting stent in patients with coronary artery disease. N Engl J Med 2004 Jan 15; 350(3):221–31.

45 Iakovou I, Schmidt T, Bonizzoni E, Ge L, Sangiorgi GM, Stankovic G, et al. Incidence, predictors, and outcome of thrombosis after successful implantation of drug-eluting stents. JAMA 2005 May 4; 293(17):2126–30.

46 Ong AT, McFadden EP, Regar E, de Jaegere PP, van Domburg RT, Serruys PW. Late angiographic stent thrombosis (LAST) events with drug-eluting stents. J Am Coll Cardiol 2005 Jun 21; 45(12):2088–92.

47 Pfisterer M, Brunner-La Rocca HP, Buser PT, Rickenbacher P, Hunziker P, Mueller C, et al. Late clinical events after clopidogrel discontinuation may limit the benefit of drug-eluting stents: an observational study of drug-eluting versus bare-metal stents. J Am Coll Cardiol 2006 Dec 19; 48(12):2584–91.

48 Nordmann AJ, Briel M, Bucher HC. Mortality in randomized controlled trials comparing drug-eluting vs. bare metal stents in coronary artery disease: a meta-analysis. Eur Heart J 2006 Dec; 27(23):2784–814.

49 Lagerqvist B, James SK, Stenestrand U, Lindback J, Nilsson T, Wallentin L, et al. Long-term outcomes with drug-eluting stents versus bare-metal stents in Sweden. N Engl J Med 2007 Mar 8; 356(10):1009–19.

50 Regar E, Lemos PA, Saia F, Degertekin M, Tanabe K, Lee CH, et al. Incidence of thrombotic stent occlusion during the first three months after sirolimus-eluting stent implantation in 500 consecutive patients. Am J Cardiol 2004 May 15; 93(10):1271–5.

51 Suzuki Y, Ikeno F, Koizumi T, Tio F, Yeung AC, Yock PG, et al. In vivo comparison between optical coherence tomography and intravascular ultrasound for detecting small degrees of in-stent neointima after stent implantation. JACC Cardiovasc Interv 2008 Apr; 1 (2):168–73.

52 Deuse T, Erben RG, Ikeno F, Behnisch B, Boeger R, Connolly AJ, et al. Introducing the first polymer-free

leflunomide eluting stent. Atherosclerosis 2008 Sep; 200 (1):126–34.

53 Prati F, Zimarino M, Stabile E, Pizzicannella G, Fouad T, Rabozzi R, *et al*. Does optical coherence tomography identify arterial healing after stenting? An in vivo comparison with histology, in a rabbit carotid model. Heart 2008 Feb 1; 94(2):217–21.

54 Capodanno D, Prati F, Pawlowsky T, Cera M, La MA, Albertucci M, *et al*. Comparison of optical coherence tomography and intravascular ultrasound for the assessment of in-stent tissue coverage after stent implantation. EuroIntervention 2009 Nov; 5(5):538–43.

55 Schinkel AF, Barlis P, van Beusekom HM, Serruys PW, Regar E. Images in intervention. Optical coherence tomography findings in very late (4 years) paclitaxel-eluting stent thrombosis. JACC Cardiovasc Interv 2008 Aug; 1 (4):449–51.

56 Regar E, van Beusekom HM, van der Giessen WJ, Serruys PW. Images in cardiovascular medicine. Optical coherence tomography findings at 5-year follow-up after coronary stent implantation. Circulation 2005 Dec 6; 112 (23):e345–e346.

57 Regar E, van Leeuwen A, Serruys PJ. Optical coherence tomography in cardiovascular research. Informa Healthcare, London: 2007, ISBN 1 84184 611 2.

58 Zhou Y, Kassab GS, Molloi S. On the design of the coronary arterial tree: a generalization of Murray's law. Phys Med Biol 1999 Dec; 44(12):2929–45.

59 Finet G, Gilard M, Perrenot B, Rioufol G, Motreff P, Gavit L, *et al*. Fractal geometry of arterial coronary bifurcations: a quantitative coronary angiography and intravascular ultrasound analysis. EuroIntervention 2007; 3:490–8.

60 Murray CD. The physiological principle of minimum work: I. The vascular system and the cost of blood volume. Proc Natl Acad Sci USA 1926 Mar; 12(3): 207–14.

61 Bassingthwaighte JB, Van Beek JH, King RB. Fractal branchings: the basis of myocardial flow heterogeneities? Ann NY Acad Sci 1990; 591: 392–401.

62 Zamir M, Chee H. Branching characteristics of human coronary arteries. Can J Physiol Pharmacol 1986 Jun; 64 (6):661–8.

63 Ramcharitar S, Onuma Y, Aben JP, Consten C, Weijers B, Morel MA, *et al*. A novel dedicated quantitative coronary analysis methodology for bifurcation lesions. EuroIntervention 2008 Mar; 3(5):553–7.

64 Medina A, Suarez de LJ, Pan M. A new classification of coronary bifurcation lesions. Rev Esp Cardiol 2006 Feb; 59(2):183.

65 Louvard Y, Thomas M, Dzavik V, Hildick-Smith D, Galassi AR, Pan M, *et al*. Classification of coronary artery bifurcation lesions and treatments: time for a consensus! Catheter Cardiovasc Interv 2008 Feb 1; 71(2):175–83.

66 Okamura T, Gutiérrez-Chico J, van Soest G, Regar E. Clinical applications of optical coherence tomography. Cardiology International. In press.

67 Barlis P, Serruys PW, Devries A, Regar E. Optical coherence tomography assessment of vulnerable plaque rupture: predilection for the plaque 'shoulder'. Eur Heart J 2008 Aug; 29(16):2023.

68 Gonzalo N, Garcia-Garcia HM, Regar E, Barlis P, Wentzel J, Onuma Y, *et al*. In vivo assessment of high-risk coronary plaques at bifurcations with combined intravascular ultrasound and optical coherence tomography. JACC Cardiovasc Imaging 2009 Apr; 2(4):473–82.

69 van SG, Goderie TP, Gonzalo N, Koljenovic S, van Leenders GL, Regar E, *et al*. Imaging atherosclerotic plaque composition with intracoronary optical coherence tomography. Neth Heart J 2009 Nov; 17(11): 448–50.

70 Barlis P, Serruys PW, Gonzalo N, van der Giessen WJ, de Jaegere PJ, Regar E. Assessment of culprit and remote coronary narrowings using optical coherence tomography with long-term outcomes. Am J Cardiol 2008 Aug 15; 102(4):391–5.

71 Barlis P, Di MC, van BH, Gonzalo N, Regar E. Novelties in cardiac imaging--optical coherence tomography (OCT). EuroIntervention 2008 Aug; 4 Suppl C:C22–C26.

72 Okamura T, Serruys PW, Regar E. Three-dimensional visualization of intracoronary thrombus during stent implantation using the second generation, Fourier domain optical coherence tomography. Eur Heart J 2010 Mar; 31(5):625.

73 Gonzalo N, Serruys PW, Okamura T, van Beusekom HM, Garcia-Garcia HM, van SG, *et al*. Optical coherence tomography patterns of stent restenosis. Am Heart J 2009 Aug; 158(2):284–93.

74 Gonzalo N, Barlis P, Serruys PW, Garcia-Garcia HM, Onuma Y, Ligthart J, *et al*. Incomplete stent apposition and delayed tissue coverage are more frequent in drug-eluting stents implanted during primary percutaneous coronary intervention for ST-segment elevation myocardial infarction than in drug-eluting stents implanted for stable/unstable angina: insights from optical coherence tomography. JACC Cardiovasc Interv 2009 May; 2(5): 445–52.

75 Gonzalo N, Serruys PW, Okamura T, Shen ZJ, Onuma Y, Garcia-Garcia HM, *et al*. Optical coherence tomography assessment of the acute effects of stent implantation on the vessel wall: a systematic quantitative approach. Heart 2009 Dec; 95(23):1913–9.

76 Gonzalo N, Serruys PW, Okamura T, Shen ZJ, Garcia-Garcia HM, Onuma Y, *et al*. Relation between plaque type and dissections at the edges after stent

implantation: An optical coherence tomography study. Int J Cardiol 2010 May 11.

77 van der Waal EC, Mintz GS, Garcia-Garcia HM, Bui AB, Pehlivanova M, Girasis C, *et al.* Intravascular ultrasound and 3D angle measurements of coronary bifurcations. Catheter Cardiovasc Interv 2009 Jun 1; 73(7):910–6.

78 Colombo A, Moses JW, Morice MC, Ludwig J, Holmes DR, Jr., Spanos V, *et al.* Randomized study to evaluate sirolimus-eluting stents implanted at coronary bifurcation lesions. Circulation 2004 Mar 16; 109(10):1244–9.

79 Pan M, de Lezo JS, Medina A, Romero M, Segura J, Pavlovic D, *et al.* Rapamycin-eluting stents for the treatment of bifurcated coronary lesions: a randomized comparison of a simple versus complex strategy. Am Heart J 2004 Nov; 148(5):857–64.

80 Okamura T, Garg S, Gutiérrez-Chico J, Shin E, Onuma Y, Garcia-Garcia HM, *et al.* In-vivo evaluation of stent strut distribution patterns in the bioabsorbable everolimus-eluting device: An OCT a*d hoc* analysis of the Revision 1.0 and Revision 1.1 stent design in the ABSORB clinical trial. EuroIntervention. 2010 Apr; 5(8):932–8.

81 Sihan K, Botha C, Post F, de WS, Gonzalo N, Regar E, *et al.* Fully automatic three-dimensional quantitative analysis of intracoronary optical coherence tomography: method and Validation. Catheter Cardiovasc Interv 2009 Dec 1; 74(7):1058–65.

82 Tanimoto S, Rodriguez-Granillo G, Barlis P, de WS, Bruining N, Hamers R, *et al.* A novel approach for quantitative analysis of intracoronary optical coherence tomography: high inter-observer agreement with computer-assisted contour detection. Catheter Cardiovasc Interv 2008 Aug 1; 72(2):228–35.

83 Gutiérrez-Chico JL, Regar E, Nüesch E, Okamura T, Wykrzykowska JJ, di Mario C, Windecker S, van Es GA, Gobbens P, Jüni P, Serruys PW. Delayed coverage in malapposed and side-branch struts with respect to well-apposed struts in drug-eluting stents: in vivo-assessment with optical coherence tomography. Circulation 2011; (In press).

84 Ormiston JA, Webster MW, El JS, Ruygrok PN, Stewart JT, Scott D, *et al.* Drug-eluting stents for coronary bifurcations: bench testing of provisional side-branch strategies. Catheter Cardiovasc Interv 2006 Jan; 67(1):49–55.

85 Tanigawa J, Barlis P, Di MC. Intravascular optical coherence tomography: optimisation of image acquisition and quantitative assessment of stent strut apposition. EuroIntervention 2007 May; 3(1):128–36.

86 Finn AVM, Kolodgie FDP, Harnek JM, Guerrero LJB, Acampado ED, Tefera KB, *et al.* Differential Response of Delayed Healing and Persistent Inflammation at Sites of Overlapping Sirolimus- or Paclitaxel-Eluting Stents. Circulation 2005 Jul 12; 112(2):270–8.

87 Räber L, Jüni P, Löffel L, Wandel S, Cook S, Wenaweser P, *et al.* Impact of stent overlap on angiographic and long-term clinical outcome in patients undergoing drug-Eluting Stent Implantation. J Am Coll Cardiol 2010 Mar 23; 55(12):1178–88.

88 Joner M, Finn AV, Farb A, Mont EK, Kolodgie FD, Ladich E, *et al.* Pathology of drug-eluting stents in humans: Delayed healing and late thrombotic risk. J Am Coll Cardiol 2006 Jul 4; 48(1):193–202.

89 Jensen JS, Galloe A, Lassen JF, Erglis A, Kumsars I, Steigen TK, *et al.* Safety in simple versus complex stenting of coronary artery bifurcation lesions. The nordic bifurcation study 14-month follow-up results. EuroIntervention 2008 Aug; 4(2):229–33.

90 Steigen TK, Maeng M, Wiseth R, Erglis A, Kumsars I, Narbute I, *et al.* Randomized study on simple versus complex stenting of coronary artery bifurcation lesions: the Nordic bifurcation study. Circulation 2006 Oct 31; 114(18):1955–61.

91 Okamura T, Serruys PW, Regar E. The fate of bioresorbable struts located at a side branch ostium: serial three dimensional optical coherence tomography assessment. Eur Heart J. 2010 Sep; 31(17):2179.

92 Barlis P, Regar E, Serruys PW, Dimopoulos K, van der Giessen WJ, van Geuns RJ, *et al.* An optical coherence tomography study of a biodegradable vs. durable polymer-coated limus-eluting stent: a LEADERS trial sub-study. *Eur Heart J* 2010; 31:165–176.

93 Barlis P, Gonzalo N, Di MC, Prati F, Buellesfeld L, Rieber J, *et al.* A multicentre evaluation of the safety of intracoronary optical coherence tomography. EuroIntervention 2009 May; 5(1):90–5.

94 Gonzalo N, Tearney G, Serruys PW, van Soest G, Okamura T, Garcia-Garcia HM, *et al.* Second generation optical coherence tomography. Rev Esp Cardiol 2010 Aug; 63(8):893–903.

95 Lansky A, Tuinenburg J, Costa M, Maeng M, Koning G, Popma J, *et al.* Quantitative angiographic methods for bifurcation lesions: a consensus statement from the European Bifurcation Group. Catheter Cardiovasc Interv 2009 Feb 1; 73(2):258–66.

CHAPTER 13

Bifurcation quantitative coronary angiography

Vivian G. Ng, MD[1] *and Alexandra J. Lansky,* MD[2]

[1]Columbia University Medical Center, New York, NY, USA
[2]Yale University School of Medicine, New Haven, CT, USA

A bifurcation lesion is a coronary artery stenosis located near and/or involves the ostium of a significant side branch [1]. For many years, there was no standard methodology for describing and analyzing these difficult to image lesions; however, new recommendations are now available to help guide interventional cardiologists and investigators. Nonetheless, despite advances in percutaneous coronary interventions, bifurcation lesions remain challenging with increased complication rates and suboptimal clinical and angiographic results. As a result, multiple stenting techniques have been developed in order to improve these outcomes; however, these techniques are difficult, time-consuming and have their own pitfalls. New stents and devices have since been developed to overcome the technical difficulties of treating these lesions and have produced variable angiographic outcomes.

Pathophysiology of bifurcation disease

The development of atherosclerotic plaques involves an interplay of endothelial dysfunction, leukocyte recruitment and lipid deposition. *In vitro* and *in vivo* studies have revealed increased intimal thickening and atherosclerosis development in areas of low shear stress within the coronary vasculature where there is a disruption of these

factors [2–6]. Low shear stress alters endothelial cell gene expression and causes upregulation of vasoactive cytokines and inflammatory mediators such as endothelin, C-reactive protein and interleukin-6 [7–9]. Furthermore, there is increased cellular adhesion molecule production along these endothelial linings [10] which, in combination with decreased flow rates and decreased transit time of circulating blood cells along the vessel wall, can increase the transmigration of leukocytes into the vessel wall. In addition, low shear stress areas may have increased lipid permeability allowing for increased atheroma size [11] and increased LDL oxidation [12]. Therefore, low shear stress can induce increased vascular tone, attraction of leukocytes to the vessel wall and lipid deposition, thus promoting atherogenesis. In contrast, high shear stress induces a protective gene profile such as increased production of nitric oxide and decreased apoptosis of endothelial cells [9,13,14]. Consequently, flow-related factors affect the endothelium at all levels of atherosclerosis development.

Within coronary artery bifurcations, blood flow patterns are altered such that there is decreased shear stress along the lateral wall of bifurcations as compared with the flow divider wall [2–5]. Furthermore, these alterations in flow patterns and shear stress can be augmented with increases

Bifurcation Stenting, First Edition. Edited by Ron Waksman and John A. Ormiston.

in the angle of side branch take-offs [15]. Pathology specimens of patients with severe coronary artery disease who passed away from sudden cardiac death revealed significantly greater intimal wall thickness and atherosclerotic plaque development along the lateral walls of bifurcations compared with flow divider walls [5,7,16,17]. This has been confirmed *in vivo* by intravascular ultrasound studies demonstrating increased plaque development in the lateral wall [16,18,19], and when a steep side branch take-off angle is present, there can be complete sparing of the flow divider wall [16]. Thus, in agreement with studies suggesting the promotion of atherogenic factors in low shear regions, atheromas within coronary bifurcations are located predominantly along the lateral wall instead of the flow divider wall.

Understanding the pathophysiology of bifurcation lesions explains in part why these lesions can be difficult to characterize using quantitative coronary angiography (QCA). Bifurcation lesions are often eccentric with increased plaque thickness along the lateral wall with sparing of the flow divider. Given the difficulty of obtaining multiple optimal images of a bifurcation in which there is minimal foreshortening of main and branch vessels and little overlap, it can be difficult to appreciate the eccentricity of these lesions. Furthermore, there can be remodeling that can compensate for the eccentric lesions which cannot be appreciated by QCA.

Classification of bifurcation lesions

Unlike lesions located in non-branching areas of coronary arteries where a single description based on the section of the coronary artery and the percent of stenosis is standard and widely understood, lesions located at coronary artery bifurcations are more difficult to describe. Bifurcation lesions can have multiple different configurations depending on which branch or combination of branches of the artery is involved (proximal parent vessel vs distal parent vessel vs side branch). Many classifications have been developed in an attempt to standardize bifurcation descriptions [20–24]. While all these classifications are able to describe the different permutations of bifurcation lesions,

many of these classifications simply assign letters or numbers to a lesion type making the classification schemes difficult to memorize. The Medina Classification, on the other hand, was developed to have an intuitive classification system with easy memorability in order to standardize descriptions of bifurcation lesions. This classification divides a bifurcation into 3 segments: (1) main branch proximal (MBP), (2) main branch distal (MBD), and (3) side branch (SB) (Figure 13.1). A binary value (0,1) is assigned to each branch in the above described order representing whether a lesion with a >50% stenosis is present (assigned 1) or not (assigned 0) (Figure 13.1). For example, a bifurcation lesion described as (0, 1, 1) would correspond to lesions in the MBD and SB regions, while the MBP region was spared. There has been some criticism of this classification system because it does not include other important prognostic and treatment information such as side branch angulation, TIMI flow and lesion length. There are other classifications which attempt to include this additional information [24]; however, the ease of a classification scheme must be balanced with the amount of information contained during reporting. Given the simplicity of this classification method, the European Bifurcation Club has endorsed the Medina classification [1].

Quantitative coronary angiography of bifurcation lesions

With the advent of new techniques and devices for the treatment of bifurcation lesions, standardized methodologies of QCA are needed to describe specific lesions and the angiographic outcomes after intervention. QCA of bifurcation lesions has not been well standardized across studies partly because current QCA programs were designed for non-bifurcating vessels and have been adapted for analyses of bifurcation lesions. Several obstacles should be considered when discussing the QCA of bifurcation lesions including image acquisition, defining vessel segments and re-defining standard QCA measurements such as reference vessel diameter.

For non-bifurcation lesions, standard QCA requires two orthogonal views which are at least 30 degrees apart. However, image acquisition of

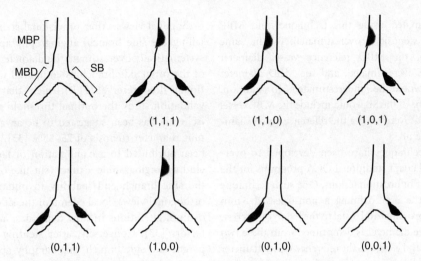

Figure 13.1 Medina classification. Simplified classification system to describe bifurcation lesions which divides the bifurcation into three segments: main branch proximal (MBP), main branch distal (MBD), and the side branch (SB).

Using 0 to indicate no lesion and 1 to indicate the presence of a lesion, each bifurcation has a number in the order (MBP, MBD, SB).

bifurcation lesions is more challenging since often there is only a single view in which the main vessel and side branches are well visualized without foreshortening of either vessel and without vessel overlap. As with any lesion, defining the lesion and the segments involved is crucial. Above we have described the Medina classification which utilizes the terms main branch proximal (MBP), main branch distal (MBD) and side branch (SB) [20]. The MBD and the SB must be clearly defined for QCA and interventions. For QCA purposes, by convention, the larger of the branches is defined as the MBD. Similar morphological descriptors of lesions are used for bifurcation lesions including lesion length, calcification, thrombus and TIMI flow in both vessel branches. In addition, other characteristics which impact outcomes should be described including ostial vs non-ostial lesions, extent, and the size of the side branch and parent vessel.

Side branch angulation, an additional parameter with important prognostic significance in bifurcation lesions, should also be described. Studies have found that side branches which are >70 degrees from the main vessel are at higher risk of abrupt vessel closure [25], side branch occlusion [26], and poorer outcomes after intervention [27] than side branches that are <70 degrees. These angles should be determined in the view with the least foreshor-

tening of the bifurcation components. Given that the main vessel itself may not be straight, two different angles should be described: the angle between the MBP and the SB and the angle between the MBD and the SB. Three-dimensional angiographic reconstruction is rapidly evolving as a better alternative to measure bifurcation lesion angulations.

Accurately determining the reference vessel diameter of the parent vessel and of the branches is a fundamental challenge to QCA analysis of bifurcation lesions. The diameters of coronary vessels decrease as the proximal main vessel bifurcates, a phenomenon well described in the coronary vasculature and defined by Murray's law $(D_1^3 = D_2^3 + D_3^3 + \ldots)$ [28–30]. This equation has been simplified for non-diseased coronary vasculature by a constant $(D_1 = 0.687(D_2 + D_3 + \ldots))$ [31,32]. Therefore, the diameter of the main vessel "steps-down" after the branch point. However, in order to determine reference vessel size, traditional QCA algorithms assume minimal vessel tapering. Thus, the traditional straight vessel QCA system would consider the main vessel as a single vessel and would not account for the "step-down" phenomenon thereby providing inaccurate bifurcation lesion measurements. As a result, the MBP reference vessel diameter is generally underestimated using this technique, and MBP diameter stenosis is overestimated. By the same reasoning, the MBD reference vessel diameter would be overestimated, and the MBD diameter stenosis would be underestimated. In addition, estimations of the SB would include the MBP vessel and would overestimate the reference vessel diameter of the SB.

User techniques have been developed to overcome and adapt traditional QCA programs for the analysis of bifurcation lesions. One such technique involves the user defining a non-diseased 5 mm segment proximal and distal to the lesion of interest. An average diameter is determined from these two segments and is used as the reference vessel diameter for the analysis. This technique is problematic when there is a long diseased segment, if there is significant vessel tapering and/or step-down, or if a lesion is located at the ostium of a side branch. In the second technique, the "interpolated reference" technique, the QCA program creates a smooth tapering vessel contour, and the user defines regions to be excluded (flagging) from the reference vessel diameter calculation such as areas of stenosis or ectasia. Again this technique does not allow for correction of a long diseased segment. Furthermore, the algorithm assumes a smooth tapering in vessel diameter and is unable to account for the step-down phenomenon in vessel diameters seen at bifurcations. Because the reference vessel diameter is determined at the site of minimal lumen diameter, the reference vessel diameter will vary depending on the location of the minimal lumen diameter at different time points of analysis (pre-procedural vs post-procedural vs follow-up). While these techniques may improve measurements of bifurcations using traditional QCA software for straight vessel segments, they are limited by high user interface, long analysis time and higher measurement variability.

Other parameters that are based on the reference vessel diameter are affected by the limitation of standard QCA programs. For example, the percent diameter stenosis [(1 − minimal lumen diameter/reference vessel diameter) × 100] can be either overestimated or underestimated as a result of systematic errors in reference vessel diameter measurements. Furthermore, the percent diameter stenosis is particularly difficult to assess for ostial lesions where it is difficult to obtain orthogonal views. After provisional stenting and jailing the side branch, angiography appears to systematically overestimate the diameter stenosis of the ostial side branch as compared with fractional flow reserve (FFR), such that in one validation study the optimal threshold to define ischemia has been suggested to be an angiographic diameter stenosis of 75–85% [33]. This has been attributed to a combination of factors including angiographic artifact (slit-like ostium of the side branch and inability to obtain a true orthogonal view), local edema of the side branch ostium, alterations in flow dynamics, and other factors [33]. Conversely, after stenting of both parent and side branch, angiography appears to systematically underestimate the diameter stenosis at the ostium of the side branch compared with intravascular ultrasound (IVUS) [34]. Thus, additional imaging modalities such as FFR and IVUS are recommended to help guide interventions of bifurcations.

At follow-up, the complexity of bifurcations dictates a systematic analysis and reporting of different regions of bifurcation lesions in order to understand the mechanism of an intervention's failure (Figure 13.2). Accurately determining the follow-up results of a bifurcation intervention is also difficult. Percent diameter stenosis and binary restenosis at follow-up has the same limitations as described above. Although, late lumen loss (LLL; post-procedural minimal lumen diameter-follow up minimal lumen diameter) is a well-validated continuous surrogate of intimal hyperplasia and target lesion revascularization (TLR) [35], this parameter is subject to possibly more variation since it is the difference in two measures of MLD obtained from two temporally different angiograms. In addition, LLL as a surrogate of TLR varies with the vessel size, which is of particular importance in bifurcation lesions given the variation in vessel size between the proximal and distal parent vessel and the side branch [36]. Furthermore, the region of MLD relocates between final procedural and follow-up images [37], leading to greater or lesser amounts of LLL due to extreme vessel taper, step-down phenomenon or vasospasm. Thus, LLL cannot be used as a single parameter to describe an entire bifurcation, but can be useful when describing pre-defined regions of a bifurcation.

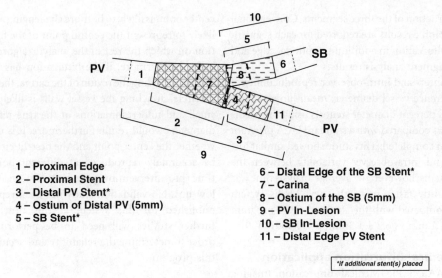

1 – Proximal Edge
2 – Proximal Stent
3 – Distal PV Stent*
4 – Ostium of Distal PV (5mm)
5 – SB Stent*

6 – Distal Edge of the SB Stent*
7 – Carina
8 – Ostium of the SB (5mm)
9 – PV In-Lesion
10 – SB In-Lesion
11 – Distal Edge PV Stent

*if additional stent(s) placed

Figure 13.2 Recommended sub-segment scheme for analysis and report of bifurcation lesions. PV= parent vessel; SB = side branch.

New QCA programs are now available to improve QCA analysis of bifurcation lesions by decreasing the amount of editing by the user, systematic and random error and processing time: the Medis medical imaging systems bifurcation application (QAngio XA V 7.2, Leiden, the Netherlands) [30] and the CAAS 5 Pie Medical Bifurcation Imaging software (Maastricht, the Netherlands) [38].

Medis bifurcation application

The Medis medical imaging systems bifurcation application utilizes two bifurcation models: a model for T-shaped bifurcations (wide angle between the distal main branch and the side branch) and a model for Y-shaped bifurcations (narrow angle between the distal main branch and the side branch). The carinal segment is either combined with the proximal vessel segment (Y-model) or the distal vessel segments (T-model). Three points are determined by the user: one start point in the proximal main branch and end points in the distal main branch and the side branch. Two path lines are created to connect the start point to the end points with automated detection of the arterial contours of all three vessel segments following a minimum cost algorithm. Thus, the outer vessel contours of the segment is defined as a whole

without interpolation across the side branch. Depending on the selected model, the carinal segment is defined differently. In the T-model, the carinal segment is defined by the program as the area between the first diameter of the distal main branch and the interpolated contour between the proximal and distal main branch. The vessel diameter is then determined for the entire main branch (proximal main branch, distal main branch and carinal segment) using the conventional Medis straight analysis approach. Because of the step-down phenomenon, the reference vessel diameter is determined for each segment of the parent vessel independently (proximal segment, distal segment and carinal region) in order to ensure that the reference vessel diameter is based on the true vessel diameters. The reference vessel of the side branch, on the other hand, is determined using a Medis ostial analysis approach to accurately determine the diameter at the ostium [39]. In the Y-model, the carinal segment is defined as the area between the distal diameter of the proximal main branch and the first diameters of the two distal segments. Three separate reference vessel diameters are calculated for the three segments (proximal main branch, distal main branch and side branch) using the conventional Medis straight analysis. The reference vessel diameter for the carinal region is determined from a reconstruction of the three segments. Conventional angiographic results are reported for each segment of the bifurcation in addition to optional edge and ostial segment analysis results.

The inter- and intra-observer reproducibility of the reference vessel diameter, mean lumen diameter and percent diameter stenosis using the Medis system as compared with a standard QCA program has been completed. This study showed similar low inter- and intra-observer variability between the two systems; however, the average analysis time was significantly faster using the new Medis system when compared with the standard QCA program $(4.7 \pm 1.1 \text{ min vs } 6.2 \pm 1.3 \text{min, p} < 0.0001)$ [30].

Pie medical bifurcation application

The CAAS 5 Pie Medical Bifurcation Imaging software similarly requires the user to define three points in the bifurcation (proximal main branch, distal main branch and side branch) and path lines are drawn to connect these points. Again the vessel contour is automatically determined using the minimal cost algorithm. However, in this model, the carinal region is defined as a best-fit circle drawn with its center located where all the centerlines meet (point of bifurcation) and with its edges touching the carina and both vessel walls. The centerlines are lines drawn through the center of each segment. A polygon of confluence is then drawn by drawing lines connecting the luminal walls bounding the circle. This defines the carinal region. Areas outside of the polygon of confluence are analyzed like single vessels. The reference linking the proximal and distal vessel segments across the bifurcation region is interpolated assuming a smooth curvature. However, the "minimum freedom" approach is utilized to estimate the diameter within the carinal region. The diameter of a particular area within the carinal region is approximated by the shortest distance from the point of bifurcation to the edge of the polygon of confluences in that location.

There are limitations to this system of analyzing bifurcation lesions. In defining the center circle to encompass the carinal region, centerlines are created through the center of each vessel segment. This can be accurately created in non-diseased vessels; however, as described above, disease in bifurcation vessels is often eccentric and identification of the

center point is likely to be more challenging and less likely to represent the central point of the bifurcation on which the rest of the analytic algorithm is built. Furthermore, if the bifurcation has diffuse disease including the region of the carina, the "best-fit circle" touching the vessel walls is likely to be small and underestimations of the true reference diameters would result. Furthermore, it is unclear whether the center point and the best-fit circle can be accurately reproduced at different points in time (pre-intervention, post-intervention and follow-up). No validation study has been reported/published for this system at this time; thus, further studies will need to be performed in order to determine the reliability and accuracy of this program.

3-dimensional angiography

As described above, current two-dimensional (2D) angiography technology has limitations at analyzing three-dimensional (3D) bifurcation vessels because of vessel overlap and vessel foreshortening during image acquisition. Interventionalists utilize multiple 2D images to mentally reconstruct the 3D morphology of a vessel; however, they are limited by the 2D images obtained. 3D angiography utilizes orthogonal 2D images (two images obtained at least 30 degrees apart and with minimal vessel overlap) and constructs 3D images which display the vessel contours. Several 3D QCA programs are now available: CardiOp-B, Paieon Medical Ltd. Park Afek, Israel; CAAS 5, Pie Medical Imaging, Maastricht, The Netherlands; as well as Medis, Leiden, The Netherlands (in beta testing). In both the Paieon and Pie systems, the user defines the area of interest by defining the proximal end, distal end and area of stenosis. However, the two systems differ in their calibration methods. CardiOp-B requires the operator to input the size of the catheter in the image into the program, whereas the CAAS 5 system automatically calibrates the images using DICOM (Digital Imaging and Communications in Medicine) information embedded in the angiographic images [40,41]. Once the image is created, operators can manipulate the images by zooming in or rotating the image. This allows the operator to have a better understanding of the bifurcation anatomy and could also help the operator find an optimal angle to image a vessel bifurcation [42,43]. The 3D QCA programs have been validated [44,45] and are now available to provide information of vessel size, bifurcation angle, percent diameter stenosis, minimal lumen diameter and other QCA values. It was thought that 3D QCA would have improved accuracy by resolving problems with vessel foreshortening and out of plane magnification. However, comparisons of 3D QCA programs to conventional 2D QCA programs have shown mixed results regarding the accuracy of this technology [41,42,45–49]. One small study has compared the two current 3D QCA programs using phantom models and has demonstrated that the CAAS 5 system may be more accurate than the CardiOp-B system [41].

The greatest benefit of 3D angiography is in analyzing bifurcation angles. 2D angiograms are unable to fully display the relationship of the bifurcation limbs within a 3-dimensional space; thus, accurate bifurcation angles are difficult to ascertain. Studies have shown that despite the problems of foreshortening and vessel overlap, 3D reconstruction of bifurcations is highly feasible with usual angiographic images, and allows for quantification of the bifurcation angles in addition to other standard angiographic parameters [50,51]. Furthermore, these studies demonstrate that the bifurcation angles change after intervention and can be followed using 3D angiography. Thus, as 3D angiography becomes more widely available, these programs may be helpful both in planning bifurcation interventions by accurately displaying bifurcation morphologies and in follow-up analysis of outcomes.

Techniques of bifurcation stenting

The simplest technique and current standard for stenting bifurcations involves a single stent within the main vessel when the side branch is small and/or supplies only a small region of myocardium. However, provisional stenting of a side branch may be necessary if there is a significant lesion within the side branch, there is poor flow through the side branch, and/or there is a side branch dissection. Multiple two-stent techniques for bifurcation lesions have been developed.

T stenting

T stenting involves introducing and deploying a stent into the side branch vessel as close to the ostium as possible without protrusion of the stent into the main vessel. A second stent is then deployed in the main vessel [52,53] (Figure 13.3A). *Modified T stenting* is very similar; however, both the main vessel and side branch stents are introduced at the same time although inflated sequentially. A *reverse T stent technique* can be utilized when a side branch is compromised after stent placement in the main vessel. In this situation, after the main vessel stent placement, another stent is introduced into the side branch through the stent struts of the main vessel's stent. In T stenting and its variations, there is often incomplete stent coverage of the proximal side branch secondary to the geometry of the side branch take off.

V stenting

In V stenting, the proximal main branch is relatively disease free while the distal main branch and the side branch are diseased. Two stents are introduced simultaneously into the distal main branch and the side branch vessels. They are sequentially inflated and the proximal ends of the stents meet to form a new small carina (Figure 13.3B). When the proximal main vessel is diseased, then a larger carina needs to be created or the simultaneous kissing stent technique can be employed.

Simultaneous kissing stents

Simultaneous kissing stents involves introducing two similarly sized stents into the distal main vessel and the side branch vessels. Both stents are deployed at the same time. The proximal ends of the stents cover the distal end of the proximal main vessel. A new carina is created in this technique [54,55] (Figure 13.3C). The proximal main vessel must be sufficiently large in order to accommodate the two stents. Hence, in general, the proximal main vessel should be at least two-thirds the sum of the two stent diameters. If the main vessel is also diseased, a modified simultaneous kissing stent technique can be used: the *trouser simultaneous kissing stent technique*. In this

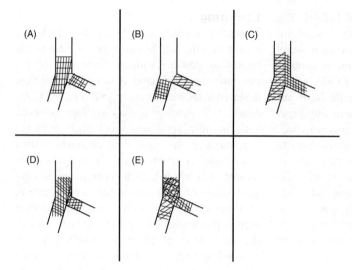

Figure 13.3 Two-stent techniques. (a) T-stent technique; (b) V-stent technique; (c) Simultaneous kissing stents technique; (d) Crush technique; (e) Culotte technique.

technique, a third stent in the proximal main vessel is also deployed.

Crush technique

In the crush technique, again two stents are introduced into the distal main vessel and the side branch. The side branch stent is deployed first with slight protrusion of the stent into the main vessel and the balloon and guide wire are removed. Next, the stent in the distal main branch is deployed and the proximal end compresses the proximal stent struts of the side branch stent. Lastly, a wire and balloon are re-introduced into the side branch vessel through the multiple layers of stent struts, and kissing balloons are inflated in the main vessel and the side branch [56] (Figure 13.3D). A *reverse crush technique* can be performed when provisional side branch stenting is required. After stent deployment in the main vessel, a stent is introduced into the side branch while a balloon is placed in the main vessel at the level of the side branch. The side branch stent is partially retracted into the main vessel and inflated. The main vessel balloon is then inflated in order to flatten the proximal aspect of the side branch stent. A balloon is reintroduced into the side branch and kissing balloon inflation is performed. A retrospective registry study containing 182 patients at two hospitals compared 1-year clinical outcomes and 6–8 month angiographic outcomes of patients receiving the T-stent technique

and those receiving the Crush technique [57]. Follow-up angiographic data was available for 79.3% of patients and showed no significant differences in overall binary restenosis rates in the main branch (16.2% vs 13.0%, p = 0.8) or in the side branch (19.2 vs 26.1%, p = 0.39) between the crush and T-stent technique. However, when specifically comparing patients who received kissing balloon post-dilatation, the crush technique had significantly lower rates of side branch binary restenosis than the T-stent technique (8.6% vs 26.5%, p = 0.04). At 1-year, MACE rates (cardiac death, acute myocardial infarction and target vessel revascularization) were similar between crush and T stenting (26.4% vs 36.1%, p = 0.23); however, patients receiving crush stenting had significantly lower target lesion revascularization rates than those receiving T stenting (14.0% vs 31.1%, p = 0.01). Thus, full coverage of the bifurcation with the crush technique with kissing balloon post-dilatation has improved angiographic results, and this technique may decrease rates of revascularization.

Culotte technique

In this technique, a stent is first deployed in the more angulated branch with the proximal end hanging within the main vessel. A second stent is then introduced into the other branch through the struts of the first stent. This stent is then deployed with an overlapping of stents within the proximal main vessel [58] (Figure 13.3E). This leads to full coverage of the bifurcation. A small retrospective single center registry study found decreased target lesion revascularization rates when this technique was compared to T stenting (8.9% vs 27.3%, p = 0.014) possibly from complete coverage of the side branch ostium. In a large multicenter randomized trial comparing the crush and culotte techniques, patients treated with the culotte technique had similar rates of MACE (cardiac death, myocardial infarction, target vessel revascularization or stent thrombosis) at 6 months (3.7% vs 4.3%, p = 0.87), but had lower rates of in-stent restenosis (4.5% vs 10.5%, p = 0.046) at 8 months than patients treated with the crush technique [59]. Thus, although the culotte technique may have improved angiographic results, it is unclear whether this is clinically significant.

Treatment with one versus two stents

As with other coronary stenoses, initially side branches were treated with balloon angioplasty; however, this led to high rates of acute closure and restenosis [60]. Treatment with bare mental stents decreased these rates of acute closure; yet, high rates of restenosis continued to persist [61–63]. Although drug-eluting stents (DES) decreased revascularization rates of bifurcation lesions, unfortunately, procedural success rates remain lower and restenosis rates remain higher in the treatment of bifurcation lesions when compared with non-bifurcation lesions [58,61,64]. Stenting the entire bifurcation using two stents would theoretically offer the best outcomes because of optimal angiographic post-procedural results. However, small randomized trials suggested that complex stenting of bifurcations with two DES stents had similar outcomes to simple stenting using only one stent with provisional side branch stenting if required [64,65]. Since then, several randomized trials have been performed comparing the one-stent with provisional side branch stenting technique versus two-stent techniques.

Three large randomized trials have been conducted to compare outcomes of the simple technique (single stent with provisional side branch stenting) and complex techniques (two-stent tech-

niques) for revascularizing bifurcations: the Nordic bifurcation study [66], the coronary bifurcations: application of the crushing technique using sirolimus-eluting stents study (CACTUS) [67] and the British bifurcation coronary study: old, new and evolving strategies (BBC-ONE) trial [68]. The Nordic bifurcation study was the first large multi-center randomized trial to look at whether the two-stent techniques (specific technique was at the discretion of the interventionalist) would have improved outcomes compared to the single stent technique with provisional stenting for TIMI flow 0 in the side branch. This study, which contained 413 patients and used sirolimus-eluting stents (SES), found similar 6-month rates of MACE (cardiac death, myocardial infarction, target vessel revascularization and stent thrombosis) and the individual component endpoints. Furthermore, 8-month QCA follow-up found similar rates of binary angiographic restenosis within the main vessel (22.5% vs 16.0%, p = 0.84) and side branch vessels (19.2% vs 11.5%, p = 0.062) between the simple and complex techniques. While the simple group had smaller minimal luminal diameter and greater percent diameter stenosis of the side branch after the index procedure and at follow-up, late lumen loss was greater in the complex group than in the simple group at 8-month follow-up. Patients receiving complex stenting required longer procedure and fluoroscopy times with increased contrast loads [66]. There are some limitations of this study. For example, it is unclear how many of the Nordic bifurcation study patients had true bifurcation lesions (*ie* lesions with >50% stenosis in both bifurcation branches). Side branch occlusions are more likely to occur if there is a true bifurcation lesion involving both bifurcation branches [69]. Thus, if a large percent of bifurcations with insignificantly diseased side branches were included in the trial, one would not expect a benefit from side branch stenting, and the results would be biased towards the null hypothesis. Furthermore, patients in the complex stenting arm may have had incomplete coverage of side branches since there was no standard technique used, and techniques such as T stenting can lead to incomplete coverage of the proximal side branch depending on the side branch angulation. This could theoretically decrease the benefits of complex stenting.

The following trial attempted to address some of the limitations of the Nordic bifurcation study. The CACTUS trial enrolled 350 patients with true bifurcation lesions and randomized them to either complex stenting with SES using the crush technique or simple stenting with provisional side branch stenting using the T-stent technique if there was residual side branch stenosis ≥50%, dissection or TIMI flow ≤2. As in the Nordic bifurcation study, there was no significant difference in the primary clinical endpoint MACE (death, myocardial infarct or target vessel revascularization), and stent thrombosis rates were similar between the two treatment arms. In addition, binary angiographic restenosis rates at 8 months in the main branch (6.7% vs 4.6%, p = NS) and side branch (14.7% vs 13.2%, p = NS) were similar between the simple and complex treatment groups [67]. Similar to the QCA findings of the previous trial, post-procedural and follow-up side branch minimal luminal diameters were smaller in the simple treatment group. Although percent diameter stenosis within the side branch was greater in the simple stenting arm after the index procedure, there was no significant difference at follow-up. There was a trend for increased late lumen loss in the complex group, but unlike the Nordic bifurcation study, this did not reach statistical significance. Thus, despite complete coverage of true bifurcation lesions, complex stenting continued to have similar outcomes to simple stenting of bifurcations. Furthermore, despite improved angiographic outcomes postprocedurally, these benefits were lost overtime. In the BBC-ONE trial, paclitaxel-eluting stents were used instead of SES when 500 patients were randomized to complex stenting with the Culotte or crush techniques or to simple stenting with provisional T stenting if there was a side branch with TIMI flow <3, stenosis >90%, or dissection. Patients were followed clinically for 9 months without angiographic follow-up. Nonetheless, they found similar results with no differences in MACE (death, myocardial infarction or target vessel revascularization), but once again found longer fluoroscopy times and increased contrast loads [68].

Recently, a meta-analysis containing six randomized controlled studies, including the three above, was performed [70]. Compared to a single stent with provisional side branch stenting technique, the two-stent technique had similar rates of 1-year overall death (RR 1.12 [0.42–3.02]), revascularization (RR 0.91 [0.61–1.35]) and stent thrombosis rates (RR 0.56 [0.23–1.35]). Furthermore, by QCA analysis, the mean percent diameter stenosis [95% CI] at follow-up was similar between the one-stent and the two-stent group (−1.08 [−2.91 to 0.74] and 1.30 [−3.35 to 5.96], p = NS). However, the two-stent technique increased the risk of one-year MI compared with provisional side branch stenting (RR 0.57 [0.37–0.87]).

Thus, current studies demonstrate that standard two-stent techniques do not have long-term clinical or angiographic benefits when compared with one-stent techniques with provisional stenting for side branch occlusions, poor flow or dissections. While QCA analysis showed initial benefit from side branch stenting in terms of minimal luminal diameters and possibly diameter stenosis, this benefit is lost within the first 6–9 months after treatment. Furthermore, complex stenting of bifurcation lesions increased X-ray radiation exposure and contrast loads. There are limitations to the current studies. Given the large variability in anatomic morphology, lesion location, side branch size and angulation, one technique is unlikely to best suit all these different possibilities. Furthermore, there is bound to be great variability in technique, even if only one technique type is allowed in the study, since adjustments will need to be made for each individual lesion and there is a learning curve for employing any of these complicated techniques. There may also be limitations with the DES currently available. Previous studies have shown that certain DES, such as the paclitaxel-eluting stent, may have increased rates of side branch occlusion compared with other DES, possibly from stent design such as stent strut size [71]. Nonetheless, these findings suggest that with the current technology available, single stent with provisional stenting of side branch lesions should be used for bifurcation lesions.

Dedicated devices

While the one-stent technique with provisional stenting of a side branch is now the convention, there are technical difficulties with this approach. Stenting of the main vessel first can lead to a jailed side branch causing difficulty to re-enter the side branch and to introduce a balloon or device through the stent struts. Furthermore, ballooning the side branch could lead to deformation of the main vessel's stent with variability of the stent's structure to withstand this distortion. In addition, there is often incomplete coverage of the side branch when the provisional approach is used. All this must be considered in addition to the technical difficulty of stenting these lesions. Thus, dedicated stents for bifurcations have been created to help overcome some of the shortcomings of the provisional stent technique.

There are several ways in which different devices are designed to ease provisional side branch stenting. In order to handle the difficulties of rewiring the side branch and introducing devices through the stent struts, several stents have been developed to maintain access to the side branch, such as the Nile Croco (Minvasys, Genevilliers, France) and the Antiares (Trireme Medical, California, USA). Other stents prepare for a second stent to be placed in order to fully treat a bifurcation lesion: Tryton (Tryton Medical, Massachusetts, USA) and Axxess plus (Devax, Irvine, California, USA).

The Nile Croco stent uses a double balloon delivery system with a stent that is crimped over the main branch balloon and the tip of the side branch balloon. The system is advanced with three markers (proximal, distal and central) on the main branch balloon to help guide placement. The central marker should be placed at the side branch ostium. The main branch balloon is inflated followed by advancement of the side branch balloon and kissing balloon inflation. The main and side branch balloons are inflated separately and require individual pressure monitoring. This device provides partial coverage of the side branch ostium and allows access to the side branch for further stenting if needed without crossing the main stent's struts or deformation of the main stent. A registry containing 93 patients with bifurcation lesions receiving the Nile Croco stent demonstrated 96% stent placement success (stent in desired location) and 99% complete angiographic success (main branch stenosis <30% and side branch residual stenosis <50%). However, despite good post-procedural angiographic results, MACE (cardiac death, myocardial infarction and target lesion revasculariza-

tion) and target lesion revascularization rates at 6 months were high in this registry. MACE occurred in 12% of patients with a 10.6% ischemia-driven target lesion revascularization rate [72]. This design has since been updated with a polymer-free paclitaxel-eluting drug (NilePAX) and is currently being studied in a prospective non-randomized multi-center study, which will look at angiographic and clinical outcomes. Preliminary 30-day results of 102 patients are promising with 99% stent placement success and no cardiac or thrombotic events [73]; however, further data are needed for this new stent.

The Antiares stent, unlike the Nile Croco, contains only one balloon. Again, there are markers in order to guide positioning of the side branch opening through which a side branch wire is advanced. The balloon is inflated, expanding the stent that contains an opening to the side branch and components which cover the side branch ostium. This dual lumen stent allows access to the side branch at all times and provides coverage of the side branch ostium.

Unlike the previous two stents described, which deliver a stent in the main vessel first with access to the side branch if needed, the Tryton side branch stent involves stenting the side branch first, and a separate stent can be delivered to the main branch afterwards. The Tryton side branch stent contains a unique design composed of three zones: side branch zone, transition zone and main vessel zone. The side branch zone is structured like a standard stent. The transition zone was designed to provide radial strength which transforms into the main zone that contains only three fronds. The main zone provides minimal coverage but allows for easy delivery of a conventional DES into the main vessel. This technique is similar to the Culotte technique; however, the new stent avoids deformation of the first stent delivered and minimizes the overlapping stent struts. This stent has been tested in a first-in-man trial containing 30 patients. At 6 months, MACE (cardiac death, stroke, MI, CABG or target lesion revascularization) was 9.9% with a target lesion revascularization rate of 3.3%. 6-month angiographic follow-up analyzed by a core laboratory showed an insignificant change in post-procedural versus follow-up percent diameter stenosis (19.2 ± 10.7 vs 18.4 ± 9.8, p = 0.36) and low amounts of proximal main branch late lumen loss (0.25 ± 0.43 mm) and side branch late lumen loss (0.17 ± 0.35 mm). Furthermore there were no events of binary restenosis in the side branch [74]. Additional trials are currently being performed to study outcomes of this device.

The above described stents are bare metal stents and require a balloon for deployment. The Axxess Plus stent is unique in that it is the only drug-eluting bifurcation stent and is self-expanding. This stent uses Biolimus-A9, which is a sirolimus derivative. The stent is placed directly over the carina of the bifurcation, and the covering sheath is pulled back. The stent straddles the two branches of the bifurcation allowing easy access if further distal stenting is required. This stent attempts to provide maximal bifurcation coverage with decreased stent strut overlap or deformation. A large prospective registry containing 302 patients found favorable results after the stent was successfully deployed in 98.3% of patients [75]. At 9 months, MACE (death, myocardial infarction, target lesions revascularization) was only 7.7% and target lesion revascularization was 4.3%. Furthermore, by QCA of 150 pre-assigned patients, in-segment binary restenosis in the bifurcation was 6.4% (3.6% parent vessel, 4.3% side branch). Late stent thrombosis occurred in 0.3% of patients. Thus, the preliminary study offers promising results for this stent that allows for easy access to the both distal bifurcation branches with acceptable MACE, target revascularization, stent thrombosis and angiographic restenosis rates. However, a randomized trial comparing this stent to current technology is needed.

Conclusions

Bifurcation stenting remains challenging because of the pathophysiology of disease and the enormous variability in anatomic and disease morphology. New recommendations and advances are being made to aid interventionalists by providing a common language, new analysis tools and new technology. Thus far, an easy-to-memorize classification has been recommended, and new QCA programs have been developed to overcome the assumptions built into current QCA programs. While there are many two-stent techniques that have been devel-

oped for bifurcations, current evidence supports a single stent approach with provisional treatment of significant side branch lesions. New devices which overcome certain obstacles in bifurcation stenting, such as side branch jailing and incomplete bifurcation coverage, have encouraging preliminary results. However, additional randomized trials are needed to test the outcomes of these stents compared to current techniques.

References

1 Louvard Y, Thomas M, Dzavik V, *et al*. Classification of coronary artery bifurcation lesions and treatments: time for a consensus! Catheter Cardiovasc Interv 2008;71: 175–83.

2 Friedman MH, Bargeron CB, Deters OJ, Hutchins GM, Mark FF. Correlation between wall shear and intimal thickness at a coronary artery branch. Atherosclerosis 1987;68:27–33.

3 Ku DN, Giddens DP, Zarins CK, Glagov S. Pulsatile flow and atherosclerosis in the human carotid bifurcation. Positive correlation between plaque location and low oscillating shear stress. Arteriosclerosis 1985;5:293–302.

4 Prosi M, Perktold K, Ding Z, Friedman MH. Influence of curvature dynamics on pulsatile coronary artery flow in a realistic bifurcation model. J Biomech 2004;37:1767–75.

5 Nakazawa G, Yazdani SK, Finn AV, Vorpahl M, Kolodgie FD, Virmani R. Pathological findings at bifurcation lesions: the impact of flow distribution on atherosclerosis and arterial healing after stent implantation. J Am Coll Cardiol 2010;55:1679–87.

6 Caro CG. Discovery of the role of wall shear in atherosclerosis. Arterioscler Thromb Vasc Biol 2009;29:158–61.

7 Cheng C, van Haperen R, de Waard M, *et al*. Shear stress affects the intracellular distribution of eNOS: direct demonstration by a novel in vivo technique. Blood 2005;106:3691–8.

8 Cheng C, Tempel D, van Haperen R, *et al*. Atherosclerotic lesion size and vulnerability are determined by patterns of fluid shear stress. Circulation 2006;113:2744–53.

9 Ziegler T, Bouzourene K, Harrison VJ, Brunner HR, Hayoz D. Influence of oscillatory and unidirectional flow environments on the expression of endothelin and nitric oxide synthase in cultured endothelial cells. Arterioscler Thromb Vasc Biol 1998;18:686–92.

10 Zhu CH, Ying DJ, Mi JH, Zhu XH, Sun JS, Cui XP. Low shear stress regulates monocyte adhesion to oxidized lipid-induced endothelial cells via an IkappaBalpha dependent pathway. Biorheology 2004;41:127–37.

11 Berceli SA, Warty VS, Sheppeck RA, Mandarino WA, Tanksale SK, Borovetz HS. Hemodynamics and low

density lipoprotein metabolism. Rates of low density lipoprotein incorporation and degradation along medial and lateral walls of the rabbit aorto-iliac bifurcation. Arteriosclerosis 1990;10:686–94.

12 Hwang J, Ing MH, Salazar A, *et al.* Pulsatile versus oscillatory shear stress regulates NADPH oxidase subunit expression: implication for native LDL oxidation. Circ Res 2003;93:1225–32.

13 Malek AM, Alper SL, Izumo S. Hemodynamic shear stress and its role in atherosclerosis. JAMA 1999;282:2035–42.

14 Kaiser D, Freyberg MA, Friedl P. Lack of hemodynamic forces triggers apoptosis in vascular endothelial cells. Biochem Biophys Res Commun 1997;231:586–90.

15 Perktold K, Peter RO, Resch M, Langs G. Pulsatile non-Newtonian blood flow in three-dimensional carotid bifurcation models: a numerical study of flow phenomena under different bifurcation angles. J Biomed Eng 1991;13:507–15.

16 Kimura BJ, Russo RJ, Bhargava V, McDaniel MB, Peterson KL, DeMaria AN. Atheroma morphology and distribution in proximal left anterior descending coronary artery: in vivo observations. J Am Coll Cardiol 1996; 27:825–31.

17 Fox B, James K, Morgan B, Seed A. Distribution of fatty and fibrous plaques in young human coronary arteries. Atherosclerosis 1982;41:337–47.

18 Badak O, Schoenhagen P, Tsunoda T, *et al.* Characteristics of atherosclerotic plaque distribution in coronary artery bifurcations: an intravascular ultrasound analysis. Coron Artery Dis 2003;14:309–16.

19 Shimada Y, Courtney BK, Nakamura M, *et al.* Intravascular ultrasonic analysis of atherosclerotic vessel remodeling and plaque distribution of stenotic left anterior descending coronary arterial bifurcation lesions upstream and downstream of the side branch. Am J Cardiol 2006;98:193–6.

20 Medina A, Suarez de Lezo J, Pan M. [A new classification of coronary bifurcation lesions]. Rev Esp Cardiol 2006; 59:183.

21 Pompa J, Bashore T. Qualitative and quantitative angiography-Bifurcation lesions. In: Topol E,ed. Textbook of interventional cardiology. Philadelphia, PA, W.B. Saunders, 1994: 1055–8.

22 Lefevre T, Louvard Y, Morice MC, *et al.* Stenting of bifurcation lesions: classification, treatments, and results. Catheter Cardiovasc Interv 2000;49:274–83.

23 Safian RD. Bifurcation lesions. In Safian RD, Freed M,eds. Manual of Interventional Cardiology. Royal Oak, Physicians' Press, 2001: 221–36.

24 Movahed MR, Stinis CT. A new proposed simplified classification of coronary artery bifurcation lesions and bifurcation interventional techniques. J Invasive Cardiol 2006;18:199–204.

25 Tan K, Sulke N, Taub N, Sowton E. Clinical and lesion morphologic determinants of coronary angioplasty success and complications: current experience. J Am Coll Cardiol 1995;25:855–65.

26 Aliabadi D, Tilli FV, Bowers TR, *et al.* Incidence and angiographic predictors of side branch occlusion following high-pressure intracoronary stenting. Am J Cardiol 1997;80:994–7.

27 Dzavik V,KR, Ivanov J, Ing DJ, Bui S, Mackie K, Ramsamujh R, Barolet A, Schwartz L, Seidelin PH. Predictors of long-term outcome after crush stenting of coronary bifurcation lesions: importance of the bifurcation angle. Am Heart J 2006;152:762–9.

28 Louvard YLT, Morice MC. Percutaneous coronary intervention for bifurcation coronary disease. Heart 2004; 90:713–22.

29 Reiber JHvdZP, Koning G, von Land CD, van Meurs B, Gerbrands JJ, *et al.* Accuracy and precision of quantitative digital coronary arteriography: observer-, short-, and medium-term variabilities. Cathet Cardiovasc Diagn 1993;28:187–98.

30 Goktekin OKS, Dimopoulos K, Barlis P, Tanigawa J, Vantankulu MA, *et al.* A new quantitative analysis system for the evaluation of coronary bifurcation lesions: Comparison with current conventional methods. Catheter Cardiovasc Interv. 2007;69:172–80.

31 S.G. Scaling laws of vascular trees: of form and function. Am J Physiol 2006;290:894–903.

32 Akira KTT. Quantitative assessments of morphological and functional properties of biological trees based on their fractal nature J Appl Physiol 2007;102:2315–23.

33 Koo BK KH, Youn TJ, Chae IH, Choi DJ, Kim HS, Sohn DW, Oh BH, Lee MM, Park YB, Choi YS, Tahk SJ. Physiologic assessment of jailed side branch lesions using fractional flow reserve. J Am Coll Cardiol 2005;46:633–7.

34 Costa RAMG, Carlier SG, Lansky AJ, Moussa I, Fujii K, Takebayashi H, Yasuda T, Costa JR, Tsuchiya Y, Jensen LO, Cristea E, Mehran R, Dangas GD, Iyer S, Collins, M, Kreps EM, Colombo A, Stone, GW, Leon MB, Moses JW. Bifurcation coronary lesions treated with the "crush" technique: an intravascular ultrasound analysis. J Am Coll Cardiol 2005;46:599–605.

35 Mauri LOE, Kuntz RE. Late loss in lumen diameter and binary restenosis for drug-eluting stent comparison. Circulation 2005;111:3435–42.

36 Pocock SJ, Lansky AJ, Mehran R, *et al.* Angiographic surrogate end points in drug-eluting stent trials: a systematic evaluation based on individual patient data from 11 randomized, controlled trials. J Am Coll Cardiol 2008;51:23–32.

37 Costa MA, Sabate M, Angiolillo DJ, *et al.* Relocation of minimal luminal diameter after bare metal and drug-eluting stent implantation: incidence and impact on

angiographic late loss. Catheter Cardiovasc Interv 2007;69:181–8.

38 Ramcharitar S, Onuma Y, Aben JP, *et al.* A novel dedicated quantitative coronary analysis methodology for bifurcation lesions. EuroIntervention 2008;3:553–7.

39 Reiber JHC TJ, Koning G, Janssen JP, Lansky A and Goedhart B. Quantitative Coronary Arteriography. Berlin, Springer-Verlag, 2008.

40 Gradaus R, Mathies K, Breithardt G, Bocker D. Clinical assessment of a new real time 3D quantitative coronary angiography system: evaluation in stented vessel segments. Catheter Cardiovasc Interv 2006;68:44–9.

41 Ramcharitar S, Daeman J, Patterson M, *et al.* First direct in vivo comparison of two commercially available three-dimensional quantitative coronary angiography systems. Catheter Cardiovasc Interv 2008;71:44–50.

42 Dvir D, Marom H, Guetta V, Kornowski R. Three-dimensional coronary reconstruction from routine single-plane coronary angiograms: in vivo quantitative validation. Int J Cardiovasc Intervent 2005;7:141–5.

43 Agostoni P, Biondi-Zoccai G, Van Langenhove G, *et al.* Comparison of assessment of native coronary arteries by standard versus three-dimensional coronary angiography. Am J Cardiol 2008;102:272–9.

44 Schuurbiers JC, Lopez NG, Ligthart J, *et al.* In vivo validation of CAAS QCA-3D coronary reconstruction using fusion of angiography and intravascular ultrasound (ANGUS). Catheter Cardiovasc Interv 2009;73:620–6.

45 Tsuchida K, van der Giessen WJ, Patterson M, *et al.* In vivo validation of a novel three-dimensional quantitative coronary angiography system (CardiOp-B): comparison with a conventional two-dimensional system (CAAS II) and with special reference to optical coherence tomography. EuroIntervention 2007;3:100–8.

46 Meerkin D, Marom H, Cohen-Biton O, Einav S. Three-dimensional vessel analyses provide more accurate length estimations than the gold standard QCA. J Interv Cardiol 2010;23:152–9.

47 Wellnhofer E, Wahle A, Mugaragu I, Gross J, Oswald H, Fleck E. Validation of an accurate method for three-dimensional reconstruction and quantitative assessment of volumes, lengths and diameters of coronary vascular branches and segments from biplane angiographic projections. Int J Card Imaging 1999;15: 339–53; discussion 355–6.

48 Tu S, Koning G, Jukema W, Reiber JH. Assessment of obstruction length and optimal viewing angle from biplane X-ray angiograms. Int J Cardiovasc Imaging 2010;26:5–17.

49 Rittger H, Schertel B, Schmidt M, Justiz J, Brachmann J, Sinha AM. Three-dimensional reconstruction allows accurate quantification and length measurements of coronary artery stenoses. EuroIntervention 2009;5:127–32.

50 Girasis C, Serruys PW, Onuma Y, *et al.* 3-Dimensional bifurcation angle analysis in patients with left main disease: a substudy of the SYNTAX trial (SYNergy Between Percutaneous Coronary Intervention with TAXus and Cardiac Surgery). JACC Cardiovasc Interv 2010;3:41–8.

51 D. Dvir HM, A. Assali, R. Kornowski. Bifurcation lesions in the coronary arteries: early experience with a novel 3-dimensional imaging and quantitative analysis before and after stenting. EuroInterv 2007;3:95–9.

52 Teirstein PS. Kissing Palmaz-Schatz stents for coronary bifurcation stenoses. Cathet Cardiovasc Diagn 1996; 37:307–10.

53 Lefevre T, Louvard Y, Morice MC, Loubeyre C, Piechaud JF, Dumas P. Stenting of bifurcation lesions: a rational approach. J Interv Cardiol 2001;14:573–85.

54 Colombo A, Gaglione A, Nakamura S, Finci L. "Kissing" stents for bifurcational coronary lesion. Cathet Cardiovasc Diagn 1993;30:327–30.

55 Sharma SK, Choudhury A, Lee J, *et al.* Simultaneous kissing stents (SKS) technique for treating bifurcation lesions in medium-to-large size coronary arteries. Am J Cardiol 2004;94:913–7.

56 Colombo A, Stankovic G, Orlic D, *et al.* Modified T-stenting technique with crushing for bifurcation lesions: immediate results and 30-day outcome. Catheter Cardiovasc Interv 2003;60:145–51.

57 Ge L, Iakovou I, Cosgrave J, *et al.* Treatment of bifurcation lesions with two stents: one year angiographic and clinical follow up of crush versus T stenting. Heart 2006;92:371–6.

58 Chevalier B, Glatt B, Royer T, Guyon P. Placement of coronary stents in bifurcation lesions by the "culotte" technique. Am J Cardiol 1998;82:943–9.

59 Erglis A, Kumsars I, Niemela M, *et al.* Randomized comparison of coronary bifurcation stenting with the crush versus the culotte technique using sirolimus eluting stents: the Nordic stent technique study. Circ Cardiovasc Interv 2009;2:27–34.

60 Pinkerton CA, Slack JD, Van Tassel JW, Orr CM. Angioplasty for dilatation of complex coronary artery bifurcation stenoses. Am J Cardiol 1985;55:1626–8.

61 Al Suwaidi J, Yeh W, Cohen HA, Detre KM, Williams DO, Holmes DR, Jr. Immediate and one-year outcome in patients with coronary bifurcation lesions in the modern era (NHLBI dynamic registry). Am J Cardiol 2001; 87:1139–44.

62 Sheiban I, Albiero R, Marsico F, *et al.* Immediate and long-term results of "T" stenting for bifurcation coronary lesions. Am J Cardiol 2000;85:1141–4, A9.

63 Yamashita T, Nishida T, Adamian MG, *et al.* Bifurcation lesions: two stents versus one stent-immediate and follow-up results. J Am Coll Cardiol 2000;35: 1145–51.

64 Colombo A, Moses JW, Morice MC, *et al.* Randomized study to evaluate sirolimus-eluting stents implanted at coronary bifurcation lesions. Circulation 2004;109: 1244–9.

65 Pan M, de Lezo JS, Medina A, *et al.* Rapamycin-eluting stents for the treatment of bifurcated coronary lesions: a randomized comparison of a simple versus complex strategy. Am Heart J 2004;148:857–64.

66 Steigen TK, Maeng M, Wiseth R, *et al.* Randomized study on simple versus complex stenting of coronary artery bifurcation lesions: the Nordic bifurcation study. Circulation 2006;114:1955–61.

67 Colombo A, Bramucci E, Sacca S, *et al.* Randomized study of the crush technique versus provisional side-branch stenting in true coronary bifurcations: the CACTUS (Coronary Bifurcations: Application of the Crushing Technique Using Sirolimus-Eluting Stents) Study. Circulation 2009;119:71–8.

68 Hildick-Smith D, de Belder AJ, Cooter N, *et al.* Randomized trial of simple versus complex drug-eluting stenting for bifurcation lesions: the British Bifurcation Coronary Study: old, new, and evolving strategies. Circulation 2010;121:1235–43.

69 Timurkaynak T, Ciftci H, Ozdemir M, *et al.* Sidebranch occlusion after coronary stenting with or without balloon predilation: direct versus conventional stenting. J Invasive Cardiol 2002;14:497–501.

70 Brar SS, Gray WA, Dangas G, *et al.* Bifurcation stenting with drug-eluting stents: a systematic review and meta-analysis of randomised trials. EuroIntervention 2009; 5:475–84.

71 Popma JJ, Mauri L, O'Shaughnessy C, *et al.* Frequency and clinical consequences associated with sidebranch occlusion during stent implantation using zotarolimus-eluting and paclitaxel-eluting coronary stents. Circ Cardiovasc Interv 2009;2:133–9.

72 Del Blanco BG, Brenot P, Royer T, *et al.* Clinical and Procedural Evaluation of the Nile Croco Dedicated Stent for Bifurcation Six month Clinical Follow-up Results of the Nile Croco Registry. Intervl Cardiol 2008;3:46–50.

73 Costa RA. BIPAX Bifurcation Study: First Results. Paris, EuroPCR, 2010.

74 Onuma Y, Muller R, Ramcharitar S, *et al.* Tryton I, First-In-Man (FIM) study: six month clinical and angiographic outcome analysis with new quantitative coronary dedicated for bifurcation lesions. EuroIntervention 2008; 3:546–552.

75 Verheye S, Agostoni P, Dubois CL, *et al.* 9-month clinical, angiographic, and intravascular ultrasound results of a prospective evaluation of the Axxess self-expanding biolimus A9-eluting stent in coronary bifurcation lesions: the DIVERGE (Drug-Eluting Stent Intervention for Treating Side Branches Effectively) study. J Am Coll Cardiol 2009;53:1031–9.

CHAPTER 14

Evaluation of a dedicated everolimus coated side branch access (SBA) system

Oana Sorop, PhD[1], Heleen M.M. van Beusekom, PhD[1], Evelyn Regar, MD, PhD, FESC[1], Li Hui-Ling, MD, PhD[1], Jurgen Ligthart, BSc[1], Katrin Boeke-Purkis, BSc, CCIR[2] and Willem J. van der Giessen†, MD, PhD[1,3]

[1]Department of Cardiology, Thoraxcentrum, Erasmus MC, Rotterdam, The Netherlands
[2]Abbott Vascular, Santa Clara, USA
[3]Interuniversity Cardiology Institute of the Netherlands, ICIN-KNAW, The Netherlands

Introduction

Coronary lesions often develop at branching points, mainly as a result of altered shear stress profiles [1,2]. However, percutaneous treatment of coronary bifurcation lesions remains challenging due to technical difficulties and long-term suboptimal clinical results [3]. There are different techniques currently used for the treatment of coronary bifurcation lesions, depending on the lesion type, mainly divided into one-stent and two-stent techniques. With the one-stent technique only the main branch (MB) is stented, while a second stent is only used when the side-branch (SB) perfusion is regarded to be jeopardized (provisional SB stenting). Using the two-stent technique the intended treatment strategy is that both the MB and SB receive a separate stent. The current consensus is that provisional SB stenting is the best strategy for the treatment of bifurcation lesions with conventional stents [4]. Provisional SB stenting consists in

stenting the main vessel across the SB, followed by the opening a stent cell with a balloon inflation in the SB and, if deemed necessary, followed by stent implantation in the proximal SB. However, this strategy is technically limited by the inability to wire the "jailed" SB or to advance the balloon or stent through the struts of the MB stent. Even in case of successful SB stenting, inadequate coverage of the SB ostium often occurs. Furthermore, the use of either stenting strategy was associated with long procedural times and high contrast utilization, contributing to a higher incidence of peri-procedural complications, need for reintervention, stent thrombosis, and other adverse clinical events [4–7].

The introduction of bare metal dedicated side-branch access systems, which have been designed to reduce most technical difficulties of treating such lesions (reduced intervention time, radiation time and contrast volume), did not translate into an improvement in the long-term clinical results [8,9]. Furthermore, while for non-bifurcation lesions the introduction of drug-eluting stents has reduced the incidence of restenosis as compared with bare

† deceased

Bifurcation Stenting, First Edition. Edited by Ron Waksman and John A. Ormiston.
© 2012 Blackwell Publishing Ltd. Published 2012 by Blackwell Publishing Ltd.

metal stents, the treatment of bifurcation lesions with conventional DES proved less effective [10]. Thus the combination of drug-elution and a dedicated system for the complex geometry of the bifurcation seems a useful approach.

The new Abbott everolimus-coated dedicated side branch access (SBA) system is one of the first platforms combining these two advantages [11]. In the present study the procedural benefit and short term (acute and 7 days follow-up) implantation efficacy of the SBA stent was evaluated in coronary bifurcations of swine. The assessment was performed using in vivo (IVUS, OCT) and ex vivo (micro CT) imaging techniques followed by histology.

Materials and methods

Animal model and preparation

Experiments were performed in Yorkshire-Landrace swine (44 ± 7 kg at implantation). The study was approved by the animal ethics committee of the Erasmus University Rotterdam and complied with the "Guide for the care and use of laboratory animals" (NIH publication 85–23, updated 1996).

After a 300 mg loading dose for both drugs, 75 mg clopidogrel and 100 mg acetylsalicylic acid were administered orally for the whole follow-up period. The animals were sedated (20 mg/kg ketamine hydrochloride and 1 mg/kg midazolam), anesthetized (12 mg/kg thiopental), and artificially ventilated. Anaesthesia was maintained with 0.5–1.5 vol% isoflurane and antibiotic prophylaxis was administered (streptomycin, penicillin procaine, 0.1 mg/kg i.m.). Under sterile conditions an introducer sheath was placed in the left carotid artery. A dose of 250 mg ASA and 10.000 i.u. heparin was administered (i.a.). After intracoronary administration of 2 mg isosorbide dinitrate, coronary angiography was performed (using a CAAS 5.5 system, Pie Medical) using a non-ionic contrast agent (iodixanol). Two orthogonal views were used in order to visualize the vascular architecture and to assess which coronary bifurcations qualify for stent implantation. To this end the MB and SB diameters as well as the distal bifurcation angle were measured.

Stents

SBA stent is a bifurcation-specific device based on the XIENCE V platform having a side portal which opens towards the SB (Figure 14.1). It is a double balloon (single shaft, single inflation) delivery system, the stent being made from a CoCr alloy, 0.0032″ strut thickness, with 100 μg/cm² everolimus in a biocompatible fluorinated copolymer coating: PVDF-HFP D:P = 1:4.9 (w/w). The stents

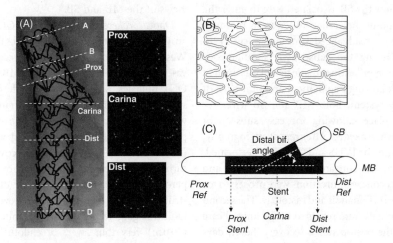

Figure 14.1 (a) Longitudinal and cross-sectional proximal, carina, and distal images of the SBA stent obtained with micro CT; the SBA stent system is based on the XIENCE V platform, but it is provided with a side portal; (b) dotted line, which opens to the side branch during the inflation of the double balloon; (c) Schematic representation of a stented bifurcation indicating the stent segments considered for analysis.

were 18 mm in length and 2.5, 3.0, and 3.5 mm in diameter.

Study groups and time-points

Acute: six SBA implants were analyzed acutely for assessment of the deployment procedure: preservation of vascular anatomy, acute stent recoil, stent symmetry, SB coverage with struts, malapposition of struts in the MB, SB, as well as vascular dissections and acute thrombus formation. QCA, in vivo (IVUS, OCT), and ex vivo (micro CT) imaging and histology techniques were performed.

7 days: seven SBA implants were analyzed both at implantation (baseline) and at 7 days follow-up for stent deployment, stent recoil, endothelialization and thrombus formation.

Stent implantation and follow-up

Under guidance of quantitative angiography, segments of 2.5–3.2 mm in diameter were selected in each of the coronary arteries in order to contain a coronary bifurcation with an SB diameter ≥1.8 mm. Stents were placed with a balloon/artery ratio of 1.1.

SBA was placed in a single procedure after wiring both the MB and SB using a technique similar to that described for the Frontier stent [9]. Briefly, with both wires in place, the device was advanced over the SB in the distal MB. After releasing the joining mandril, the device was withdrawn to allow the SB associated wire to enter the SB. At this point the earlier SB wire was removed and the device readvanced simultaneously in SB and MB. During the subsequent simultaneous double balloon inflation the side portal was opened to the SB. Following deployment and pull-back of the delivery system, both MB and SB wires remained in place, allowing for easy subsequent treatment, when needed. After repeat angiography, in vivo imaging by IVUS and OCT was performed.

Thereafter, the acute animals were sacrificed and the stented coronary bifurcations were processed for ex vivo micro CT analysis and histology. The second group of animals were returned to the animal care facility for the postoperative recovery. Seven days later, follow-up angiography and imaging of the stented arteries by IVUS and OCT were carried out followed by sacrifice of the animals and processing of the arteries for micro CT and histology.

The stent segments (proximal, distal, carina) considered in all analyses are schematically presented in Figure 14.1C.

In vivo imaging

Angiography: angiographical images were obtained repetitively, in multiple projections: 0° and 30°, 45° left and right anterior oblique. The measurements were always performed in two different orientations >45° apart, chosen such as the vessels including the side-branches were best visible. An offline 3D reconstruction of the stented bifurcation was computed in order to better assess the anatomy of the coronary bifurcation.

Intravascular ultra-sound(IVUS) imaging: this was performed using the Boston Scientific Atlantis SR pro system (40 MHz) with an automatic continuous pullback at a rate of 0.5 mm/s. The gray scale IVUS analysis was performed both at baseline and follow-up. Each target bifurcation was divided in three segments, proximal from the bifurcation, the carina (bifurcation point) and distal from the bifurcation. Stents were assessed for stent deployment, strut apposition, vessel trauma (dissections), and preservation of the bifurcation angle.

At follow-up, the stent recoil and tissue coverage of the carina (neointima) was also assessed. Neointimal area was as the area between the stent and the lumen area. The distal bifurcation angle was calculated from two different frames with clear views of the MB and SB.

Optical coherence tomography (OCT) imaging: an OCT wire (ImageWire, LightLab Imaging Inc., Westford, Massachusetts), was advanced through the vascular lumen 5 mm distal to the MB stent and an OCT pullback was performed inside the deployed stent (pullback rate of 3.0 mm/s, 15 frames/s). Stents were assessed for stent expansion, strut apposition, presence of intraluminal tissue, and vessel trauma (dissections). At follow-up, tissue coverage of the carina was also assessed, and data are presented as percentage of covered struts from the total number of struts visible in the section. However, since the OCT imaging technique has a limited resolution (20 μm) very thin layers of endothelium will be missed. Furthermore, since not always all struts at the carina could be carefully assessed for malapposition or thrombus, the stent was scored as positive when at least one strut was malapposed or showed thrombus presence. Therefore, these data should be interpreted with caution.

Ex vivo imaging

Following in vivo imaging the animals were sacrificed, the hearts were flushed with saline, and pressure-perfusion fixed in situ (approximately 100 mmHg) with formaldehyde. The stented arterial segments including 0.5–1 cm proximal and distal to the stent were excised from the epicardial surface and studied by micro computed tomography (micro CT). Thereafter, vessels were embedded in methylmethacrylate (MMA) and prepared for histological analyses.

Micro CT imaging: the 3D reconstruction of the stented bifurcation was performed following scanning with a computer tomography micro-scanner (35 μm resolution). A fly-through 3D reconstruction of the vessel could be computed in order to assess the stent deployment parameters (symmetrical deployment and proximal and distal stent tapering and positioning of the SB opening in relation to the stent length). Proximal tapering was assessed by dividing the calculated cross-sectional stent area at point (A)/area(B), while distal tapering was calculated as stent area (D)/stent area(C), (see Figure 14.1A). Proximal and distal symmetry was calculated as minimal/maximal diameter at the proximal and distal points indicated on Figure 14.1A. A symmetry coefficient cut-off value of 0.8 was considered acceptable. The positioning of the SB opening was considered proximal if the opening was in the first seven strut rings (the total stent had 13–14 rings) of the stent.

Histology: en-block toluidine blue staining was performed on both longitudinal and perpendicular (cross-sections) sections through the branching point (carina) for the assessment of the MB and SB coverage with stent struts, presence of struts in the lumen, malapposition, and distal branching angle. Furthermore a qualitative and quantitative assessment of endothelial coverage of the struts (at 7 days FU), thrombus formation at the struts (in the carina) both in MB and SB, injury and inflammation score, malapposition (both acutely and at 7 days) was performed.

The injury score was defined as follows: 0 = no injury, 1 = media intact, 2 = media rupture, 3 = media and adventitia rupture per strut, while the score per vessel was the average of all struts analysed. The inflammation and thrombus presence were scored as 0 if no inflammatory cells/thrombus were present around the strut and 1 if present; even very small thrombi being scored. The mean score for each artery was calculated as percentage struts showing thrombus or malapposition from the total number of struts in the section.

Statistical analysis

Data are presented as mean ± SD and were analyzed with SPSS (SPSS Inc. version 11.5.0). Differences were assessed using two-way ANOVA. In case of differences between groups or methods, further testing was performed using linear regression analysis. Statistical correlations between bifurcation angle measurements performed with different methods were assessed by Pearson's correlation tests. Statistical significance was considered for P < 0.05.

Results

Procedural characteristics: on average, 26.5 ± 19.0 ml contrast was used for the implantation of a SBA stent.

QCA analysis: the angiographic images analyzed in the same two orientations using both the standard 2D software as well as the new 3D analysis method, indicate no differences in MB or SB diameters pre- or post- stent implantation or at follow-up, between the acute and 7 days animals (Table 14.1). Furthermore, no differences were seen in the distal branching angles either between groups or pre- or post- stent implantation.

The distal angle measurements by 2D and 3D QCA showed a good correlation of the two methods. The linear correlation analysis indicated that all data were situated between the 95% confidence intervals. Further testing by Pearson's correlation test showed a significant coefficient P < 0.001. Also no differences in acute gain or late loss in the SB were seen between the two methods (P = NS by ANOVA).

IVUS analysis: indicates similar vascular diameters of both the MB and SB between groups, both at baseline and follow-up (Table 14.2). Also similar and very small neointima areas were seen. Furthermore, no tissue deposition, no dissections

Table 14.1 2D and 3D QCA measurements of SBA (N = 6 implants acute and 7 at 7 days FU)

2D QCA	Acute	7 days
Pre		
MB prox (mm)	3.07 ± 0.24	3.21 ± 0.22
MB dist (mm)	2.61 ± 0.26	2.69 ± 0.24
SB (mm)	1.98 ± 0.27	1.91 ± 0.33
Distal branching angle (°)	54 ± 17	51 ± 28
Post		
MB prox (mm)	3.50 ± 0.40	3.53 ± 0.45
MB dist (mm)	2.95 ± 0.51	3.08 ± 0.45
SB (mm)	1.94 ± 0.21	2.02 ± 0.29
Distal branching angle (°)	52 ± 19	49 ± 18
Acute gain MB prox	0.44 ± 0.31	0.33 ± 0.35
Acute gain MB dist	0.34 ± 0.32	0.39 ± 0.31
Acute gain SB	−0.04 ± 0.17	0.13 ± 0.09
FU		
MB prox (mm)		3.33 ± 0.37
MB dist (mm)		2.93 ± 0.31
SB (mm)		1.70 ± 0.32
Distal branching angle (°)		48 ± 19
LL MB prox		0.21 ± 0.14
LL MB dist		0.14 ± 0.18
LL SB		0.32 ± 0.18
3D QCA		
Pre		
MB (mm)	2.98 ± 0.27	2.89 ± 0.30
SB (mm)	2.12 ± 0.24	1.86 ± 0.26
Distal branching angle (°)	67 ± 28	47 ± 28
Post		
MB (mm)	3.57 ± 0.46	3.31 ± 0.58
SB (mm)	2.15 ± 0.25	1.98 ± 0.30
Distal branching angle (°)	54 ± 22	48 ± 23
Acute gain MB	0.57 ± 0.21	0.41 ± 0.56
Acute gain SB	0.06 ± 0.19	0.10 ± 0.27
FU		
MB (mm)		3.20 ± 0.56
SB (mm)		1.68 ± 0.43
Distal branching angle (°)		46 ± 13
LL MB		0.13 ± 0.12
LL SB		0.26 ± 0.14

and no malapposition of the stent struts could be detected by IVUS, suggesting that this technique might not be sensitive enough to detect small malappositions. The symmetry indexes were above 0.8 both in the MB and SB. However, measurements of distal bifurcation angles by IVUS showed significantly lower values than those measured by both 2D

and 3D QCA (P = 0.02 IVUS vs 2D QCA and P = 0.006 IVUS vs 3D QCA by ANOVA).

OCT analysis: examples of the OCT images including normal strut coverage, presence of intraluminal tissue (possibly thrombus) on the struts, and media dissections are presented in Figure 14.2 (6,7,8). Each vessel was divided in three segments (proximal, carina, distal), and the data are presented in Table 14.2. Since in some vessels the large diameter in the carina did not allow for a resolution high enough for reliable measurements, data are not presented when less than three animals/group are available. Stent diameters proximal and distal to the carina for the vessels measured, both at implantation and follow-up, show a very good reproducibility by OCT. Three of the 12 stents showed proximal dissection, one showed dissection in the carina and one showed a distal dissection at implantation. One dissection in the proximal reference segment was still present at 7 days follow-up. All other dissections seen in the chronic group were repaired at follow-up.

Micro CT analysis: the 3D reconstruction of the stented segments was used for the assessment of the symmetry of the stent cells (longitudinal view, Figure 14.1A), tapering and symmetry of the proximal and distal segments of the MB (cross-sectional view, Figure 14.1A) as well as the positioning of the branching point in relation to the total stent length. Data from both follow-up times were pooled. No proximal or distal *tapering* was seen, as indicated by a tapering coefficient (minimal/maximal diameter ratio) of 0.96 ± 0.12 in the proximal part of the stent and 1.00 ± 0.08 distally. *Symmetry* assessment indicated symmetric deployment in all stents, since the minimal/maximal diameter ratio was close to 1 (0.96 ± 0.05 proximally and 0.95 ± 0.04 distally). By design the *SB positioning* was always at ring eight (from distal to proximal, 14 rings in total).

Histology: endothelial coverage at 7 days was similar in the MB and SB (~40%). Low levels of inflammation and low injury scores were observed in all stents, irrespective of follow-up time. Most vessels had an intact media, although the intima was sometimes very compressed and intima ruptures could be eventually seen. Data are summarized in Table 14.3.

A good support of the SB ostium was seen, as 5 ± 2 struts were counted in SB, being positioned

Table 14.2 IVUS and OCT data obtained both in the acute and 7 days groups

IVUS		Acute	7 days	
		Baseline	Baseline	7 days
MB Stent diameter (mm)	Prox.	3.46 ± 0.50	3.97 ± 0.71	3.57 ± 0.68
	carina	3.73 ± 0.74	4.13 ± 0.82	3.61 ± 0.67
	Dist.	3.04 ± 0.55	3.42 ± 0.65	3.21 ± 0.61
MB Stent symmetry index	Prox.	0.81 ± 0.08	0.85 ± 0.05	0.85 ± 0.05
	carina	0.79 ± 0.02	0.79 ± 0.06	0.79 ± 0.05
	Dist.	0.89 ± 0.05	0.91 ± 0.03	0.90 ± 0.03
SB Lumen diam. (mm)		2.22 ± 0.23	2.42 ± 0.38	2.11 ± 0.17
SB Lumen symm.		0.90 ± 0.00	0.87 ± 0.05	0.89 ± 0.05
Angle (°)		37 ± 11	24 ± 12	37 ± 23
OCT				
Stent diameter (mm)	Prox.	3.23 ± 0.25	3.37 ± 0.31	3.34 ± 0.36
	carina	3.96 ± 0.32	NA	3.60 ± 0.38
	Dist.	3.17 ± 0.32	3.22 ± 0.33	3.27 ± 0.29
Strut coverage with tissue (carina) (% struts)		–	–	32 ± 46
Malapposition carina (% stents)		67%	80%	67%
Thrombus carina (% stents)		17%	0%	33%

mostly distal to the flow divider. Limited malapposition of stent struts in the MB was observed, however, a higher percentage malapposition was observed in the stent struts placed in the SB, $41 \pm 26\%$ of the total number of struts were malapposed (Figure 14.2). In the 7 days group, the percentage malapposed struts were similar in both MB and SB. In total 33% of the stents in SBA acute

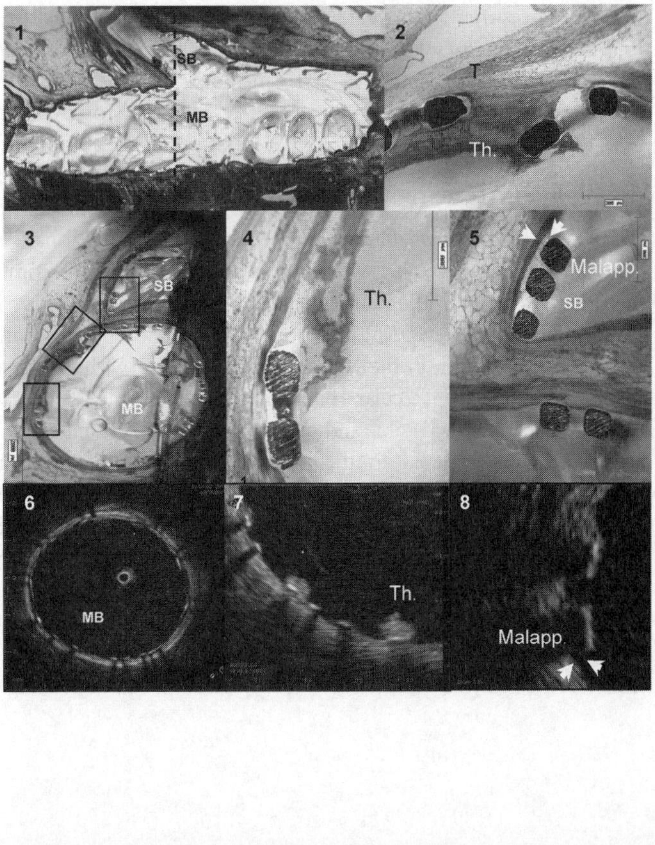

Figure 14.2 Overview and details of a longitudinal (**1**) and cross-section (**3**) of a coronary artery receiving a SBA stent. The dotted line in the longitudinal view shows the location of the cross-section, showing the MB and SB. Medial tearing by the stent struts (T) with adherent thrombus (Th) and placement of the struts in the side branch are clearly visible (**2, 4**). Arrows indicate malapposition of stent struts in the SB (**5**). The same features could also be seen in the OCT images (**6, 7, 8**).

Table 14.3 Macroscopic assessment of the percentage endothelial coverage of the stent struts, injury and inflammation scores, malapposition, thrombus presence around the struts in the cross-section through the vessel bifurcation (carina) and distal bifurcation angles in both acute and 7 days group

Stent	Thrombus (%)	EC %	Injury score	Inflammation score	Malapposition (%)	Distal bifurcation angle (°)
Acute group	11 ± 11	0.00 ± 0.00	1.22 ± 0.15	0.05 ± 0.00	5 ± 8	47 ± 11
7 days group	40 ± 34	42.90 ± 13.10	1.03 ± 0.16	0.13 ± 0.00	14 ± 23	47 ± 17

and 43% in SBA chronic group showed at least one malapposed strut on histology.

In the acute group, 10–15% of the struts showed signs of thrombus formation with no differences being seen between MB and SB (Figure 14.2). In the 7 days group, slightly higher percentage of thrombus formation were seen (40–50% of the struts) although the differences did not reach statistical significance due to the small sample size.

Presence of stent struts in the lumen of the carina was assessed at both follow-up times. In the acute group 33% of the vessels showed ostial stent jailed SB versus 57% in the 7 days group.

The measurement of distal bifurcation angles on the longitudinal en-block sections correlated with the same measurements by 2D and 3D QCA as indicated by Pearson's correlation tests, (P = 0.002 en-block vs 2D QCA, and P = 0.002 en-block vs 3D QCA).

Discussion

The present study shows that the new Abbott SBA stent can be safely deployed with good procedural outcome. The main findings are that the SBA stent shows good results regarding the preservation of luminal diameter both in the MB and SB, and the preservation of the vascular branching angles. The side branch was accessible and most of the stent struts were well apposed to the luminal surface without major modification of the stent pattern during deployment. The stents were uniformly deployed and supported well the ostium as shown by the coverage of the SB with stent struts, mainly opposite to the flow divider. An additional positive aspect is the rather low volume of contrast agent needed for the implantation of the SBA stent.

However, the results also indicate that bifurcation stenting remains accompanied by vascular damage as shown by the presence of thrombus and vascular dissections. Further studies, including histology of longitudinal sections of the stented vessels are required in order to assess the chronic neointimal response to the stents.

Implantation technique

Percutaneous coronary intervention on ostial lesions carry technical challenges related to the size of the SB and its orientation relative to the MB (bifurcation angle) [12], as well as the position of the plaque and possible obstruction of the SB due to plaque shift. Provisional stenting of the MB across the branching point confers an additional level of complexity to the percutaneous treatment of the SB since the stent struts may jail the SB and impede the access of the guide wire or balloon to the SB. Moreover, potential complications of balloon dilatation of side branches through stent struts include device entrapment as well as deformation of the stent cells in the parent vessel, resulting in additional vessel trauma. Most of these problems are overcome by the SBA stent since its deployment requires a single inflation of a double balloon opening both the MB and SB at the same time without the need of rewiring the SB. Furthermore, the SB is easily accessible for imaging and if necessary extra treatment. The stent cells remained uniform in size and stent deformation or tapering was hardly seen, suggesting good uniform deployment of the SBA stents.

Technically demanding procedures, such as stenting of coronary bifurcations or percutaneous revascularization of total occlusions, are associated with the use of large volume of contrast-medium and prolonged X-ray exposure. This may result in an increased risk for contrast-induced nephropathy associated with a prolonged recovery period and a poor prognosis in these patients [13,14]. Although the X-ray exposure was not quantified, one important advantage of the SBA stent implantation technique is the low amount of contrast used at implantation, lowering the probability of contrast-induced nephropathy occurrence.

Stent deployment and patency

No statistical differences were observed in the vascular diameters and bifurcation angles pre- or post-implantation or at follow-up, indicating that the SBA stent preserves well the vascular geometry of the bifurcation.

It has been shown that a wide bifurcation angle ($>50°$) was one of the predictors for restenosis at the bifurcation ostium [15] after crush stenting technique, while a small bifurcation angle ($<40°$) predicted a higher SB compromise during the provisional MB stenting [12]. The data reported here showed no correlation between the stent area in the MB or SB and the distal bifurcation angle in the SBA stent indicating that the device is effective over a range of bifurcating angulations. The SBA stent showed a good coverage with stents struts in the SB, the struts being seen mainly opposite to the flow divider. This is beneficial as it has been shown that low shear stress areas opposite to the flow divider correspond to the areas showing most plaque development in human coronary bifurcations [16].

Imaging methods

The present study employed different imaging techniques, aside the standard histology, to give a wide description of the deployment parameters and the effects of stenting on the vessel wall. While comparison of the results obtained with the different methods was not always possible, some advantages or pitfalls became clear indicating that each study parameter is best assessed by a different technique as not all techniques are equally sensitive.

Thus, the 3D QCA analysis provides a more reliable assessment of the vascular architecture than the classical 2D QCA. Although a good correlation was seen between both methods and the histology in branching angle measurement, the 3D method takes into account the 3D branching architecture of the stented coronary, which is underestimated by the 2D method.

Strut malapposition and dissection was best identified by OCT in vivo, since IVUS was not sensitive enough to detect these parameters. Malapposition assessment by OCT did not always correlate with histology indicating less overall malapposition (total number of stents showing malapposed struts) than OCT. A possible explanation for this discrepancy may be the tissue shrinkage post-fixation, which can affect the histology results. In contrast, OCT has a lower resolution than histology in detecting early endothelial coverage and thrombus around the stent struts. The stent symmetry, tapering, and the positioning of the opening towards the SB is best assessed by micro CT, due to the high resolution of this imaging technique.

In conclusion, the new Abbott dedicated SBA stent is safe, shows good preservation of the vascular architecture, including the SB ostium and is potentially superior to the clinical DES on long term in preventing restenosis due to the easy implantation procedure and good SB coverage.

Acknowledgements

The article is dedicated to Wim van der Giessen who sadly passed away in June 2011.

References

1 Gijsen FJ *et al.* A new imaging technique to study 3-D plaque and shear stress distribution in human coronary artery bifurcations in vivo. J Biomech 2007;40 (11):2349–57.

2 Helderman F *et al.* Effect of shear stress on vascular inflammation and plaque development. Current Opinion Lipidol 2007;18(5):527–33.

3 Lefevre T *et al.* Stenting of bifurcation lesions: classification, treatments, and results. Catheter Cardiovasc Interv 2000;49(3):274–83.

4 Stankovic G *et al.* Percutaneous coronary intervention for bifurcation lesions: 2008 consensus document from the fourth meeting of the European Bifurcation Club. EuroIntervention 2009;5(1):39–49.

5 Steigen TK *et al.* Randomized study on simple versus complex stenting of coronary artery bifurcation lesions: the Nordic bifurcation study. Circulation 2006;114 (18):1955–61.

6 Sheiban I *et al.* Very long-term results comparing a simple versus a complex stenting strategy in the treatment of coronary bifurcation lesions. Catheter Cardiovasc Interv 2009.

7 Jensen JS *et al.* Safety in simple versus complex stenting of coronary artery bifurcation lesions. The Nordic bifurcation study 14-month follow-up results. EuroIntervention 2008;4(2):229–33.

8 Radke PW *et al.* Evaluation of the dedicated Frontier coronary bifurcation stent: A matched pair analysis with drug-eluting and bare metal stents. Clin Res Cardiol 2008;97(4):260–5.

9 Lefevre T *et al.* The Frontier stent registry: safety and feasibility of a novel dedicated stent for the treatment of bifurcation coronary artery lesions. J Am Coll Cardiol 2005;46(4):592–8.

10 Colombo A *et al.* Randomized study to evaluate sirolimus-eluting stents implanted at coronary bifurcation lesions. Circulation 2004;109(10):1244–9.

11 Sheiban I *et al.* Update on dedicated bifurcation stents. J Intervent Cardiol 2009;22(2):150–5.

12 Gil RJ *et al.* The carina angle-new geometrical parameter associated with periprocedural side branch compromise and the long-term results in coronary bifurcation lesions with main vessel stenting only. J Intervent Cardiol 2009.

13 McCullough PA *et al.* Acute renal failure after coronary intervention: incidence, risk factors, and relationship to mortality. Am J Med 1997;103(5):368–75.

14 Aguiar-Souto P *et al.* Frequency and predictors of contrast-induced nephropathy after angioplasty for chronic total occlusions. Int J Cardiol 2008.

15 Dzavik V *et al.* Predictors of long-term outcome after crush stenting of coronary bifurcation lesions: importance of the bifurcation angle. AmHeart J 2006;152(4): 762–9.

16 van der Giessen AG *et al.* Plaque and shear stress distribution in human coronary bifurcations: a multislice computed tomography study. EuroIntervention 2009;4(5):654–61.

CHAPTER 15

Devices: TriReme

Ricardo A. Costa, MD[1,2]*, Gary Binyamin,* PhD[3]*,*
Eitan Konstantino, PhD[3] *and Alexandre Abizaid,* MD, PhD[1,2,4]

[1]Instituto Dante Pazzanese de Cardiologia, São Paulo, SP, Brazil
[2]Cardiovascular Research Center, São Paulo, SP, Brazil
[3]TriReme Medical, Inc., Pleasanton, CA, USA
[4]Columbia University Medical Center, New York, NY, USA

Introduction

Percutaneous coronary intervention (PCI) in bifurcation lesions generally attempts to obtain an optimal result in the main vessel (MV) while maintaining adequate patency of the side branch (SB) [1]. The provisional stenting technique in particular has been supported by several clinical trials, as general outcomes favoring the simpler, staged approaches have been concordant [2–5]. In selected lesions, clinical outcomes with provisional stenting have been similar to, or better than, more complex procedures where stenting of both the MV and SB was mandated [6]. Nevertheless, single or provisional stenting procedures with conventional (straight or tubular) stents require access through the MV stent struts to the SB; potentially requiring multiple passages of wires and balloons, with the risk of SB access loss [7]. Inability to cross the MV stent struts and losing SB access poses challenges for performing SB procedures [8]. Stent manipulations resulting from SB access may lead to unpredictable strut distribution, strut malapposition, cell distortion, and multiple metal layers. Mechanical manipulation of tubular stents, to fit bifurcation anatomy, poses a risk of local vascular injury in the transition zone between the MV and SB, in addition to the unknown performance of altered stents and potential deleterious impact to drug-eluting

coatings [9–12]. These challenges increase both procedural risks and patient outcomes; including an increased risk of dissection, perforation, or SB occlusion. It is reported that SB compromise due to MV stenting, at the location of a major SB, occurs in 12–16% of cases [13–15]. Persistent major SB compromise is associated with increased myocardial necrosis and peri-procedural myocardial infarction. Thus, even though SB stenoses are not always hemodynamically significant by physiological assessment [16], their compromise during the procedure is still a matter of concern for interventionalists.

Anatomic characterization of coronary bifurcations

The morphology of a bifurcation has been demonstrated to be complex and can impact the local flow dynamics [1,17]. A study by Russell *et al.* reported an ex-vivo characterization of coronary bifurcation lesions, evaluating the intersections by measuring diameters, angles, and shapes at the SB ostium in human coronary arteries. In this analysis, a complex and asymmetric geometry was demonstrated at the MV-SB transition zone (carina) of the bifurcation. In particular, polymer casts of the human coronary tree in 23 human adult cadavers were used to characterize the morphology of the SB

Bifurcation Stenting, First Edition. Edited by Ron Waksman and John A. Ormiston.
© 2012 Blackwell Publishing Ltd. Published 2012 by Blackwell Publishing Ltd.

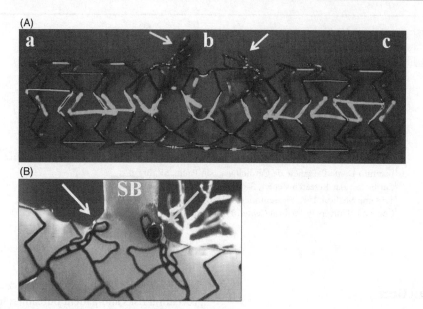

Figure 15.1 (a) Longitudinal view of the bifurcation dedicated TMI Antares stent: [a] proximal end of the stent; [b] SB aperture including the proprietary OP (Ostial Preservation) structure matching bifurcation morphology, localized in the middle of the stent; and [c] distal end of the stent. Dotted arrow indicates the proximal wing of the OP structure (with radiopaque markers), solid arrow indicates the distal wing. The OP structure is designed to adapt to the asymmetric geometry of the bifurcation carina as well as to provide optimal scaffolding of the SB ostium; (b) Image of the TMI Antares stent deployed within a porcine coronary bifurcation (cast model). The proximal wing taking the proximal "transition" angle (dotted arrow) and distal wing taking the distal "transition" angle (solid arrow). By design, the asymmetric OP structure allows treatment of bifurcation lesions with any angulations between the two distal branches. SB = side branch.

vessels relative to the MV, and results demonstrated SB with increased vessel tapering compared to the MV within the bifurcation length, and relative reductions in vessel diameter from proximal MV to distal MV and SB. Regarding bifurcation angles, the mean proximal and distal angles (intersection angles commonly assessed by angiography) for non-LM locations were $136.4 \pm 22.0°$ and $57.5 \pm 24.7°$, respectively. Interestingly, analysis of the transition of the SB take-off depicted a curvilinear geometry, rather than a bisecting angle represented by two straight tubes intersecting, given that the mean proximal and distal "transition" angles (consisting of a proximal and distal angle measured from the MV at the SB take-off level) in non-LM locations were obtuse (150.1 ± 21.2 degrees and 111.3 ± 29.6 degrees, respectively) as opposed to complimentary (proximal) obtuse and (distal) acute intersection angles. In addition, SB ostial lumen cross-sectional areas demonstrated asymmetry, presenting with an actual elliptical shape in the majority of cases rather than round [18].

Dedicated bifurcation devices may address some of the unmet needs for bifurcation PCI including: continuous access to the SB; optimal shape within the bifurcation anatomy; SB ostium scaffold; and a modular approach for different lesion complexity [10].

Device description

The TriReme Medical Inc (TMI) (Pleasanton, CA, USA) Antares® Coronary Stent System is a CE Mark approved, low-profile, dedicated bifurcation stent that incorporates a balloon expandable, stainless steel stent with a proprietary Ostial Preservation (OP) structure in the center of the stent (Figure 15.1a). The system is designed to provide continuous access to the SB throughout the stenting procedure as well as scaffold to the SB ostium. The OP structure was developed to adapt to the asymmetric ostial anatomy found in coronary bifurcations and includes a proximal wing and a shallower distal wing; both of which are deployed into the SB on expansion of the stent through the inflation of a single balloon (Figure 15.1b).

The TMI Antares Coronary Stent delivery system is a torqueable, RX (rapid-exchange), one-balloon, two-wire catheter compatible with standard 0.014″ coronary guide wires and high flow 6F guiding catheters (the usable length is approximately 135 cm). Two radiopaque markers are inside the balloon with additional markers at the center of the stent, to allow for positioning and orientation of the stent at the junction. An important feature of the TMI Antares Coronary Stent System is the side wire management system, which includes a pre-loaded 0.014″ SB wire within a dedicated SB wire lumen having peel-away access in the shaft of the delivery system; this prevents wire-to-wire tangling and allows for continuous access to the SB throughout a procedure. Prior to stent deployment, the stent system is advanced to the bifurcation and rotated into alignment, so that the OP structure is facing the SB. The SB wire is then advanced into the SB and the stent is deployed with single balloon inflation. Following stent deployment, the SB wire is released from the proximal end of the delivery system and the delivery system is removed. SB access is constant without the need to "jail" a wire or cross through the side of the stent with a wire due to the OP structure deployment. Preservation of SB access allows modular SB treatment options, including post-dilatation and, if required, SB stent placement following the Antares stent deployment.

The Antares® Coronary Stent System was designed to facilitate provisional stenting by overcoming the acute procedural and mechanical challenges posed by using conventional straight stents at or near a major SB. It is available in size range of 3.0–3.5 mm for the MV, and 2.5 and above for the SB, and in length of 14 mm. Its indication includes lesions in non-left main locations involving coronary vessels 3.0–3.5 mm in diameter with or without significant involvement of a major SB (≥2.5 mm).

Procedure

Figures 15.2 and 15.3 depict two cases with technical details regarding positioning, deployment and procedure.

Clinical trials

First-in-human study

The preliminary clinical evaluation of the Antares technology for bifurcation lesions included a subset of patients treated at Institute Dante Pazzanese of Cardiology, São Paulo, Brazil. Overall, nine patients with single, *de novo* coronary lesion with >50% stenosis involving a bifurcation in non-left main location were consecutively enrolled in this first-in-human trial. The objective of this study was to investigate the safety, feasibility and performance of the Antares stent including procedural and early (30-day) outcomes. Angiographic criteria were: lesion length in the MV ≤10 mm; and vessel size 3.0–3.5 mm in the MV, and 2.0–3.0 mm in the SB. Angiographic analysis was performed by an independent angiographic core laboratory following the recommendations of the European Bifurcation Angiographic Subcommittee [19]. The majority of lesions (5/9) were located in the LAD/Diagonal, with two lesions found in both LCx and distal RCA (i.e. PDA/PLSA). By the Medina classification [20], 67% of lesions (6/9) had significant involvement of the SB ostium (type 1,1,1 in three cases; 1,0,1 in two cases, and 0,1,1 in one case), and 33% (n = 3) were classified as Medina 1,1,0; also, the mean intersection (proximal) angle was 137.7°, and the "carina" (distal) angle was 65.1°. Regarding procedure, MV and SB predilatation were performed in 8/9 cases, and the Antares stent was successfully implanted in all cases; an additional stent in the SB was implanted in two cases, and final kissing-balloon (FKB) inflation was performed in 56% (5/9). At final procedure, both branches had TIMI 3 flow, and procedural success (residual stenosis <50% in the MV with maintenance of SB access) was achieved in all cases. By QCA, preprocedural lesion length, reference diameter and percent diameter stenosis (DS) were: 11.85 mm, 2.71 mm, and 61.3% in the MV, and 4.32 mm, 2.14 mm, and 47% in the SB, respectively. At post-procedure, mean in-lesion percentage DS was 19.1% in the MV and 35% in the SB. Up to 30-day follow-up, there was neither death nor myocardial infarction. At 6-month angiographic follow-up, performed in eight cases, there was one restenosis in the MV, and mean late lumen loss was 0.79 mm in the MV and 0.43 mm in the SB 5 mm ostium [21].

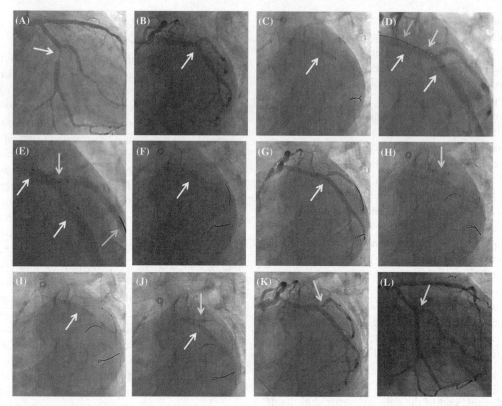

Figure 15.2 Coronary bifurcation lesion involving the mid-LCx/1st OM branch with significant involvement of the distal MV (RAO/caudal view; (a) and mild disease involving the SB ostium (LAO/caudal view; (b) with distal (carina) angle ~90°; (c) Predilatation of the MV; (d) Advancement of the dedicated bifurcation TMI Antares stent into the bifurcation lesion site: solid arrows indicate the proximal and distal markers of the delivery balloon located at the proximal and distal ends of the stent; dotted arrow indicates the stent markers delimiting the SB aperture with the OP preservation structure in the middle of the stent; dashed arrow indicates the SB wire encapsulated in the SB wire lumen (system prevents wire-to-wire tangling); (e) TMI Antares stent placed in the bifurcation lesion site. The dedicated stent is delivered with a single balloon expandable delivery system, which allows for active alignment and rotation to align the central opening of the stent (SB aperture) with the SB ostium. At this point, optimal positioning of the system is achieved by rotating the catheter and advancing a preloaded SB guidewire into the distal SB. The middle marker positioned at the SB (dotted arrow) and the distal wire in the SB (dashed arrow) indicate adequate positioning of the device (solid arrows indicate proximal and distal ends of the stent); (f) Implant of the TMI Antares stent. Of note is the fact that the OP structure is automatically deployed as the main body of the stent expands, with elements (wings, Figure 15.1) protruding approximately 2 mm into the SB to optimize scaffold at the ostium; (g) Angiographic result after TMI Antares stent deployment; (h) Single postdilatation of the SB ostium, which can be performed by advancing the balloon-catheter into the SB over the SB guidewire; without the need for wire re-crossing; (i) Single postdilatation of the TMI Antares stent in the MV; (j) Performance of final kissing-balloon inflation; (k) Final angiographic result with optimal SB scaffold (LAO/caudal view); (l) Final angiographic result with optimal SB scaffold (LAO/caudal view). LAO = left anterior oblique; MV = main vessel; OP = ostial preservation; RAO = right anterior oblique; SB = side branch.

TMI ostial preservation trial

Following, in the prospective, multicenter, single-arm TOP (TMI ostial preservation) study, 56 non-left main bifurcation lesions involving vessels with diameter 3.0–3.5 mm in the MV, and 2.0–3.0 mm in the SB were included. Overall, 62.4% of lesions had significant involvement of both MV and SB (Medina type 1,1,1 in 48.2%, and 0,1,1 in 7.1%), with remaining Medina lesion types as follows: 1,1,0 in 23.2%, 1,0,0 in 7.1%, 1,0,1 in 7.1%, 0,1,0

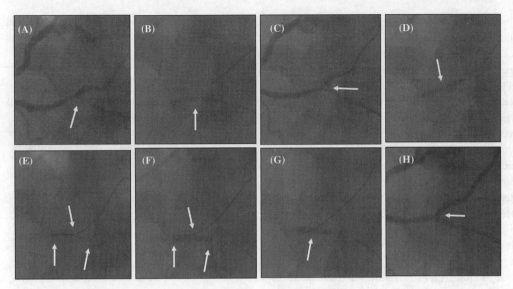

Figure 15.3 (a) Coronary bifurcation lesion involving the distal RCA (PDA/PLSA) with significant involvement of the MV (Medina 1,1,0) (cranial view); (b) Predilatation of the MV; (c) Angiographic result after MV predilatation demonstrating significant compromise of the SB due to plaque (or carina) shift; (d) Predilatation of the SB; (e) TMI Antares stent positioned at the site of the bifurcation lesion – dotted arrow indicates the middle marker with optimal positioning at the SB; solid arrows indicate proximal and distal ends of the stent; (f) Implant of the TMI Antares stent (OP structure automatically deployed during stent implant in the MV); (g) Single post dilatation of the TMI Antares stent in the PV; (h) Final angiographic result with optimal SB scaffold. MV = main vessel; OP = Ostial Preservation; SB = side branch.

in 5.4% and 0,0,1 in 1.8%. Regarding procedure, the Antares stent was successfully implanted in 100% of cases as there was no failure to reach the lesion site due to wire-wrap. After deployment of the Antares stent in the MV, wire access was evidenced in all SB, and treatment (in the SB) was performed as follows: 12.5% no further treatment, 67.9% balloon postdilatation only, 19.6% (additional) stent implanted (Taxus® Liberté® mandatory by protocol), and FKB in 69.6%; at the end, all lesions had <50% DS in the MV and 55/56 SBs had final TIMI 3 flow. Three patients had major adverse cardiac events (MACE) during index hospitalization, and only five patients experienced MACE up to 30 days follow-up [22].

Post-marketing evaluation

Lastly, a post-marketing (PM) evaluation of the Antares stent included 48 patients treated by 17 operators in multiple clinical sites. In this study, 62.5% of lesions were located in LAD/diagonal, 18.8% in LCx/OM, and 16.7% in RCA (i.e. PDA/ PLSA), and lesion complexity according to the Medina classification was: 1,1,1 in 39.6%, 1,0,1 in 10.4%, 0,1,1 in 12.5%, 1,1,0 in 18.8% 1,0,0 in 4.2%, 0,1,0 in 8.3%, and 0,0,1 in 6.3%. During procedure, SB wire access was successfully maintained in 91.1% of cases (41/45), and SB treatment included: 37.5% no further treatment, 62.5% balloon post-dilatation only, and 14.6% (additional) stent implanted; also, post-procedural TIMI 3 in the MV and SB was reported in all cases. Regarding procedural duration, the total procedure time from Antares insertion to completion of the intervention was 22.4 ± 12.2 minutes, including MV post-dilatation and/or further treatment in the SB (post-dilatation, stent implantation, FKB).

Technical considerations

Recent randomized clinical trials comparing simple (provisional) versus complex approach in selected bifurcation lesions demonstrated cross-over rates of 3–31% from single to double stenting in order to optimize results in the SB [2–5].

Furthermore, double stenting strategies have been reported in about 36–45% of cases in real world clinical series [23,24]. With the Antares technology, an additional stent in the SB was needed in 14–20% of cases [21,22]. In general, SB stenting is required when SB is compromised (significant residual stenosis, dissection, impaired flow and/or vessel occlusion) during bifurcation PCI, which appears to be directly related to the degree of anatomic/morphologic complexity of the lesion [25]. Importantly, with provisional approach using conventional (straight) coronary stents, further treatment in the SB tends to add complexity (more material, contrast, cost) and unpredictability as re-access to the SB may be laborious (sometimes unfeasible) despite having skilled operators and training [2,4]. In addition, inadequate SB ostial coverage, incomplete stent apposition at the carina, significant ostial underexpansion, strut deformation, poor SB accessibility, and wire tangling are frequently encountered with current double stenting techniques, which have been associated with PCI failure even with drug-eluting stents [11,12,26]. The TMI Antares stent design allows for modular treatment of bifurcation lesion, with a primary provisional approach, but without penalty for further treatment in the SB if needed. In the provisional arms of the NORDIC, BBC ONE (British bifurcation coronary study: old, new, and evolving strategies), BBK (bifurcations Bad Krozingen), and CACTUS (coronary bifurcations: applications of the crushing technique using sirolimus-eluting stents) trials, SB stent was implanted in 4.3%, 3%, 18.8%, 31%; and FKB was performed in 32%, 29%, 100%, 90.2%, respectively [2–5]. Of note is the fact that, to date, no consensus has been reached regarding the optimal SB result with provisional approach, as exemplified by the different criteria used in these trials (Table 15.1). With TMI Antares stent, successful SB access post-MV stenting was 100%, 100%, and 98% for Dante Pazzanese, TOP, and PM studies, respectively; also, SB single post-dilatation was performed in 61.5% (TOP) and 67% (PM); SB stenting was performed in 22.2% (Dante Pazzanese), 17.9% (TOP), and 14% (PM); and FKB was performed in 56% (Dante Pazzanese) and 71.8% (PM), given that all cases achieved final TIMI 3 flow in both branches. Furthermore, the

Table 15.1 Criteria to stent the SB in lesions primarily approached with single (provisional) stenting in previous randomized clinical trials

Study	Criteria
NORDIC [2]	After MV stenting, SB dilatation was recommended if TIMI flow <3. Further treatment with stenting was performed if TIMI flow = 0 after SB dilatation.
CACTUS [3]	After MV stenting, SB was stented if residual stenosis ≥50%, dissection ≥type B, or TIMI flow ≤2.
BBC-ONE [4]	After MV stenting, SB was not treated unless TIMI flow <3, severe ostial pinching (>90%), threatened (SB) vessel closure, or dissection >type A. If one of these criteria existed, kissing-balloon inflation was performed. The SB was not further treated unless TIMI flow <3, persisted ostial pinching (>70%), threatened (SB) vessel closure, or dissection >type A. If one of these criteria remained, SB stenting was performed.
BBK [5]	After MV stenting, post-dilatation with kissing balloon was recommended. Further treatment with stenting was performed if presence of flow limiting dissection or residual stenosis of ≥75%.

MV = main vessel; SB = side branch; TIMI = thrombolysis in myocardial infarction

provisional stenting with the TMI Antares stent appears to simplified the procedure as demonstrated by the relatively shorter mean procedural time (22.5 ± 12.6 minutes) [22] versus NORDIC (62 ± 51 vs 76 ± 40 minutes) [2], BBC ONE (57 vs 78 minutes) [4], and BBK (51 ± 23 vs 56 ± 25 minutes) [5], for provisional versus double stenting groups, respectively.

Finally, a qualitative analysis assessed the overall performance of the Antares stent compared against conventional provisional stenting approach considering eight parameters, including: (a) overall ease of use, (b) predictable outcome, (c) ability to complete SB treatment, (d) SB access, (e) wire management, (f) maintain SB access, (g) MV lesion cross, and (h) tracking. Overall, operators found the Antares stent significantly better in regard to predictable outcome, SB access, wire management, and maintaining SB access; also, there was a non-significant trend favoring the Antares stent in regard to overall ease of use and ability to complete SB treatment, but similar performance considering MV lesion cross and tracking [22].

Considerations and future directions

Even with a single stent approach, maintenance of SB access during bifurcation PCI remains critical. Provisional stenting is a multi-step procedure that can be protracted if recurrent passes into SB with various wires and balloons and/or stents are required. The Antares Coronary Stent System provides continuous SB access without jailed wires, wire tangling or need for re-wiring. Overall, it has been demonstrated to be highly effective on maintaining SB access during PCI in complex bifurcation morphology. Preliminary clinical data have shown that treatment success and clinical outcomes are reasonable with the Antares Coronary Stent System. Continued accumulation of clinical experience will provide necessary information on the long-term outcomes of the device.

References

1 Costa RA, Kyono H, Costa M, Russell M, Moussa ID. Coronary artery bifurcation lesions: Anatomy. In Moussa ID, Colombo A, eds. Tips and Tricks in Interventional Therapy of Coronary Bifurcation Lesions. 1st ed. London, Informa Healthcare, 2010.

2 Steigen TK, Maeng M, Wiseth R, Erglis A, Kumsars I, Narbute I, et al. Randomized study on simple versus complex stenting of coronary artery bifurcation lesions: the Nordic bifurcation study. Circulation 2006;114(18): 1955–61.

3 Colombo A, Bramucci E, Sacca S, Violini R, Lettieri C, Zanini R, et al. Randomized study of the crush technique versus provisional side-branch stenting in true coronary bifurcations: the CACTUS (Coronary bifurcations: application of the crushing technique using sirolimus-eluting stents) Study. Circulation 2009;119(1):71–8.

4 Hildick-Smith D, de Belder AJ, Cooter N, Curzen NP, Clayton TC, Oldroyd KG, et al. Randomized trial of simple versus complex drug-eluting stenting for bifurcation lesions. The British Bifurcation Coronary Study: Old, New, and Evolving Strategies. Circulation 2010;121(10):1235–43..

5 Ferenc M, Gick M, Kienzle RP, Bestehorn HP, Werner KD, Comberg T, et al. Randomized trial on routine vs. provisional T-stenting in the treatment of de novo coronary bifurcation lesions. Eur Heart J 2008;29(23):2859–67.

6 Brar SS, Gray WA, Dangas G, Leon MB, Aharonian VJ, Brar SK, et al. Bifurcation stenting with drug-eluting stents: a systematic review and meta-analysis of randomised trials. EuroIntervention 2009;5(4):475–84.

7 Lefèvre T, Darremont O, Albiero R. Provisional side branch stenting for the treatment of bifurcation lesions. EuroIntervention 2010;6(Supplement J): J65–J71.

8 Burzotta F, De Vita M, Sgueglia G, Todaro D. How to solve difficult side branch access? EuroIntervention 2010;6(Supplement J): J72–J80.

9 Mortier P, De Beule M, Dubini G, Hikichi Y, Murasato Y, Ormiston J. Coronary bifurcation stenting: insights from in vitro and virtual bench testing. EuroIntervention 2010;6(Supplement J): J53–J60.

10 Lefèvre T, Chevalier B, Louvard Y. Is there a need for dedicated bifurcation device? EuroIntervention 2010;6 (Supplement J): J123–J129.

11 Ormiston JA, Currie E, Webster MW, Kay P, Ruygrok PN, Stewart JT, et al. Drug-eluting stents for coronary bifurcations: insights into the crush technique. Catheter Cardiovasc Interv 2004;63(3):332–6.

12 Costa RA, Mintz GS, Carlier SG, Lansky AJ, Moussa I, Fujii K, et al. Bifurcation coronary lesions treated with the "crush" technique: an intravascular ultrasound analysis. J Am Coll Cardiol 2005;46(4):599–605.

13 Prasad N, Seidelin PH. Sidebranch compromise during percutaneous coronary interventions. J Invasive Cardiol 2002;14(3):138–45; quiz 146.

14 Kralev S, Poerner TC, Basorth D, Lang S, Wolpert C, Haghi D, et al. Side branch occlusion after coronary stent implantation in patients presenting with ST-elevation myocardial infarction: clinical impact and angiographic predictors. Am Heart J 2006;151(1):153–7.

15 Chaudhry EC, Dauerman KP, Sarnoski CL, Thomas CS, Dauerman HL. Percutaneous coronary intervention for major bifurcation lesions using the simple approach: risk of myocardial infarction. J Thromb Thrombolysis 2007;24(1):7–13.

16 Koo BK, Park KW, Kang HJ, Cho YS, Chung WY, Youn TJ, et al. Physiological evaluation of the provisional side-branch intervention strategy for bifurcation lesions using fractional flow reserve. Eur Heart J 2008;29(6): 726–32.

17 Yazdani SK, Nakano M, Otsuka F, Kolodgie FD, Virmani R. Atheroma and coronary bifurcations: before and after stenting. EuroIntervention 2010;6(Supplement J): J24–J30.

18 Russell ME, Binyamin G, Konstantino E. Ex vivo analysis of human coronary bifurcation anatomy: defining the main vessel-to-side-branch transition zone. EuroIntervention 2009;5(1):96–103.

19 Lansky A, Tuinenburg J, Costa M, Maeng M, Koning G, Popma J, et al. Quantitative angiographic methods for bifurcation lesions: a consensus statement from the European Bifurcation Group. Catheter Cardiovasc Interv 2009;73(2):258–66.

20 Medina A, Suarez de Lezo J, Pan M. [A new classification of coronary bifurcation lesions]. Rev Esp Cardiol 2006; 59(2):183.

21 Costa RA, Abizaid A, Abizaid A, Feres F, Staico R, Mattos LA, et al. Preliminary Results of the Novel TMI (TriReme Medical Inc.) Antares Side Branch Adaptive System (Antares SAS™ Stent) for the Treatment of De Novo Coronary Bifurcation Lesions. J Am Coll Cardiol 2008;51:B51.

22 Di Mario C. The TriReme Medical Antares Stent: Design Evolution and Results from the Ongoing TOP First-In-Man Study. In Transcatheter Cardiovascular Therapeutics; 2008 October, 13; Washington, DC, Cardiovascular Research Foundation, 2008, p 46.

23 Routledge HC, Morice MC, Lefevre T, Garot P, De Marco F, Vaquerizo B, et al. 2-year outcome of patients treated for bifurcation coronary disease with provisional side branch T-stenting using drug-eluting stents. JACC Cardiovasc Interv 2008;1(4):358–65.

24 Latib A, Cosgrave J, Godino C, Qasim A, Corbett SJ, Tavano D, et al. Sirolimus-eluting and paclitaxel-eluting stents for the treatment of coronary bifurcations. Am Heart J 2008;156(4):745–50.

25 Latib A, Moussa I, Sheiban I, Colombo A. When are two stents needed? Which technique is the best? How to perform? EuroIntervention 2010;6(Supplement J): J81–J87.

26 Colombo A, Moses JW, Morice MC, Ludwig J, Holmes DR, Jr., Spanos V, et al. Randomized study to evaluate sirolimus-eluting stents implanted at coronary bifurcation lesions. Circulation 2004;109(10):1244–9.

CHAPTER 16

Dedicated bifurcation stents: The petal stent

Frederic De Vroey, MD[1]*, John A. Ormiston,* MBChB[1,2]
and Mark Webster, MBChB[2]
[1]Auckland City Hospital, Auckland, New Zealand
[2]Mercy Angiography, Auckland, New Zealand

Introduction

Coronary bifurcation disease remains one of the outstanding challenges in the field of percutaneous coronary intervention (PCI), accounting for at least 20% of lesions encountered in daily practice [1]. Coronary bifurcation sites are particularly susceptible to developing obstructive atherosclerotic disease due to turbulent blood flow and change of shear stress. Despite improvements in the immediate and long-term outcomes of bifurcation stenting since the introduction of drug eluting stents [2] and greater attention given to deployment techniques, treatment of bifurcation stenoses has been associated with a lower procedural success rate, a higher likelihood of restenosis and a higher incidence of major adverse events [3] than treatment of other lesions. Achieving optimal angiographic and long-term clinical results in patients with this particular lesion cohort remains difficult. Randomised trials [1,4–6] evaluating standard tubular stents in patients with bifurcation lesions, have mostly shown that a provisional one-stent strategy achieves a better outcome than elective stenting of both branches. Two-stent methods are more likely to produce multiple layers of distorted and malapposed stent struts, leading to increased turbulent flow, thrombosis and restenosis. However, large, complex bifurcation lesions are under-represented in the randomised trials; many of these are unsuited to a single stent approach, and there are risks associated with loss of side branch access during provisional stenting. Therefore, dedicated stents have been developed to overcome some of the shortcomings associated with current bifurcation stenting techniques.

Rationale for dedicated bifurcation stenting system

Regardless of the technique used, strategies for treating bifurcation lesions with standard stents remain technically demanding and time consuming. First, tubular stents' shape must be distorted to conform to a non-tubular bifurcation. Second, a tubular stent across a bifurcation may have struts compromising the branch vessel ostium, and not provide optimal coverage and scaffolding where needed. Third, most conventional approaches require recrossing through the struts of the stent with a guide wire and then with a balloon; with the culotte technique this must be done twice. Jailing a guide wire aids rewiring by maintaining a path into the branch vessel and by narrowing the angle between the downstream branches, at a small risk of guide wire entrapment. In some bifurcation lesions with particular anatomical configurations or bifurcation angles, two-stent techniques are

Bifurcation Stenting, First Edition. Edited by Ron Waksman and John A. Ormiston.
© 2012 Blackwell Publishing Ltd. Published 2012 by Blackwell Publishing Ltd.

needed. These cause greater stent distortion resulting in possible malapposition and vessel turbulence, which combined with multiple layers of stent struts, may predispose to stent thrombosis and in-stent restenosis.

Dedicated bifurcation stents, both BMS and DES, have been designed to overcome those difficulties. The devices to date have limitations related to high profile, limited ability to be rotated in the coronary artery, guide wire wrap, and problems associated with branch vessel alignment [7]. The wide variety of vessel sizes, bifurcation angles, disease location and lesion length also represent a major issue in designing the perfect device. To date, none have gained widespread clinical acceptance.

Taxus Petal stent

The Taxus Petal stent (Boston Scientific, Natick, Massachussetts, USA) is designed to scaffold the upstream and downstream main vessel, with maintained guide wire access in the branch vessel to facilitate deployment of a second standard stent in the branch, if necessary (Figure 16.1). The stent has a side aperture located mid-stent with balloon-expandable "petals", which provide some coverage, mechanical scaffolding and drug delivery to the side branch ostium [8].

Device description

This paclitaxel-eluting stent has a platinum chrome backbone, and is an improved version of the bare metal, stainless steel Advanced Stent Technologies (AST) Petal [9]. The platinum chromium alloy gives the stent greater radial strength despite thinner stent struts than if made from stainless steel or a cobalt chrome alloy. The stent is also more radio-opaque. The Taxus Petal uses the same drug and polymer as the Taxus Express and Taxus Liberté stents [10]. The stent delivery system is a dual-side exchange catheter with a main branch (MB) wire lumen and a side branch (SB) wire lumen. Four radiopaque markers assist with proper alignment of stent and petal (Figure 16.1). A standard cylindrical-shaped balloon deploys the stent into the MB while a secondary teardrop-shaped balloon

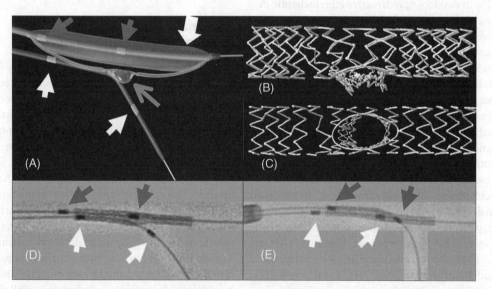

Figure 16.1 Expanded deployment balloons, deployed Petal stent and rotational alignment. In (a), the cylindrical main branch balloon is indicated by the open black triangle and the tear-drop shaped balloon that deploys the petal elements is indicated by the white triangle; (b) and (c) are microcomputed tomographic images of the deployed petal stent from the side (b) and from within the stent looking towards the side-branch (c). In (a), (d) and (e), the main branch lumen is indicated by the black arrows and the side-branch lumen by the white arrows; (d) and (e) are cineangiographic recordings of bench deployments. Separation of the markers in (d) indicates correct rotational alignment of the petal elements to the side-branch. In contrast, in (e) the markers are not separated indicating failure of rotation and mal-alignment with the side-branch.

connected to the same inflation lumen deploys the petal into the ostium of the SB. The petals extend up to 2 mm into the branch vessel.

Potential clinical advantages of this device include complete SB ostial coverage and drug delivery, a frequent site of restenosis following percutaneous intervention in bifurcation lesions. The SB ostial support by the petal elements facilitates placement of a second stent in the SB, if needed. Provisional stenting is made safer because SB access is maintained throughout the procedure. Carina shift during intervention may also be reduced.

First-in-human study

The first-in-human experience with this dedicated bifurcation stent was recently reported by Ormiston and colleagues [11]. The safety and feasibility of the device was studied in a prospective, single-arm, multi-centre study. The primary endpoint was a composite of death, myocardial infarction (MI), and target vessel revascularisation (TVR) at 30 days. Angiographic and intravascular ultrasound follow-up was at six months, with clinical follow-up through 5 years. A total of 28 patients were enrolled at three sites worldwide (New Zealand, France and Germany). Patients were aged 61 ± 9 years, and 18% had medically-treated diabetes. The lesion length was 13.8 ± 5.9 mm in the main branch (MB) and 4.4 ± 2.5 mm in the side branch (SB). A Taxus Petal stent was successfully implanted in 25 of 28 (89%) patients. On a per device basis, 25 of 34 (74%) of Petal deployments were successful. The primary endpoint occurred in one patient (4%, in-hospital non–Q-wave MI). Through one year, TVR was 11%, target lesion revascularisation was 7%, and there were no deaths, Q-wave MIs, or stent thromboses. In-segment late loss (assessed in 21 patients) was 0.47 ± 0.45 mm, 0.41 ± 0.57 mm and 0.18 ± 0.39 mm in the proximal MB, distal MB, and SB, respectively.

This study showed that treatment of bifurcation lesions using the Boston Scientific Taxus Petal stent is feasible, although the requirement for rotation of the device in the coronary to align the petal with the side branch ostium made delivery more challenging than with conventional stents. A combination of wire wrap (twisting together of the wires which prevented further stent advance-

ment), wire bias (wire position guiding the stent SB component away from the SB), and the oval cross-sectional shape of the device made correct rotational alignment difficult. The higher profile of the device than that of a standard stent was a particular limitation during intervention in tortuous and calcified vessels.

On the other hand, in cases where successful delivery was achieved, wire access to the side branch was maintained after deployment and there was little difficulty deploying further stents in either branch vessel, when necessary. The 1-year clinical follow-up and 6-month QCA and IVUS outcomes with the Taxus Petal stent were very satisfactory.

The study showed that the Petal design has promise, although the delivery difficulties must be overcome. An improved version of the Taxus Petal stent with a modified delivery system incorporating a torquable catheter shaft is under development. Preliminary evaluation of this device in a bifurcation phantom model and in pig coronary arteries suggest that clinical performance will be much better and procedural success rates will be high.

Conclusion

In summary, when using standard stents a provisional MB stenting strategy is the best approach in the majority of bifurcation lesions. This strategy has limitations, and is not possible in all lesions. Dedicated bifurcation devices have yet to fulfil their clinical promise, largely because the devices have been difficult to consistently deliver to the bifurcation. The Taxus Petal has achieved encouraging first-in-human clinical results. Insights from benchtop testing and from the clinical first-in-man study have led to design improvements that appear to have overcome the limitations of the device. Clinical evaluation of the next-generation delivery system is warranted, and may lead to the Taxus Petal dedicated bifurcation stent being widely used in bifurcation lesions.

References

1 Steigen TK, Maeng M, Wiseth R, Erglis A, Kumsars I, Narbute I, Gunnes P, Mannsverk J, Meyerdierks O, Rotevatn S, Niemelä M, Kervinen K, Jensen JS,

Galløe A, Nikus K, Vikman S, Ravkilde J, James S, Aarøe J, Ylitalo A, Helqvist S, Sjögren I, Thayssen P, Virtanen K, Puhakka M, Airaksinen J, Lassen JF, Thuesen L; Nordic PCI Study Group. Randomized study on simple versus complex stenting of coronary artery bifurcation lesions: the Nordic bifurcation study. Circulation 2006; 114(18):1955–61.

2 Thuesen L, Kelbaek H, Kløvgaard L, Helqvist S, Jørgensen E, Aljabbari S, Krusell LR, Jensen GV, Bøtker HE, Saunamäki K, Lassen JF, van Weert A; SCANDSTENT Investigators. Comparison of sirolimus-eluting and bare metal stents in coronary bifurcation lesions: subgroup analysis of the Stenting Coronary Arteries in Non-Stress/Benestent Disease Trial(SCANDSTENT). Am Heart J 2006;152(6):1140–5.

3 Stankovic G, Darremont O, Ferenc M, Hildick-Smith D, Louvard Y, Albiero R, Pan M, Lassen JF, Lefèvre T. Percutaneous coronary intervention for bifurcation lesions: 2008 consensus document from the fourth meeting of the European Bifurcation Club. EuroIntervention 2009;5(1):39–49.

4 Hildick-Smith D, de Belder AJ, Cooter N, Curzen NP, Clayton TC, Oldroyd KG, Bennett L, Holmberg S, Cotton JM, Glennon PE, Thomas MR, Maccarthy PA, Baumbach A, Mulvihill NT, Henderson RA, Redwood SR, Starkey IR, Stables RH. Randomized trial of simple versus complex drug-eluting stenting for bifurcation lesions: the British Bifurcation Coronary Study: old, new, and evolving strategies. Circulation 2010;121(10):1235–43.

5 Ferenc M, Gick M, Kienzle RP, Bestehorn HP, Werner KD, Comberg T, Kuebler P, Büttner HJ,

Neumann FJ. Randomized trial on routine vs. provisional T-stenting in the treatment of de novo coronary bifurcation lesions. Eur Heart J 2008;23:2859–67.

6 Grube E, Buellesfeld L, Neumann FJ, Verheye S, Abizaid A, McClean D, Mueller R, Lansky A, Mehran R, Costa R, Gerckens U, Trauthen B, Fitzgerald PJ. Six-month clinical and angiographic results of a dedicated drug-eluting stent for the treatment of coronary bifurcation narrowings. Am J Cardiol 2007;99(12):1691–7.

7 Latib A, Colombo A, Sangiorgi GM. Bifurcation stenting: current strategies and new devices. Heart 2009;95 (6):495–504.

8 Johnson TW, Kay IP, Ormiston JA. A novel paclitaxel-eluting dedicated bifurcation stent: a case report from the first human use Taxus Petal trial. Catheter Cardiovasc Interv 2009;73(5):637–40.

9 Ormiston J, Webster M, El-Jack S, McNab D, Plaumann SS. The AST petal dedicated bifurcation stent: first-in-human experience. Catheter Cardiovasc Interv 2007;70(3):335–40.

10 Colombo A, Drzewiecki J, Banning A, Grube E, Hauptmann K, Silber S, Dudek D, Fort S, Schiele F, Zmudka K, Guagliumi G, Russell ME; TAXUS II Study Group. Randomised study to assess the effectiveness of slow- and moderate- release polymer-based paclitaxel-eluting stents for coronary artery lesions. Circulation 2003;108(7):788–94.

11 Ormiston JA, Lefevre T, Grube E, Allocco DJ, Dawkins KD. First human use of the TAXUS Petal paclitaxel-eluting bifurcation stent. Eurointervention 2010;6(1):46–53.

CHAPTER 17
The Sideguard Side branch stent

Eberhard Grube, MD

Medizinische Klinik und Poliklinik II, University Hospital Bonn, Germany

One of the more challenging subsets facing interventional cardiologists in the post-balloon angioplasty era is the use of conventional coronary stents for the treatment of coronary bifurcation disease.

In the bare-metal stent (BMS) era, the use of two conventional coronary stents at bifurcation points was associated with high restenosis rates, particularly at the ostium of the side branch. As coronary stenting evolved and became the gold standard of percutaneous coronary intervention (PCI) for bifurcation lesions, two-stent use increased and with it, so did restenosis rates, as well as other complications [1].

Historically, there have been two schools of thought regarding how coronary bifurcation disease should be approached and treated: (1) the simple approach of using one stent in the main vessel and then waiting to see the outcome (or provisional T-stenting); or (2) taking a more systematic approach to treating bifurcation disease using two stents. In recent years however, primarily due to the publication of the Nordic 1 study in 2006, provisional T-stenting – where the main vessel is treated with a conventional tubular coronary stent and the option to treat the side branch vessel is determined by the operator afterwards – has become the default approach for coronary bifurcation disease. The systematic approach is generally reserved for cases when disease is present in all three segments of the bifurcation and where the disease in the side branch is determined to be significant enough to merit a second stent. Problems exist with both strategies, but particularly with provisional stenting when the side branch is left untreated or unstented. Provisional T-stenting provides less than optimal coverage of the ostium of the branch and places the side branch at risk of side branch loss while the systematic strategy provides only somewhat better acute hemodynamic results and increases the risk of restenosis, repeat vascularization, and thrombotic events. Nevertheless, the use of a systematic strategy for treating bifurcations might be the more appropriate approach, particularly in situations when there is concern about whether a second stent is needed from the start.

The two-stent approach, whereby the side branch and parent vessel are stented in a sequential fashion, is beneficial, since it reduces the incidence of plaque shifting and lumen loss. But conventional two-stent techniques are difficult to perform, distort and damage the stents themselves, and alter the native anatomy within the bifurcation segment [1]. This can lead to intravascular turbulences and flow dynamics issues, which, in turn, can lead to thrombotic events. Moreover, long-term angiographic results where two-stent use has been evaluated in randomized clinical trials and observational studies restenosis rates have approached 40%.

To address the problems associated with conventional two-stent bifurcation techniques, Antonio Colombo, MD, Chief of Invasive Cardiology at San Raffaele Hospital in Milan, Italy, co-founded Cappella Inc. (Boston, MA) in 2004. Cappella's flagship product is the Sideguard Side branch Stent system, a stent that is designed

Bifurcation Stenting, First Edition. Edited by Ron Waksman and John A. Ormiston.
© 2012 Blackwell Publishing Ltd. Published 2012 by Blackwell Publishing Ltd.

to treat the ostium of the side branch and the lesion extending into the side branch from the vessel's origin. The Sideguard Side branch Stent was introduced in Europe in May 2009. Cappella believes the Sideguard stent has at least two distinguishing characteristics that may address the limitations of existing stent technology and thereby provide an effective alternative to conventional two-stent approaches:

1 A self-expanding nitinol ostium protection device that is designed to conform to the shape of the bifurcation at the ostium
2 A proprietary balloon-delivery system specifically designed to deliver and deploy self-expanding devices.

Cappella completed the human clinical trials in Europe to evaluate the Sideguard stent's safety and efficacy in the treatment of coronary bifurcations, receiving CE Mark in April 2009.

This chapter introduces the Sideguard stent for the treatment of ostial-bifurcation lesions by:

- Reviewing the challenges associated with conventional main vessel stent use to treat bifurcations
- Examining the optimality of current bifurcation stenting techniques
- Presenting the advantages of the Cappella approach and technology over conventional techniques and technologies.

Challenges of bifurcation stenting

In a DES era, where restenosis and repeat revascularization rates are below 10%, why are outcomes following bifurcation procedures so poor? It is likely that the answer lies with the technologies and techniques being used to treat these types of lesions, which, although efficient and innovative when used in the treatment of straightforward lesions, have fallen short of solving the ostial-bifurcation problem.

Conventional approaches and technologies are not always suited for the treatment of less common lesion subsets, such as bifurcations. In many cases, conventional technologies are not designed to address these types of problems, which present themselves in a small percentage of patients being treated and can ultimately impact outcomes.

In contrast, conventional technologies are developed to cater to a broader cross-section of patients. As a result, operators are required to devise ways to adapt technologies developed for broader use and use them in unconventional ways (i.e. using conventional tubular stents at a bifurcation point).

Challenge #1: lesion length and size

One of main challenges associated with conventional bifurcation stenting is the disparity in vessel size and lesion length. Compared to main vessel diameters and lesion lengths, side branch diameters are typically narrower and the lesions shorter. Despite good acute results, when conventional stents are used, long-term patency issues remain a problem at the ostium of the side branch. A common trend often observed with the various bifurcation stenting techniques (provisional, crush, V, T, culotte) is the frequency of angiographic recurrences at the ostium. This has been attributed to poor lesion preparation and poor stent expansion and stent distortion at this location [1,2].

Stent under-expansion, which may be associated with disparity in vessel size, is difficult to detect angiographically [3]. Restenosis occurring at the side branch ostium can be attributed to chronic stent recoil, under-expansion, and intimal hyperplasia. Stent under-expansion may be the catalyst of restenosis with drug-eluting stents (DES). Costa et al. indicates that even smallest amounts of intimal hyperplasia can lead to restenosis when a DES is under-expanded, regardless of the bifurcation technique used [3]. Restenosis, resulting from stent under-expansion has been observed to systematically occur at the side branch ostium. Furthermore, final kissing balloon dilation does not guarantee optimal apposition or lumen patency of the side branch and ostium and can impact the main vessel stent, resulting in incomplete main vessel wall apposition [3].

The advantages of self-expanding stents include increased flexibility, less barotrauma to the vessel wall, and differential expansion capabilities [4].

Table 17.1 Sideguard stent IVUS findings at the side branch carina

Doi et al. [4]	Post-intervention	Follow-up	P-value
Stent area, mm²	3.9 +/− 1.2	4.6 +/− 1.1	0.04
Lumen area, mm²	3.9 +/− 1.3	4.0 +/− 1.2	0.77

The self-expanding characteristics of the Sideguard stent eliminates the side branch stent under-expansion problem at the ostium of the side branch and the side branch's disparity in vessel size issue. When evaluated by intravenous ultrasound (IVUS), even with the presence of intimal proliferation at 6-month follow-up, the chronic expansion properties of the Sideguard stent preserved lumen patency at the side branch ostium by compensating for the neointimal hyperplasia.

Doi *et al.* reported the results of the Sideguard stent IVUS pilot study involving 11 patients on the Sideguard stent's dynamic responsiveness characteristics. Intravenous ultrasound was performed post-intervention and during 6-month angiographic follow-up in all 11 patients. At 6-months follow-up, an increase in stent area at the carina was observed in all patients, in addition to an increase in lumen area in six patients [5] confirming the dynamic apposition characteristics of the Sideguard in the side branch. The results reported by Doi's group are consistent with the results observed in other self-expanding stent trials [4,6,7] (Table 17.1).

Challenge #2: remodeling

Negative remodeling contributes to bifurcation lesions more frequently than non-bifurcation lesions, particularly when only the main vessel is stented and balloon angioplasty is performed on the side branch [8]. Negative remodeling has been reported as being a dominant contributor of significant coronary bifurcation remodeling.

Compensatory remodeling has been observed in non-bifurcation lesions. However, this is not always the case with bifurcation lesions. Negative remodeling (or non-compensatory remodeling) has been reported to contribute to the development of bifurcation lesions. Although the mechanism as to why the incidence of negative remodeling is

higher at bifurcation points is unknown, Fujii *et al.* [8] reported that it is possible that the origin of the side branch may play a role by impeding positive remodeling. As a result, the natural lack of positive remodeling at the side branch may place an unstented side branch at higher risk of compromise following bifurcation percutaneous coronary intervention (PCI). This cannot be achieved with the use of only one stent, as reported Timurkaynak, because the single stent approach provides less than 25% coverage of the ostium [9]. As a result, this contributes to a significantly increased risk of side branch occlusion, anywhere from 12% to 41% [10–13].

Using the Sideguard stent to open and protect the origin of a side branch prior to the placement of the main vessel stent, even in moderately diseased lesions (40–70% diameter stenosis), may provide both long-term clinical and angiographic advantages. Glagov *et al.* reported that compensatory remodeling delays luminal loss until the atherosceloris plaque occupies 40% of the luminal area [14]. IVUS assessment at 6-month follow-up following the Sideguard stent implantation revealed an increase in both luminal and stent area (positive remodeling at the ostium). This positive remodeling effect is associated with the Sideguard stent's dynamic apposition properties, which allows the stent to dynamically respond to the artery as the vessel heals. Gains typically not observed with conventional coronary stents.

Challenge #3: conventional stent use

Bifurcation type should also be taken into consideration when selecting a bifurcation treatment strategy [15]. T-shaped bifurcations are better treated than Y-shaped bifurcations when using conventional coronary stents. This is because in T-shaped bifurcations, the side branch stent can be positioned at the ostium of a branch in a perpendicular fashion, providing better coverage of the ostial area.

In contrast, Y-shaped bifurcations are more difficult to treat using conventional coronary stents because ostial coverage is incomplete and leaves excess metal at the carina. This is caused by the cylindrical, symmetrical design of tubular stents. Conventional stents used in Y-shaped bifurcations also can be compromised and collapse the side branch stent's lumen once the main vessel stent is implanted. As a result, treating lower angle bifurcations using conventional tubular stents can be difficult, particularly for less experienced operators. This often leads to suboptimal clinical and angiographic results.

For example, adverse cardiac events were higher in patients treated for Y-shaped bifurcations when compared to patients treated for T-shaped bifurcations (83.6% vs 30.4%; p = 0.004) when conventional tubular coronary stents were used [16].

The poorer outcomes associated with Y-shaped bifurcation stenting is linked to the amount of metal or stent-to-stent overlap needed to cover the proximal side branch wall in order to compensate for the shallower angle. As a result, this leads to a larger amount of excess metal being crushed at the carina.

This excessive metal overlap at Y-shaped bifurcation points, coupled with the amount of additional trauma caused to the artery during conventional stent delivery and multiple post-stenting balloon dilations has been associated with stimulating the formation of neointimal hyperplasia and triggering luminal loss. As a result, this can lead to severe ischemic events caused by higher restenosis rates and lead to more frequent repeat revascularizations.

By contrast, the Sideguard stent's trumpet design, which is quite different from tubular stents, affords complete coverage to the ostium and carina by the stent. Tubular stents have to be manipulated to fit the different geometries of bifurcation and ostial lesions, reflecting poor results, both clinically and from a device deployment perspective. This can cause poor wall apposition and struts protruding into the main branch and can complicate the procedure and impact outcomes. These problems can be avoided with the Sideguard stent because of the Sideguard's trumpet-shaped design.

Additionally, the self-expanding nature and the trumpet shape of the Sideguard stent provide the stent with a margin of tolerance, which means that if the stent is not exactly positioned at the side-branch ostium, the Sideguard stent will still conform (or moulds) to the bifurcation's anatomy. Furthermore, the ease of which the proximal trumpet-shaped end of the stent flares outwards and can be flattened against the main vessel wall once the main vessel stent is implanted.

The Sideguard stent's anatomic-shaped design and super-elastic frame makes the device particularly well-suited to address Y-shaped bifurcations. Again, its unique trumpet section allows the stent to be used in shallow angles without placing excess metal at the carina.

The trumpet section also leaves a small footprint at the ostium once the main vessel stent is implanted. Moreover, unlike conventional tubular coronary stents there is no deformation and protrusion of stent struts in the main vessel lumen, because during implantation the main vessel stent flattens the Sideguard's trumpet section instead of crushing it.

The Sideguard stent strikes a balance between maintaining good wall apposition and circumferential coverage of the ostium. The Sideguard stent maintains lumen patency both at high and shallow angles, as low as 45°.

Challenge #4: side branch occlusion

An issue associated with the single stenting strategy is side branch occlusion and loss of side branch access. Leaving the side branch untreated (or unstented), particularly in circumstances where there is disease or plaque burden at the ostium, puts the side branch at increased risk of side branch occlusion and loss of future side branch access due to a lack of ostial scaffolding.

Factors predictive of side branch target lesion revascularization (TLR) reported by Brunel et al. include light to moderate calcification and absence of jailed wires [17].

Of 186 patients treated in the TULIPE study [17], a French multicenter study, 60% of bifurcations treated were classified as "true" bifurcation, having disease in all-three bifurcation segments. The mean take-off angle was 60° (a typical Y-shaped bifurcation).

The cross-over rate to two stents from one stent was reported in more than one-third (34%) of the cases with a TLR PCI rate of nearly 20%. Furthermore, the TULIPE investigators enumerated the lengthy steps required to prepare the bifurcated segment in order to perform side branch stenting following failed one stent procedures. Plaque shift was also reported as a predictor of loss of side branch, which necessitated the use of extra wires

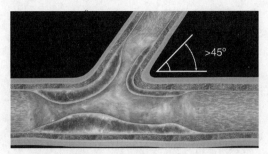

Figure 17.1 Minimum bifurcation take-off angle suitable to the Sideguard Side branch stent.

and wire jailing in order to preserve the side branch access using a single stent approach.

The Sideguard stent is well suited to a range of bifurcation lesions and angles. The stent is rated for use in bifurcations with take-off angles as low as 45° (Figure 17.1). The Sideguard approach can be performed in fewer steps than conventional T-stenting and a typical case requires less equipment to complete the procedure, resulting in low TLR rates (∼6%).

In contrast to the TULIPE study, where three guide wires were used per case in nearly 100 patients – in order to jail one of the wires to preserve side branch access – the Sideguard approach requires only two guide wires and does not require jailing of the wire following Sideguard placement. Moreover, removing the wire prior to main vessel stent implantation eliminates any damage to the abluminal main vessel surface (or to the polymer coating when the guide wire is extracted) that may result.

Selecting the Sideguard approach as the intent to treat strategy in bifurcations where disease is present in both the main vessel and the side branch, and in situations where there is a probability of plaque shift from the main vessel into the side branch, eliminates the loss of branch associated with plaque shift by trapping plaque between the stent and the vessel was at the ostium. Furthermore, the Sideguard eliminates the need for jailed wires in order to preserve access, because Sideguard is designed to maintain ostial patency once implanted.

Challenge # 5: current bifurcation stenting techniques

Many approaches have been created specifically to treat bifurcation lesions using two stents. Most fall short of the intended goal: preventing restenosis and repeat revascularizations.

Historical target lesion revascularization (TLR) rates with conventional bare-metal coronary stents have been reported between 16% and 38% [18]. The availability of drug-eluting stents and the routine use of post-dilation kissing balloon inflation have reduced TLR rates in bifurcation lesions in recent years.

Anecdotally, Colombo *et al.* [19] was one of the first to experiment with stents in the treatment of ostial-bifurcation lesions. His group's earliest experiences with bifurcation lesions involved the use of various stents, cutting and shaping the devices to provide scaffolding to the ostium of the side-branch. This concept would come to be referred to as "rebuilding the bifurcation."

Other approaches involved techniques with multiple stents. These approaches include the crush, culotte technique, simultaneous kissing stent technique, and the skirt stent technique. However, performing some of these conventional two-stent procedures may be too complex for the less experienced bifurcation operator, further complicating issues such as procedural and clinical outcomes.

Ormiston *et al.* sought to identify methods for appropriate strategy selection and the potential pitfalls associated with using single and dual-stent strategies for bifurcations [1]. They noted that many interventionalists are unaware of the intricacies involving coronary stent use for the treatment of bifurcations, which has lead to suboptimal stent deployments and poor results.

The crush technique, has been widely studied in both randomized and observational studies, and as a result, has been widely adopted as preferred bifurcation stenting technique after provisional T-stenting and T-stenting [20]. Colombo *et al.* evaluated the crush technique in 20 consecutive patients with true bifurcation disease [19]. Their approach was to protrude the side branch stent up to 5 mm proximal of the ostium into the main vessel in order to compensate for the gap in coverage that would have been left with T-stenting. There are two additional concerns with the crush technique: (1) risk of thrombotic events high metal density at the carina; and (2) further compromise of the side branch stent luminal integrity. Hoye *et al.*

reasoned that the higher incidences of stent thrombosis is likely to be associated with the increased complexity bifurcation techniques, such as the crush technique when conventional stents are used for treating bifurcations [18]. Increases in thrombotic events due to the triple layer of stent struts, polymer, and drug concentration at the ostium also have been reported [18].

When performed by an experienced bifurcation operator, the Crush technique is a relatively straightforward bifurcation strategy. However, re-accessing the side branch following Crush stenting can be difficult due to the multi-layer of struts covering the ostium. Furthermore, it may require several post-dilations in both branches in order to achieve the desired post-procedural result. This unnecessarily prolongs the procedure, increases fluoroscopy time, and places the patient at risk of procedural complications [1]. Moreover, achieving good stent-to-vessel apposition with the crush technique is also highly dependent on the bifurcation angle. In higher bifurcation angles (closer to 90°), post dilation may not properly expand the side branch stent enough in order to provide coverage of the carina.

Conversely, in bifurcation angles less than 90°, a balance between achieving full-expansion of the side branch stent and preventing main vessel stent distortion [1] can be challenging. This can be even more difficult for the less experienced bifurcation operators, because of the intricacies that involve choosing the right balloons, using the appropriate inflation pressures, and post-dilation sequences, which can further complicate the procedure.

Crush stenting, even following final kissing balloon dilation, does not guarantee optimal lumen patency at the side branch ostium and can impact the main vessel stent, resulting in incomplete main vessel wall apposition. Costa *et al.* indicates the findings are consistent with reported side branch ostium restenosis in other studies [3].

The Sideguard strategy approaches the treatment of the bifurcation point in a compartmentalized fashion. Once the Sideguard's in place, the operator can focus their efforts on treating the main vessel without being concerned for the loss of branch and side branch re-access. Re-accessing the side branch is facilitated because only one layer of struts needs to be re-crossed. Furthermore, in order to restore

side branch access, once the main vessel is in place, a single-post-dilation kissing balloon inflation is required to open the struts of the main vessel stent at the ostium.

Approaching bifurcation from the side branch first

Cappella approaches bifurcations from the side branch first with similarities to T-stening. The Sideguard stent is a dedicated, self-expanding nitinol side branch ostium protection device that works seamlessly with any conventional tubular stent implanted in the main vessel.

The Sideguard stent's low profile design is compatible with 6F guide catheters (allowing it to be used for both transradial and femoral access), and Cappella believes its multi-segment design (Figure 17.2) provides superior scaffolding within the side branch, radial strength at the ostium, and minimal stent-strut overlap in the main branch.

The Sideguard stent provides complete apposition and scaffolding to the ostium. It is mounted onto a semi-compliant, 2 mm diameter balloon catheter and is secured into place by Cappella's proprietary Split-Sheath Technology (Figures 17.3a and 17.3b). The sheath keeps the stent in place until it is ready to be implanted. The Sideguard delivery system tracks over a standard 0.014″ guide wire to the ostium of the side branch and has no need for rotation when positioning the delivery system prior to deploying the stent.

Bench tests have demonstrated that the Sideguard stent is highly trackable through tortuous anatomies and luminal diameters as low as 1.25 mm. Furthermore, in the clinical setting, the Sideguard stent is not hindered by calcification in

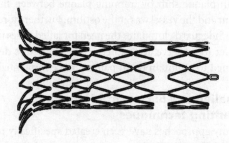

Figure 17.2 The Sideguard stent's multi-segment design.

(A)

(B)

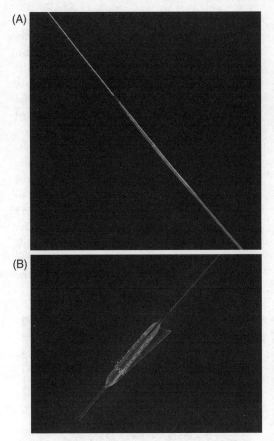

Figure 17.3 (a) Sheathed Sideguard stent; (b) Unsheathed Sideguard stent.

the proximal segment of a bifurcation because the stent is short (∼10 mm crimped), flexible, because it is made from nitinol, and sheathed. The sheath prevents the Sideguard stent's struts from catching obstructions while it is tracking through severely narrowed artery segments.

The difficulty of using conventional dual-stent techniques in the treatment of bifurcations is trying to maintain adequate luminal geometry and wall apposition throughout the side branch, the transition zone, and the main vessel segment. The Sideguard stent is unique because the device is self-expanding. Its design conforms to the luminal geometry, provides continuous access to the side branch, and, more importantly, adapts to the vessel as it remodels. While the elastic properties of nitinol provide the Sideguard stent with its self-expanding characteristics, the Sideguard stent's

unique design provides the conformability, flexibility, and apposability.

Advantages of the Sideguard First approach in the treatment of bifurcations

The advantage to using the Sideguard First approach is that the technique is familiar to interventional cardiologists because it is performed like T-Stenting. Operators utilize the same devices and instruments they would to perform a standard PCI. The Sideguard stent can be accurately and easily positioned at the side branch ostium over one wire and then once implanted, any conventional coronary stent can be positioned and implanted in the main branch.

The Sideguard stent is a dedicated side branch stent system that approaches bifurcations in a compartmentalized way without placing excess metal in the main vessel lumen. The Sideguard allows the operator to treat each limb independently as opposed to being limited to using a dedicated main vessel biurcation stent that supplies guide wires to both branches, which can end up braiding or twisting together.

Another advantage of the Sideguard stent, is the complete coverage afforded to the ostium and carina by the stent (Figure 17.4). This is attributed to the Sideguard stent's trumpet-shape design, which is quite different from conventional stents. As an example, poor wall apposition and struts protruding into the main vessel lumen are commonplace with conventional stents and other dedicated bifurcation stents. These problems are

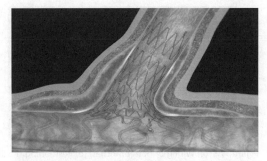

Figure 17.4 Complete ostial coverage of the side branch following side branch stent implantation.

avoided with the Sideguard stent because of the Sideguard's trumpet-shape design.

Performing a Sideguard First procedure

The procedure begins with the placement of two guide wires: one in the side branch and the other in the main vessel (Figure 17.5a). The lesion in the side branch is pre-dilated. Once the side branch lesion is prepared the operator may choose to pre-dilate the lesion in the main vessel.

This is followed by the removal of the balloon catheters and the Sideguard stent is advanced over the side branch guide wire. Radiopaque markers located at the proximal ends of the Sideguard stent and the delivery system overlap to create the Sideguard stents integral ostial-positioning mark-

er. The integrated ostial-positioning marker is used to position the Sideguard stent's delivery system at the side branch ostium (Figure 17.5b).

The Sideguard stent is deployed using the nominal pressure balloon to which it is mounted, which initiates the sheath-splitting process that keeps the Sideguard stent in place until deployed (Figure 17.5c). The Sideguard stent's balloon catheter is inflated using a conventional angioplasty inflator to 12 atmospheres, releasing the stent. Once released from the sheath (the proximal end of the sheath remains attached to the proximal end of the Sideguard stent's delivery catheter), the Sideguard self-expands into place. The Sideguard stent's anchor section embeds itself in the vessel, preventing the Sideguard stent from migrating during the retraction of the

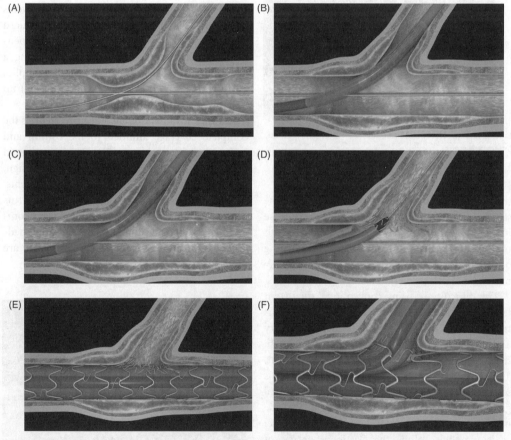

Figure 17.5 (a) Wiring of both branches; (b) Positioning the Sideguard stent at the ostium using the ostial positioning marker; (c) Sideguard stent delivery split-sheath technology; (d) Retraction of Sideguard stent delivery system and guide wire; (e) Implantation of main vessel stent; (f) Final kissing balloon inflation.

delivery catheter following deployment. Once the Sideguard stent is implanted, the delivery system and the guide wire are then removed from the side branch (Figure 17.5d).

Any conventional balloon-expandable main vessel stent is advanced over the main vessel guide wire, easily bypassing the Sideguard's trumpet-shaped proximal end, and deployed into place (Figure 17.5e). The procedure is completed with kissing-balloon inflation (Figure 17.5f). The final kissing balloon inflation is performed not so much to alter the shape of the Sideguard stent, but to open the struts of the main vessel stent into a more circular configuration surrounding the side branch ostium.

Early experience: animal studies

Cappella carried out studies in 60 animals to evaluate the Sideguard stent and its delivery system. Due to the novel method of delivery, acute animal studies were required to ensure the functionality of both delivery and removal of the delivery system. The animal studies were undertaken before initiation of the first-in-man (FIM) bare-metal stent trial in November 2006.

The Sideguard stent demonstrated ease of delivery, favorable acute angiographic results, and seamless apposition (as observed by both intravascular ultrasound and histology) validated the Sideguard stent as a potential alternative to current bifurcation practices.

Animal studies were also conducted to define the ratio between radial force and stent oversizing, an important characteristic for self-expanding stents. Because the Sideguard stent is self-expanding, it exerts a chronic expansive force over time. Too much radial force could trigger intimal proliferation [6]. Conversely, too little radial force would not allow the stent to work optimally. Radial force is a function between stent oversizing and stent geometry. As a result, it was important for Cappella to carefully design a stent that exerted the appropriate amount of radial force and that was optimally oversized.

There's a direct relationship between radial force and the amount of stent oversizing. A self-expanding stent does not begin to lose its radial strength until it reaches 90% of its free-diameter. The fol-

lowing points concerning oversizing and radial force were learnt from successive bench testing and animal studies.

Oversizing

- Significantly oversizing an SE has been demonstrated to cause more injury [6] and will result in lumen loss due to intimal hyperplasia
- Early animal histology studies with the Sideguard revealed an increase in lumen occlusion when the amount of stent oversizing exceeded 50%
- Further animal histology studies with the Sideguard revealed a reduction in lumen occlusion when the amount of stent oversizing was less than 40%

Radial force

- It was determined that more radial force would be needed at the ostium than in the distal part of the stent. As a result, cell-strut combinations were adjusted accordingly: higher radial force and a tighter cell-strut combination at the ostium, while a more open cell-strut combination with less radial force distally.
- Radial force was also determined based on the minimal amount of force needed to the following deployment for contact between the Sideguard and the vessel wall. But, not so much force where the stent would cause excessive injury to the vessel wall, compromising luminal patency.

Elastic properties of nitinol provide the Sideguard self-expanding characteristics, while the design provides the conformability, flexibility, and apposability.

Pivotal CE clinical trial

Following the completion of the Sideguard first-in-man study (known as Sideguard 1 or SG1), Cappella initiated the Sideguard 2 (SG2) trial, a non-randomized prospective study to evaluate the safety and effectiveness of the Sideguard stent in *de novo* coronary bifurcation lesions.

Sixty-nine (69) patients with de novo coronary bifurcation lesions requiring stenting from multiple centers throughout Europe were enrolled into SG2. The primary endpoint was major cardiac adverse events (MACE) – cardiac death, MI or ischemia-driven TLR – evaluated at six months.

Secondary endpoints included total procedure time, total fluoroscopy time, volume of contrast used, technical success of the Sideguard stent, lesion success, procedural success, incidence of stent thrombosis as well as angiographic criteria at six months.

Statistical hypothesis testing was performed to compare the results of SG2 to an objective performance criteria of 38% defined in the clinical protocol. A non-inferiority delta of 19% was pre-selected as a reasonable margin. Non-inferiority testing was performed to compare the rate of composite MACE at six-month follow-up in the Sideguard stent cohort to the reference rate.

Patients were assessed at 1 month with a clinical assessment and at 6 months with both angiographic and clinical assessments. The study also requires a telephone assessment at 12 months.

Dual antiplatelet therapy (aspirin and clopidogrel) was give by protocol post-procedure (aspirin is required indefinitely and clopidogrel required for a minimum of 12 months).

The study enrolled 50 men and 19 women with a mean age of 66.2 years; 15 patients (21.7%) presented with diabetes. Side branch lesion length was 6.53 ± 3.03. Baseline in segment MLD was 0.9 ± 0.4 mm for the main branch and 0.7 ± 0.4 for the side branch pre-procedure and 2.4 ± 0.4 mm and 2.0 ± 0.3 mm post-procedure for the main branch and side branch, respectively (Table 17.2). Percent diameter stenosis reduced in the main branch from 67.9 ± 10.2% pre-procedure to 20.9 ± 6.2% post procedure; and in the side branch was reduced from 68.5 ± 13.5% pre-procedure to 16.5 ± 8.8% post-procedure.

Of the 69 patients who were enrolled in the SG2 study, 44 were implanted with stents using the Sideguard stent's original delivery system (SG2 "A") and 25 with new delivery system (SG2 "B"). Of the entire SG2 group, eight subjects were not implanted with a Sideguard stent: seven subjects from the SG2 "A" group and one subject from the SG2 "B" group.

The overall technical success in the SG2 group was 80.8% by device and 85.5% by patient

Table 17.2 Sideguard 2 baseline patient demographic and angiographic values

	N = 69
Demographic values	
Age (mean)	66.2
Male gender (%)	72.5%
Baseline angina	
No ischemia	1
Stable angina	53
Unstable angina	8
Baseline ejection fraction	66.3
Diabetes (%)	21.7
Smoking (%)	46.4
Previous MI (%)	21.7
Previous CAGB (%)	4.3
Previous PCI (%)	36.2
Angiographic values	
Medina classification (%)	
1,1,1	85.5
1,0,1	2.9
0,1,1	7.2
0,0,1	1.4
1,1,0	2.9

	MV	SB
MLD (mm)	0.9 ± 0.4	0.7 ± 0.4
RVD (mm)	2.9 ± 0.4	2.3 ± 0.3
Lesion length (mm)	14.0 ± 5.8	6.5 ± 3.0
% Diameter stenosis	67.9 ± 10.2	68.5 ± 13.5

Location of bifurcation (%)	
LAD	79.7
LCx	17.4
RCA	2.9

Source: Cappella Medical Devices Ltd., Galway, Ireland

(Table 17.3). The lower overall rate of procedural success was attributed to a problem the operators reported with the delivery system's sheath in SG2 "A." As a result, SG2 "A" was temporarily halted in order to look into the problem.

The necessary enhancements to the Sideguard stent's delivery catheter were completed in April of 2008 with improvements to the sheath and the delivery catheter's profile (no modification was made to the stent itself). The enhancements fixed the problem.

With the new delivery system however, technical success improved to 92.3% (24/26) by device and 96% (24/25) by patient. Notably, improvements in

Table 17.3 Summary of Sideguard stent technical success for SG2

Sideguard stent technical success	SG2-A	SG2-B	All SG2 group
by device	74.5%	92.3%	80.8%
by patient	79.5%	96.0%	85.5%

Note: Technical success was defined as successful delivery, deployment and implantation of the Sideguard stent at the intended lesion location
Source: Cappella Medical Devices Ltd., Galway, Ireland

procedural and fluoroscopy times were also observed with the introduction of the new delivery system (Table 17.4).

For this reason, of the 37/69 patients who were treated using the original delivery system 36 had passed through the 6-month follow-up point at the time the data was submitted for CE Mark. No patients enrolled from May 2008 onward in the SG2 "B" study, with the new delivery system, were eligible for the 6-month follow-up assessment.

Sixty-seven (67) of 69 patients (97%) completed 1-month follow-up (two patients having withdrawn from the study prior to that time-point). Thirty-six (36) of 61 subjects had been followed through the 6-month follow-up, which was sufficient for submitting the data for CE Mark.

Cumulative MACE in the primary analysis cohort through 30 days was 3.3% (2/61) based on one MI and one TLR. At 6 months the cumulative MACE rate for the primary analysis cohort was 11.8% (4/61); one MI, two ischemia-driven TLRs, and one cardiac death (Table 17.5).

The angiographic results demonstrate the robustness of the device through 6-month follow-up and are summarized below (Table 17.6). All analyses that

Table 17.4 Procedural information

	SG2-A	SG2-B	All SG2 group
Mean procedural times (min)	83.3 ± 24.2	62.0 ± 21.0	70.4 ± 24.4
Mean fluoroscopy times (min)	21.6 ± 8.5	18.1 ± 6.7	19.7 ± 8.4

Source: Cappella Medical Devices Ltd., Galway, Ireland

Table 17.5 Summary of clinical data

	N = 61
30-day MACE	2 (3.3%)
Cardiac death	0 (0.0%)
Myocardial infarction	1 (1.6%)
Target lesion revascularization (ischemia driven)	1 (1.6%)
	N = 34
180-day MACE	4 (11.8%)
Cardiac death	1 (2.9%)
Myocardial infarction	1 (2.9%)
Target lesion revascularization (ischemia driven)	2 (5.9%)

Note:
Two (2) cases of stent thrombosis: (1) peri-procedure and (2) 10 days following the procedure which led to a TLR. Both cases were treated
One (1) cardiac death occurred in a subject that was hospitalized due to renal insufficiency six months after the index procedure. The renal insufficiency was associated with a pre-existing condition and not related to the study stent or the study procedure
Source: Cappella Medical Devices Ltd., Galway, Ireland

were performed as in stent assessments within the side branch are summarized by the Sideguard stent only and also by including all stents.

The side branch was noted to have a final percent diameter stenosis (in-stent Sideguard) at the completion of the procedure of 5.5% +/− 8.1,

Table 17.6 Summary of angiographic data

	MV (36)	SB (36)
MLD (mm)		
In-stent	2.6 ± 0.6	1.8 ± 0.5
In-segment	2.2 ± 0.6	1.7 ± 0.5
% Diameter stenosis		
In-stent	14.2 ± 17.6	19.8 ± 20.8
In-segment	28.1 ± 16.7	27.0 ± 17.5
Late loss (mm)		
In-stent	0.3 ± 0.5	0.4 ± 0.5
In-segment	0.2 ± 0.6	0.4 ± 0.4
Binary restenosis		
In-stent	2 (6.3%)	2 (6.3%)
In-segment	3 (9.4%)	2 (6.3%)

Source: Cappella Medical Devices Ltd., Galway, Ireland

which was maintained relatively stable through 6 months where the percent diameter stenosis was 19.8% +/− 20.8.

Similar results were noted in the main vessel where the post procedure present diameter stenosis (in-stent) was 6.6% ± 6.7 post-procedure and 14.2% ± 17.6. These results are confirmed by the determination of MLD.

The late loss results demonstrate the favorable vessel interface that the stent provides through the follow-up phase. The main vessel in-stent late loss was 0.3 ± 0.5 and the late loss for the Sideguard stent was 0.4 ± 0.5 mm. In-stent restenosis by Core Lab Assessment was 6.3% for both the main and side branch. There was no additional in-segment restenosis in the side branch.

Conclusion

All of the techniques to treat bifurcations using two stents, while creative and in many cases successful have resulted in poor long-term outcomes, including thrombotic events and restenosis at the sites of bifurcations.

It remains debatable as to the cause(s) of these clinical failures. However, it is thought that excessive trauma to the vessel at sites where the combination of conventional stents and employing dual stenting techniques, are causing more damage to the ostium, carina, and the bifurcation point than is true elsewhere. This might initiate the cascade leading up to a thrombotic event and restenosis, making the Sideguard stent a viable alternative to current technologies and approaches. When a self-expanding stent is placed at the carina, the impact it has in terms of decreasing the trauma to the vessel wall and lessening the cascade that follows is potentially less than when using a conventional stent.

The Sideguard stent maintains good luminal geometry throughout the bifurcated area and because it provides good wall apposition, it is demonstrated to reduce restenosis rates, particularly when combined with drug-eluting technology.

An important factor of placing a stent at the ostium of a side branch is to dilate the end of the stent protruding in the lumen of the side branch like a trumpet. The Sideguard stent echoes this concept.

The only difference is that the Sideguard already comes pre-shaped and is ready for use. No special techniques are required except for positioning the stent at the side branch ostium, for which the Sideguard's delivery systems come equipped with the integral Ostium Positioning Marker.

Furthermore, the Sideguard stent's nitinol, self-expanding construction eliminates uncertainties as to stent deformation and enhances stent deliverability. The nitinol material provides unsurpassed flexibility, enabling the treatment of a wide variety of anatomical angles.

Sideguard provides continuous access to the side branch, even with a main vessel stent in place. This leaves the side branch free for distal stenting. More importantly, once the Sideguard stent is deployed, the operators can stent the parent vessel with any conventional coronary stent or DES. Moreover, the Sideguard stent ensures a seamless transition to the side branch without obstructing normal vessel flow at the bifurcation point.

Future developments

The Sideguard stent platform is suitable for drug delivery. Cappella is exploring the use of biodegradable polymer carriers for a Sideguard DES system.

References

1 Ormiston JA, Currie E, Webster MWI, et al. Drug-eluting stents for coronary bifurcations: Insights into the crush technique. Catheter Cardiovasc Interv 2004;63:332–6.

2 Moussa I, Costa R, Leon M, et al. A prospective registry to evaluate sirolimus-eluting stents implanted at coronary bifurcation lesions using the "crush technique". Am J Cardiol 2006;97:1317–21.

3 Costa RA, Mintz GS, Carlier SG, et al. Bifurcation coronary lesions treated with the "crush" technique: An intravascular ultrasound analysis. J AM Coll Cardiol 2005;46:599–605.

4 Kandzari DE, Goldberg S, Schwartz RS, et al. Clinical and angiographic efficacy of a self-expanding nitinol stent in saphenous vein graft atherosclerotic disease: The Stent Comparative Restenosis (SCORES) Saphenous Vein Graft Registry. Am Heart J 2003;145:868–74.

5 Doi H, Maehara A, Mintz GS, et al. Serial intravascular ultrasound analysis of bifurcation lesions treated using

the novel self-expanding Sideguard side branch stent. J AM Coll Cardiol 2009;104:1216–21.

6 Tanaka S, Watanabe S, Matsuo H, *et al.* Prospective randomized trial comparing a nitinol self-expanding coronary stent with low-pressure dilatation and a high-pressure balloon expandable bare metal stent. Heart Vessels 2008;23:1–8.

7 Kobayashi Y, Honda Y, Christie L, *et al.* Long-term vessel response to a self-expanding coronary stent: A serial volumetric intravascular ultrasound analysis from the ASSURE trial. J AM Coll Cardiol 2001;37:1329–34.

8 Fujii K, Kobayashi Y, Mintz GS, *et al.* Dominant contribution of negative remodeling to development of significant coronary bifurcation narrowing. J AM Coll Cardiol 2003;92:59–61.

9 Timurkaynak T, Ciftci H, Ozdemir M, *et al.* Sidebranch occlusion after coronary stenting with or without balloon predilation: direct versus conventional stenting. J Invas Cardiol 2002;14:497–501.

10 Meier B, Gruentzig AR, King SB III, *et al.* Risk of side branch occlusion during coronary angioplasty. Am J Cardiol 1984;53:10–14.

11 Vetrovec GW, Cowley MJ, Wolfgang TC, *et al.* Effects of percutaneous transluminal angioplasty in lesion associated branches. Am Heart J 1985;109:921–5.

12 Ciampricutti R, El Gamal M, Van Gelder B, *et al.* Coronary angioplasty of bifurcation lesions without protection of large sidebranches. Catheter Cardiovasc Diag 1992;27:191–6.

13 Renkin J, Wijns W, Hanet C, *et al.* Angioplasty of coronary bifurcation stenosis. Catheter Cardiovasc Diag 1991;22:167–73.

14 Glagov S, Weisenberg E, Zarins CK, *et al.* Compensatory enlargement of human atherosclerotic coronary arteries. NEJM 1987;316:1371–5.

15 Lefevre T, Louvard Y, Morice MC, *et al.* Stenting of bifurcation lesions: classification, treatment, and results. Catheter Cardiovasc Interv 2000;49:274–83.

16 Al Suwaidi J, Berger PB, Rihal CS, *et al.* Immediate and long-term outcome of intracoronary stent implantation for true bifurcation lesions. J AM Coll Cardiol 2000;35:929–36.

17 Brunel P, Lefevre T, Darremont O, *et al.* Provisional T-stenting and kissing balloon in the treatment of coronary bifurcation lesions: Results of the French multicenter "TULIPE" study. Catheter Cardiovasc Interv 2006;68:67–73.

18 Hoye A, Iakovou I, Ge L, *et al.* Long-term outcomes after stenting of bifurcation lesions with the "crush technique: predictors of an advanced outcome. J Am Coll Cardio 2006;47:1949–58.

19 Colombo A, Stankovic G, Orlic D, *et al.* Modified T-stenting technique with crushing for bifurcation lesions: immediate results and 30-day outcomes. Catheter Cardiovasc Interv 2003;60:145–51.

20 Latib A and Colombo A. Bifurcation disease: What do we know, what should we do. JACC: Cardiovasc Interv 2009;1:218–26.

CHAPTER 18

XIENCETM side branch access system for the treatment of bifurcation lesions (XIENCE SBA)

Gary M. Idelchik, MD *and David G. Rizik,* MD, FACC, FSCAI

Division of Interventional Cardiology, Scottsdale Healthcare Hospitals, Scottsdale, Arizona, USA

Coronary bifurcation lesions are present in approximately 10–15% of patients undergoing diagnostic angiography and remain a challenging subset of coronary artery disease (CAD) to treat by a percutaneous approach [1,2]. The complexity of this lesion subgroup arises from the morphology of the affected vessels and the limitations of the current generation of stents to effectively treat the disease variability and the angulations encountered in bifurcation lesions. Specifically, the extent of atherosclerosis affecting the main branch (MB) and side branch (SB), the diameters of the MB and SB absolutely and relative to one another, the amount of calcific and fibrocalcific disease in each vessel, the extent and location of lesions affecting both vessels, and the geometric relationship of the MB to the SB all affect treatment success [3]. These factors contribute to higher rates of procedural complications, restenosis, and target vessel revascularization (TVR) following percutaneous intervention of coronary bifurcation lesions compared with non-bifurcated lesions, independent of stent platform evaluated [2,4–6]. Despite these anatomic considerations, the successful treatment of bifurcation lesions clinically depends in part on the ability of the interventionalist to maintain continued access to the side branch and achieve adequate coverage of the side branch ostium, thereby reducing the

incidence of restenosis and/or occlusion of the side branch vessel [4,7].

Many techniques have been proposed to treat coronary bifurcation lesions, including deployment of a single stent in the main vessel followed by balloon angioplasty of the side branch alone. A variety of two-stent methodologies have also been studied, including provisional T-stenting with or without crush, V-stenting, simultaneous kissing stents, the culotte technique, and more recently, a variation called balloon alignment T-stenting [3].

Several recent randomized studies suggest that provisional T-stenting provides outcomes comparable to those seen with a dedicated two-stent approach, as well as offering procedural advantages [8,9]. The Nordic bifurcation study randomized 413 patients with a bifurcation lesion and demonstrated a statistically significant reduction in procedure time (76 vs 62 mins, P < 0.001), fluoroscopy time (21 vs 15 mins, P < 0.001), and contrast volume (283 vs 233 mL, P < 0.001) with a provisional T-stenting approach compared with planned use of two sirolimus-eluting stents [8]. However, clinical outcomes did not differ between these two strategies; the primary end-point of major adverse cardiac events (MACE: cardiac death, myocardial infarction, TVR, or stent thrombosis) occurred in 2.9% and 3.4% (P = NS) of

Bifurcation Stenting, First Edition. Edited by Ron Waksman and John A. Ormiston.
© 2012 Blackwell Publishing Ltd. Published 2012 by Blackwell Publishing Ltd.

patients at 6 months with provisional T-stenting and the planned two-stent strategy, respectively, and in 9.5% and 8.2%, respectively, at the 14-month follow-up (P = NS) [10]. Similar results were reported in the 350 patient, randomized coronary bifurcation application of the crush technique using sirolimus-eluting stents (CACTUS) trial, in which the incidence of MACE, in-segment restenosis, and stent thrombosis at 6 months did not differ between provisional T-stenting and a dedicated two-stent strategy (15% vs 15.8%, P = NS) [9]. Moreover, angiographic follow-up did not differ between.

The Nordic bifurcation study further evaluated 307 patients with follow-up angiography 8 months after the index procedure (151 patients with provisional T-stenting, 156 with planned T-stenting). The combined angiographic end point of diameter stenosis >50% of the main vessel and occlusion of the side branch was seen in 5.3% of patients who underwent provisional T-stenting and 5.1% in patients who received two sirolimus-eluting stents (P = NS) [8]. The CACTUS trial also evaluated patients 6 months after revascularization with angiographic follow-up (173 patients with provisional T-stenting and 177 patients with planned two-stent strategy) and demonstrated similar restenosis rates between provisional T-stenting (6.7% and 14.7% in the main branch and side branch, respectively) and placement of two sirolimus-eluting stents (4.6% and 13.2% in the main branch and side branch, respectively; P = NS) [9]. On the basis of these observations, provisional T-stenting has been recommended as the initial treatment strategy for bifurcation lesions.

The similarities in clinical and angiographic outcomes between provisional T-stenting and a planned two-stent approach seen in the Nordic bifurcation study and CACTUS arise from the limitations of stents to treat bifurcation lesions. Indeed, all of the proposed two-stent strategies to treat bifurcation lesions attempt to overcome the design limitations of current stents to effectively treat the complexity of disease seen in bifurcation lesions [3]. Designed to treat lesions in a single, uniform tubular vessel, stents were not intended to overcome the structural and lesion complexities encountered in branching vessels. Currently available drug-eluting stents (DES) are similarly limited

in their efficacy to treat bifurcation lesions and are currently not approved for this CAD subgroup.

Several design factors limit the use of standard DES in bifurcation lesions [3,11]. The cell architecture of current generation of DES may be distorted when manipulated to conform to the branching geometry of bifurcation lesions, increasing the risk of dissection, mal-apposition, disruption of the polymer-drug interface, and strut fracture. The uniform design of available DES, moreover, prevents access to the SB vessel due to coverage of the SB ostium with the struts of the MB stent. This limitation of current generation DES increases the procedural complexity of bifurcation lesions and increases the incidence of incomplete SB preservation and occlusion. The SB vessel must be accessed, and SB stent ultimately delivered, through the struts of the MB stent, invariably disrupting the polymer-drug interface of both the MB and SB DES. Moreover, coverage of the SB by the MB stent obscures the anatomical location of the SB ostium, which may result in either protrusion of the SB stent into the MB vessel or incomplete coverage of the SB ostium; increasing the risk for restenosis and stent thrombosis in both arteries (Figure 18.1). In addition, multiple guide wires are required to deliver stents to both the MB and SB arteries, irrespective of bifurcation treatment strategy employed, increasing the risk of wire entanglement (wire wrap) in the MB artery (Figure 18.2). Wire wrap in turn may prevent device delivery to the SB vessel and require removal of the undeliverable device and subsequent re-accessing of the SB. Attempts at accessing or re-accessing the SB may further be confounded by the inability to freely advance the guide wire within the delivered MB stent without having the wire following a course through one of the struts in the body of the MB stent proximal to the ostium of the SB artery. Moreover, depending on the degree of occlusion of the SB vessel from the MB DES, the delay in successfully accessing the SB with a guide wire and freely delivering a device to preserve the ostium of the SB vessel may increase the risk of SB occlusion.

The design limitations of current DES to treat bifurcation lesions emphasizes the need for a stent device that allows for: the continued and controlled access to the SB vessel both during and after delivery of the MB stent; treatment of the MB artery without obstruction of the SB ostium by the struts

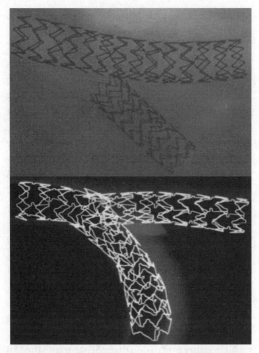

Figure 18.1 Ostial side branch stent gap (top panel) and overlap of the side branch stent into the main branch (bottom panel) are demonstrated in these Faxitron images taken from swine model, using a standard provisional T-stenting methodology.

of the MB stent; and localization of the anatomic SB ostium. The XIENCETM Side Branch Access System (XIENCETM SBA Abbott Vascular, Santa Clara, CA) is an everolimus-eluting SBA stent (EE-SBAS) designed to overcome the design limitations of current DES and therefore effectively treat bifurcation lesions. The EE-SBAS incorporates the drug, polymer, and scaffolding technology of the currently available XIENCETM V everolimus-eluting coronary stent. However, it differs from the commercially available XIENCETM V EES by incorporating design elements that provide the ability to access the SB artery through a dedicated wire port, placement of the MB artery stent without obstructing the SB artery ostium, and preservation as well as localization of the anatomic SB ostium (Figure 18.3).

The EE-SBAS was based on the bare metal Multi-Link Frontier coronary bifurcation stent system, which is currently only available in Europe. In the FRONTIER stent registry, which involved 105 patients with coronary bifurcation lesions, the bare metal Multi-Link Frontier stent system was successfully deployed in 96 patients (91%) and was associated with a low rate of acute procedural complications with an in-hospital MACE rate of

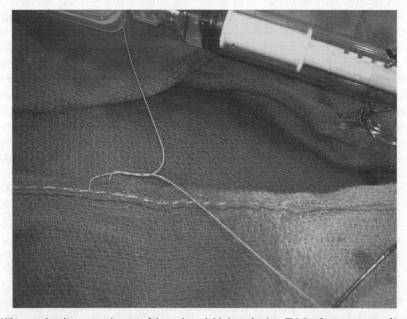

Figure 18.2 Wire wrap involves entanglement of the main and side branch wires. This is a frequent cause of inability to pass coronary devices beyond the carina of the vessel.

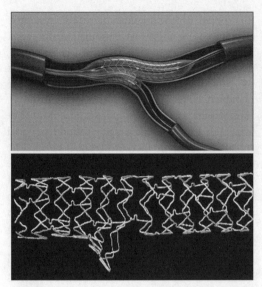

Figure 18.3 The Xience SBA system shown in fully expanded profile.

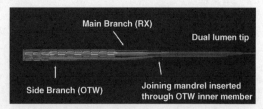

Figure 18.4 Deployment profile of the Xience SBA system. Until released, the joining mandrel maintains the main and side branch ports a single-tip delivery system.

2.9% [6]. However, the incidence of MACE at 6 months was 17.1%, primarily due to a TVR rate of 13.3%. Quantitative coronary angiography at 6 months revealed main branch in-stent and in-segment restenosis rates of 25.3% and 29.9%, respectively, and side branch in-segment restenosis incidence of 29.1%. Overall, the rate of restenosis for any branch artery (main or side) was 44.8%. The high rate of restenosis observed in the FRONTIER stent registry was due to the use of a bare metal device as well as lack of a clear consensus on the optimal side branch treatment strategy.

The EE-SBAS was designed to address the MB and SB restenoses seen with a bare metal stent platform like the FRONTIER stent, while similarly preserving access to the SB artery. Composed of radio-opaque cobalt chromium with struts only 0.0034 inches in thickness, the EE-SBAS is coated with a biocompatible fluoropolymer containing everolimus, which allows release of the drug at a dose and rate similar to that in the XIENCE™ V DES. The EE-SBAS delivery catheter contains a unique joining mandrel that holds the main branch and side branch tips together, thereby helping to avoid wire wrap (Figure 18.4). This also allows for a lower delivery profile in that main and side branch ports are advanced to the bifurcation as a single-tip delivery system. The delivery catheter has a two

guide wire lumens and two balloons attached to the distal end. The MB balloon is attached to the rapid-exchange (RX) lumen, while the SB balloon is attached to the over-the-wire (OTW) lumen. The bifurcation stent is crimped on both balloons, allowing for the SB balloon to exit the stent at the portal opening located in the center of the stent. Proximal to the two balloons, the two inflation lumens are joined into a single common inflation lumen that can be pressurized with a single inflation device. The side branch OTW lumen is occupied by a joining mandrel that exits the side branch balloon and immediately enters a pocket alongside the extended main branch balloon, effectively joining the two balloon tips together and thereby allowing for easy delivery using the RX lumen wire only. The design of the EE-SBAS allows for treatment of the MB artery with an EES while providing simple access into the SB. In this regard, the device remains identical in strut architecture, strut thickness, polymer, and drug elution kinetics to the commercially available EES with the simple addition of a SB access wire port.

The similarities in design of the EE-SBAS to the XIENCE™ V EES may also improve preservation of the side-branch independently of the ability to access the SB provided by the EE-SBAS. The SPIRIT III trial evaluated 1,002 patients that were randomized to either EES or to the TAXUS Express-2™ stent (paclitaxel-eluting stent, PES) [12]. Although true bifurcations were excluded, MB lesions with an involved SB <2 mm in diameter and having an ostial stenosis of <50% were enrolled and characterized as having a SB jailed by the MB stent (113 EES and 63 PES). EES was associated with a 64.2% reduction in MACE at 2 years (6.8% vs 19.0%, P = 0.03) and a 48.3% decrease in the incidence of TVR (10.7% vs 20.7%, P = 0.10). There was also a trend in the reduction of MI (2.9% vs 10.3%, P = 0.07) as well as stent thrombosis (1.0% vs 3.5%, P = 0.30) in patients treated with EES relative to PES. The recently published COMPARE trial randomized 1,800 patients to either EES or to the second-generation TAXUS LiberteTM stent (PES) and evaluated the combined primary endpoint of all-cause mortality, MI, and TVR at 12 months [13]. Of the patients randomized, approximately18% were classified as having bifurcation lesions in each treatment arm. The absolute reduction in the primary endpoint associated with EES was 3% (6% vs 9% incidence, P = 0.02). The difference was attributable to a lower incidence of stent thrombosis (<1% vs 3%, P = 0.002), MI (3% vs 5%, P = 0.007), and TVR (2% vs 6%, P = 0.0001). The incidence of cardiac death, non-fatal MI, and TVR occurred in 5% of patients treated with EES compared with 8% of patients treated with PES (P = 0.005).

The deployment sequence of the EE-SBS is basic (Figure 18.5). Logistically, the EE-SBAS is delivered to the target site via the main branch RX wire only. Following wiring of the main branch artery, the main branch stent RX balloon tip of the XIENCETM SBA stent is back-loaded onto the wire in the main branch. With the two balloon tips joined by the mandrel wire, the system is advanced to a point just proximal to the target bifurcation. The joining mandrel wire is subsequently removed by unlocking the mandrel wire at the proximal adapter hub, and withdrawing the mandrel wire from the OTW lumen (Figure 18.4). A new wire is then introduced into the OTW lumen to exit the side branch balloon tip, and carefully placed in the side branch vessel. The system is advanced into the bifurcation until gentle resistance is encountered and forward progress of the device is stopped. With a single inflation device, both the main and side branch balloons are pressurized, deploying the stent in the main branch and opening a portal into the side branch. Following deflation, the delivery system is retracted over both the RX and the OTW wires, preserving access to both the main and side branch arteries and allowing for post-dilation of the stented segments and additional treatment of the side-branch artery if warranted. Bifurcation lesions requiring pre-treatment of both main and side branches prior to EE-SBAS placement and deployment, are treated in a similar manner, with the additional steps of pre-wiring of both arteries, pretreatment of the stenotic segments in the main and side branch vessels, advancement of the device as described

1. System is advanced into the main branch over conventional RX wire

2. Joining mandrel is released allowing advancement into the side-branch tip

3. Positioning of guide wire in the side branch. Entire system is advanced to the carina

4. Stent is deployed with a simultaneous inflation of both balloons through a single inflation port

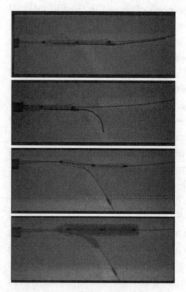

Figure 18.5 Deployment sequence of the Xience SBA system.

over the RX wire alone while maintaining the SB wire (if warranted), removal of the mandrel wire from the EE-SBAS OTW lumen, introduction of a third wire through the OTW lumen of the EE-SBAS into the side branch, removal of the previously placed side branch wire, and subsequent deployment of the EE-SBAS and removal of the delivery device as described.

Recently the EE-SBAS has been evaluated against provisional T-stenting with Multi-Link Vision stents using an in vitro bench-top, perfused, synthetic coronary artery model with SB angulations of 30°, 50°, 70° and 90° [14]. The deployment of both the EE-SBAS and provisional T-stenting with Multi-Link Vision stents was performed under fluoroscopic guidance and stent positioning was analyzed using high-resolution 2D Faxitron imaging to evaluate deployment accuracy of the side branch stent relative to the main branch. The primary endpoints evaluated were: (1) total procedure time until kissing balloon post-dilatation; (2) elapsed time until MB stent deployment, and additional elapsed time to SB stent deployment; (3) total fluoroscopy time; (4) total contrast media volume used; (5) delivery and deployment accuracy of the stents in the MB and SB, including evaluation of SB stent overlap, protrusions, and gaps; (6) incidence, severity, and impact of guide wire wrap during procedure; and (7) incidence of out-of-phase deployment of the bifurcation DES.

A total of 18 procedures, nine using the EE-SBAS and nine using provisional T-stenting with Multi-Link Vision stents, were performed. Deployment of the EE-SBAS was accomplished in a similar total time as the Multi-Link Vision stents deployed by a provisional T-stenting approach (14.9 vs 14.6 minutes). The time required to achieve stent deployment in the MB, however, was less with the to EE-SBAS (4.0 vs 6.6 minutes), and as a result, total contrast usage (49.4 vs 69.4 cm³) and fluoroscopy time (5.1 vs 6.2 minutes) was lower in the EE-SBAS arm. The EE-SBAS had a lower incidence of wire wrap (22% vs 89%) and less distal protrusion of the SB stent into the MB (0.54 vs 1.21 mm) relative to the provisional T-stenting arm and there was a trend for less proximal protrusion with the EE-SBAS (0.43 vs 0.59 mm). Significant

gaps in ostial SB coverage were not seen in either study group.

The differences in fluoroscopy time and total contrast administered are relevant when considering the risk-versus-benefit of treating bifurcation lesions percutaneously. Iodinated contrast media, known to cause nephrotoxicity, is the third leading cause of hospital-acquired acute renal failure [15–17]. The use of lower contrast volumes would therefore be expected to reduce risk of contrast-induced nephropathy. Fluoroscopy may be associated with radiation exposure at a rate as high as 0.2 Gy (20 rads) per minute and can lead to radiation-related complications [18,19]. A decrease in fluoroscopy time would reduce radiation exposure during the stenting procedure. With increasing tortuosity and angulations of both the main and side branch arteries proximal and distal to the areas of stenoses seen in vivo, the difference in contrast administration, fluoroscopy time, as well as total procedure time between the EE-SBAS and provisional T-stenting would likely be even more significant.

The outcome of one- and two-stent strategies in the treatment of bifurcation coronary lesions has been extensively evaluated [3,5]. Although numerous techniques have been proposed, no single approach completely circumvents the limitations of the current DES platforms to treat the complex lesions and geometries encountered in bifurcation lesions [5,15]. Secondary to the inherent limitations of current DES platforms, provisional T-stenting has demonstrated clinical and angiographic outcomes comparable to more complex, multi-stent approaches.

The EE-SBAS possesses many of the features desired in an optimal device for bifurcation lesions. The side branch portal of EE-SBAS provides scaffolding to the ostium of the side branch, thereby minimizing ostial gaps and MB overlap (Figures 18.1 and 18.6). Access to the SB is preserved following deflation and retraction of the delivery device, as well as a reduction in MB over-lap compared to slotted tube stents used in a provisional T-stenting approach. Together, these features contribute to a reduction in contrast usage and fluoroscopy time seen in the synthetic anatomical model described by Rizik *et al.* [14].

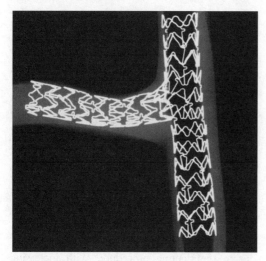

Figure 18.6 Faxitron image (taken form a swine model) of the optimal deployment of the Xience SBA system with additional side branch stent deployed. The side branch ostium is optimally covered in this model at a side branch angle of 90°.

Although the clinical endpoints of TVR, MI, stent thrombosis, and cardiac death are lacking for the EE-SBAS, the efficacy of the EES demonstrated by SPIRIT III and COMPARE in patients with jailed SB vessels and bifurcation lesions, respectively, strongly suggests that the added ability of accessing the SB provided by the EE-SBAS would further result in improved outcomes in the treatment of coronary bifurcation lesions relative to a provisional T-stenting approach [12,13]. Further evaluation of the EE-SBAS in both animal models and clinical trials is needed.

References

1 Al Suwaidi J, Yeh W, Cohen HA, et al. Immediate and one-year outcome in patients with coronary bifurcation lesions in the modern era (NHLBI dynamic registry). Am J Cardiol 2001;87:1139–1144.

2 Garot P, Lefevre T, Savage M, et al. Nine-month outcome of patients treated by percutaneous coronary interventions for bifurcation lesions in the recent era. A report from the Prevention of Restensosis with Tranilast and its Outcomes (PRESTO) trial. J Am Coll Cardiol 2005;46: 606–12.

3 Rizik DG, Klassen KJ, Hermiller JB. Bifurcation coronary artery disease: Current techniques and future directions (Part 1). J Invasive Cardiol 2008;20:82–90.

4 Colombo A, Moses JW, Morice MC, et al. Randomized study to evaluate sirolimus-eluting stents implanted at coronary bifurcation lesions. Circulation 2004;109: 1244–9.

5 Iakovou I, Colombo A. Contemporary stent treatment of coronary bifurcation. J Am Coll Cardiol 2005;46: 1446–55.

6 Lefevre T, Ormiston J, Guagliumi G, et al. The FRONTIER stent registry. Safety and feasibility of a novel dedicated stent for the treatment of bifurcation coronary artery lesions. J Am Coll Cardiol 2005;46:592–8.

7 Costa RA, Mintz GS, Carlier SG, et al. Bifurcation coronary lesions treated with the "crush" technique. An intravascular ultrasound analysis. J Am Coll Cardiol 2005;46:599–605.

8 Steigen TK, Maeng M, Wiseth R, et al. Randomized study on simple versus complex stenting of coronary artery bifurcation lesions. The Nordic bifurcation study. Circulation 2006;114:1955–61.

9 Colombo A, Bramucci E, Sacca S, et al. Randomized study of the crush technique versus provisional side-branch stenting in true coronary bifurcations. The CACTUS (Coronary Bifurcations: Application of the Crushing Technique Using Sirolimus-Eluting Stents) Study. Circulation 2009;119:71–8.

10 Jensen JS, Galløe A, Lassen JF, et al. Safety in simple versus complex stenting of coronary artery bifurcation lesions. The Nordic Bifurcation Study 14-month follow-up results. EuroIntervention 2008;4:229–33.

11 Rizik DG, Klassen KJ, Hermiller JB. Bifurcation coronary artery disease: Current techniques and future directions (Part 2). J Invasive Cardiol 2008;20:135–41.

12 Stone GW, Midei M, Newman W, et al. for the SPIRIT III Investigators. Randomized Comparison of Everolimus-Eluting and Paclitaxel-Eluting Stents: Two-year clinical follow-up from the clinical evaluation of the Xience V everolimus eluting coronary stent system in the treatment of patients with de novo native coronary artery lesions (SPIRIT) III trial. Circulation 2009;119; 680–6.

13 Kedhi E, Joesoef KS, Eugene McFadden E, et al. Second-generation everolimus-eluting and paclitaxel-eluting stents in real-life practice (COMPARE): a randomised trial. Lancet Published Online January 8, 2010;1–6.

14 Rizik DG, Klag JM, Tenaglia A, et al. Evaluation of a bifurcation drug-eluting stent system versus provisionl T-stening in a perfused synthetic coronary artery model. J Interven Cardiol 2009;22:537–46.

15 Tsuchida K, Colombo A, Lefevre T, et al. The clinical outcome of percutaneous treatment of bifurcation lesions in multi-vessel coronary artery disease with the sirolimus-eluting stent: Insights from the Arterial Revascularization

Therapies Study part II (ARTS II). Eur Heart J 2007;28: 433–42.

16 Schneider LM, Roubin GS. Minimal contrast use in carotid stenting: avoiding contrast pitfalls. J Invasive Cardiol 2007;19:37–8.

17 Schweiger MJ, Chambers CE, Davidson CJ, *et al.* Prevention of contrast-induced nephropathy: Recommendations for the high-risk patient undergoing cardiovascular procedures. Catheter Cardiovasc Interv 2007;69:135–40.

18 Mettler FA Jr, Koenig TR, Wagner LK, *et al.* Radiation exposure after fluoroscopic procedures. Semin Ultrasound CT MR 2002;23:428–42.

19 Rehani MM, Ortiz-Lopez P. Radiation effects in fluoroscopically guided cardiac interventions–keeping them under control. Int J Cardiol 2006;109:147–51.

CHAPTER 19

The spherical balloon: A new tool to optimize bifurcation treatment

Remo Albiero, MD

Emodinamica, Istituto Clinico San Rocco, Ome (Brescia), Italy

Introduction

Bifurcation lesions are frequent in routine practice, accounting for up to 20% of all coronary disease treated by percutaneous coronary intervention [1]. Based on the results of six randomized controlled trials (RCTs) [2–7], a stepwise provisional side branch (SB) stenting strategy with drug-eluting stents is consensually considered [8] a preferable technique to deliberate double stenting in bifurcation lesions. The spherical balloon is a post-dilatation balloon, very useful to optimize the provisional SB T-stenting technique in the treatment of coronary bifurcations with minimal or no disease at the ostium of the SB (i.e. in type 1,1,0 or 0,1,0 bifurcations as described by the simple and well accepted Medina classification [9,10]) or with disease in the SB ostium only (i.e. type 0,0,1 by Medina). In order to understand the usage of the spherical post-dilation balloon to optimize the results of the provisional SB T-stenting strategy in these types of lesion it is useful first to describe an important anatomical characteristic of coronary bifurcations (i.e. plaque distribution) and briefly review the technique.

Plaque distribution in coronary bifurcations

Atherosclerotic plaques and wall thickenings in human coronary arteries are localized almost exclusively on the outer wall of one or both daughter vessels at major bifurcations, where the flow is either slow or disturbed with the formation of slow recirculation and secondary flows and where wall shear stress (WSS) is low. Pathologic studies in coronary arteries show that the atherosclerotic plaques are located mainly along the inner side of the curved coronary arteries, close to the areas of low shear stress. Regions exposed to the non-uniform low shear stresses develop early atherosclerotic lesions while areas exposed to uniform high shear stresses are protected [11–18]. Consequently, atherosclerotic plaque usually develops in both branches opposite of the flow divider [19–22], which is almost always free of disease, due the atheroprotective effect of high shear stresses [23–26]. In an intravascular ultrasound (IVUS) study in left main bifurcations in 73 patients [27], angiography suggested that the flow divider (carina) was involved in 61%, while IVUS showed that the carina was spared in all 73 patients. Current IVUS observations confirm these findings (Figure 19.1). Understanding the patterns of plaque distribution in coronary bifurcations has led to technique modification and the idea of using a post-dilatation spherical balloon in order to increase the likelihood of success when adopting the provisional SB T-stenting technique in coronary bifurcations with minimal or no disease at the ostium of the SB or with disease in the SB ostium only.

Bifurcation Stenting, First Edition. Edited by Ron Waksman and John A. Ormiston.

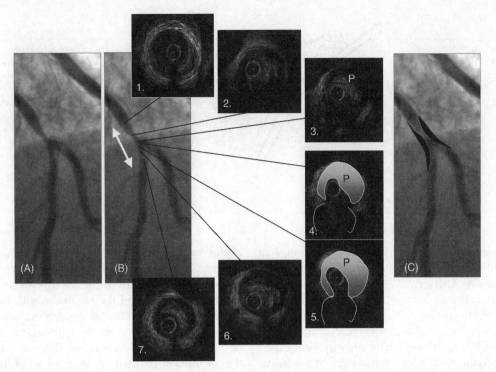

Figure 19.1 Carina is not involved by atherosclerosis. (a) True bifurcation lesion (Medina 1,1,1) in the mid LAD involving the ostium of diagonal branch; (b) IVUS performed before stenting shows that the flow divider (carina) (images 4 and 5) is not involved by the atherosclerotic plaque (P), which is localized; (c) on the outer wall of one or both daughter vessels, where wall shear stress (WSS) is low.

Review of the provisional SB T-stenting technique

Provisional T stenting consists of stenting the main branch (MB) first, followed, if necessary, by the delivery of a second stent in the SB through the main branch stent in a classic T [28] or TAP (T and small protrusion) [29] configuration. The advantage of this approach is that the use of a second stent is only provisional. Provisional SB T-stenting strategy begins with wiring of both branches. The MB is then pre-dilated if required. Predilation of the SB is not required in coronary bifurcations with minimal or no disease at the ostium of the SB. A stent with a diameter sized according to the distal reference segment is then implanted in the MB, leaving the SB wire outside the stent ("jailed" guide wire technique). After MB stenting, the carina (almost always free of disease) is displaced/shifted toward the SB ostium. At this point a decision is required regarding the need for kissing balloon inflation. If the angiographic results in the MB and in the SB are satisfactory with normal flow and with residual diameter stenosis <50–75% [4,5,30], the jailed SB wire is removed and the procedure is complete [31]. If the result at the SB ostium is not satisfactory or if the operator performs systematic final kissing balloon inflation, the SB should be rewired. Side branch rewiring is generally performed by "guide wire exchange", using the MB wire pulled back slowly from the main vessel with its tip pointed toward the SB ostium with the intention to cross into the SB through the distal strut closest to the tip of the flow divider. After the MB wire has crossed into the SB, the "jailed wire" is withdrawn from the SB and pushed distally in the MB. For most operators who do not perform a systematic kissing balloon inflation after MB stenting, the treatment of bifurcations with minimal or no disease at the ostium of the SB (Medina 1,0,0 or 1,1,0 or 0,1,0 as shown in Figure 19.2A; also called

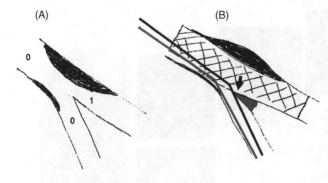

Figure 19.2 The case of false bifurcation (Medina 0,1,0). (a) Atherosclerotic plaque is mainly located on the outer wall of the mother vessel; (b) After main branch stenting the carina is shifted (short arrow) and there is the possibility (due to the absence of disease in the side branch ostium) to rewire the side branch through a proximal or a distal strut (proximal versus distal cross).

"pseudo-bifurcations") seems easier compared to the treatment of bifurcation with a SB lesion (Medina 1,1,1 or 0,1,1 or 1,0,1; also called "true bifurcations") because they stop the procedure after MB stenting, without performing the "guide wire exchange", dilatation of the SB ostium and/or final kissing balloon. On the contrary, more expert operators who adopt the strategy of systematic kissing balloon after MB stenting [8,10,32], are faced with the problem of a "proximal" versus "distal cross" during "guide wire exchange" before kissing balloon (Figure 19.2B). In other words, although SB rewiring is done taking care to pull the wire back slowly from the main vessel and pointing the tip toward the SB ostium with the intention to cross into the SB through the distal strut closest to the tip of the flow divider, this is not certain. Only a "distal cross" (i.e. rewiring the SB through the stent strut at the tip of the flow divider, Figure 19.3C) will guarantee an optimal SB ostium scaffolding after subsequent kissing balloon inflation (Figure 19.3D). A "proximal cross"

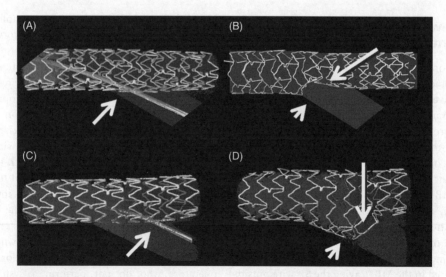

Figure 19.3 Proximal versus distal cross and result after kissing balloon inflation. (a) The case of proximal cross (arrow); (b) After kissing balloon: poor side branch ostium scaffolding (short arrow) associated with strut displacement inside the main branch stent (long arrow); (c) The case of distal cross (arrow); (d) After kissing balloon: good side branch ostium scaffolding (short arrow) associated with expansion of the main branch stent at the carina level (long arrow).

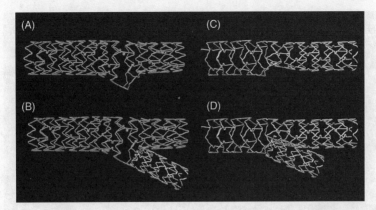

Figure 19.4 The case of "proximal cross" with and without the use of a spherical balloon during provisional T stenting. (a) Final result with the use of the spherical balloon post-dilation strategy; (b) If an additional stent is required in the side branch, T stenting without neo-carena can be performed; (c) Risk of final result without the use of the spherical balloon post-dilation strategy; (d) In case of provisional T stenting, the TAP (T and protrusion) with a neocarena should be done to completely cover/scaffold the side branch ostium. This could increase the risk of subsequent restenosis and/or stent thrombosis.

(i.e. rewiring the SB through a stent strut proximal to the flow divider, Figure 19.3A) may lead to deformation of the MB stent during subsequent kissing balloon inflation (Figure 19.3B) and increases the odds of needing provisional stent implantation. In this latter scenario, to optimally scaffold the SB ostium, the provisional SB stent typically protrudes into the MB, creating a neocarena in the main vessel (Figure 19.4D), with potentially increased risk of stent thrombosis.

A new tool: the spherical balloon

To assist operators in identifying a wrong "proximal cross" versus a correct "distal cross" in coronary bifurcations with minimal or no disease at

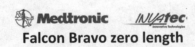

Falcon Bravo zero length

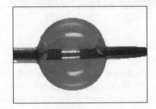

Shaft length	145 cm
Balloon material	FLEXITEC™ HF
Balloon diameter	3.0, 3.5, 4.0, 4.5, 5.0 mm
Coating	LFC Hydrophilic Coating
Shaft diameter	RX: 2.5F (dist), 2.0F (prox)
Marker	1 swaged Platinum Iridium
RBP (bar)	15

Specifications

Ref N°.	Balloon diameter (mm)	Balloon lenght (mm)	OTW / RX	Usable shaft lenght (cm)	N° of markers
FLC 030 000 B11	3.00	0	RX	145	1
FLC 035 000 B11	3.50	0	RX	145	1
FLC 040 000 B11	4.00	0	RX	145	1
FLC 045 000 B11*	4.50	0	RX	145	1
FLC 050 000 B11*	5.00	0	RX	145	1

* Sizes not yet available

Compliance Chart

Pressure (bar)	Balloon diameter 3.00	3.50	4.00
5	2.90	3.40	3.90
6	2.95	3.45	3.95
7(nominal)	3.00	3.50	4.00
8	3.03	3.54	4.05
9	3.07	3.58	4.10
10	3.11	3.62	4.15
11	3.15	3.66	4.20
12	3.19	3.70	4.25
13	3.23	3.75	4.30
14	3.27	3.80	4.35
15	3.31	3.85	4.40

☐ in vitro results   ▨ do not exceed RBP

Not available for sale in US

Figure 19.5 Technical specifications of the spherical balloon available for sale in Europe (by Medtronic-Invatec) with the commercial name of "Falcon Bravo zero length".

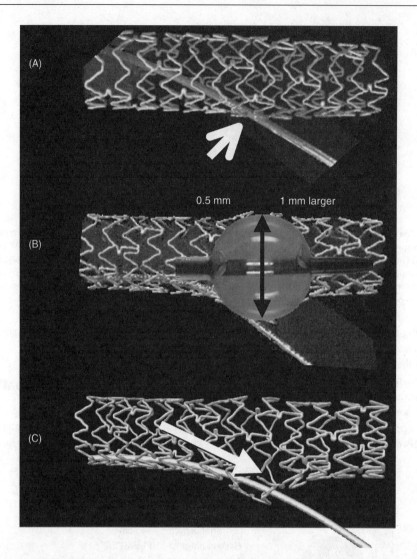

Figure 19.6 Utility of a very short (spherical) oversized, post-dilation balloon to discover a proximal cross. (a) The case of proximal cross (arrow); (b) Inflation of the spherical oversized balloon (with a diameter 0.5 mm larger than the proximal reference and 1 mm larger than the distal reference diameter) with the central marker positioned 1 mm proximal to the flow divider. After spherical balloon inflation, the guide wire will be jailed and the balloon used for the subsequent kissing inflation will not cross easily in the side branch; (c) Due to protrusion of struts into the side branch ostium induced by the spherical balloon inflation, it will be easy to reposition the wire between distal struts where the wire will cross now on a wide front.

the ostium of the SB (i.e. type 1,1,0 or 0,1,0 by Medina) or with disease in the SB ostium only (i.e. type 0,0,1 by Medina), a new tool is currently being used: a spherical balloon (Figure 19.5), which is inflated at the carina after guide wire exchange and before the kissing balloon inflation (Figure 19.6). This spherical balloon is sized 0.5 mm larger than the proximal reference main branch diameter and 1 mm larger than the distal main branch diameter,

as illustrated in Figure 19.6B. After inflation of this spherical balloon with the central marker positioned 1 mm proximal to the flow divider (Figure 19.7D), two tests are performed: (1) a check of the free movement of the guide wire in the SB; (2) a check of the free passage into the SB of the balloon selected for the kissing (Figure 19.7F). If one or both the tests fail, there is still the chance to rewire the SB before performing the final kissing

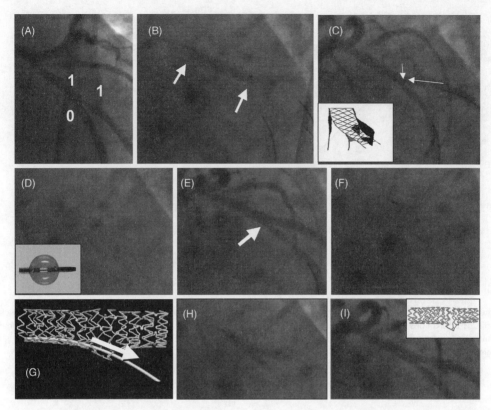

Figure 19.7 Stent implantation in a false bifurcation (Medina 1,1,0). (a) Baseline angiogram of the LCx-OM bifurcation; (b) 3.0 × 23 mm drug eluting stent implantation at 12 atm with a jailed wire in the side branch; (c) The flow divider (carina) is mildly shifted; guide wire exchange is performed trying to cross into the side branch through the more distal strut closest to the carina (short arrows); (d) Spherical 3.5 mm balloon inflation at 18 atm with the central marker of the balloon positioned 1 mm proximal to the flow divider; (e) Angiogram after spherical balloon inflation; (f) A 2,0 × 15 mm new Maverick balloon failed to cross into the side branch; (g) The side branch guidewire (probably jailed after the prior proximal cross) was removed and easily repositioned in the distal struts where it crossed on a wide front; (h) Final kissing balloon; (i) Final result after kissing balloon with good side branch ostium scaffolding associated with expansion of the main branch stent at the carina level.

balloon inflation. During the next SB rewiring, the probability to rewire the wrong proximal strut ("proximal cross") is minimized because with the prior spherical balloon inflation the proximal stent strut was apposed against the outer wall of the SB. There is therefore a very high probability to cross into the SB through the "right" distal strut ("distal cross") (Figure 19.7G).

The need of a final kissing inflation

The final kissing balloon inflation is mandatory after the spherical balloon inflation (Figure 19.7H)

in order to correct the MB stent deformation at the edges of the balloon that results after inflation of this slightly oversized and not cylindrical balloon. The final kissing balloon inflation, when done correctly after a "distal cross" (Figure 19.7I), not only corrects the MB stent deformation, but also provides a better scaffolding of the SB ostium and facilitates future access to the SB [33,34]. Kissing balloon inflation should be performed with two balloons that are matched to the MB distal reference and to the SB diameters (Figure 19.7H). Furthermore, the final kissing balloon inflation in Medina (0,1,0) lesions, guarantees a good vessel wall apposition of the proximal stent segment (Figure 19.8).

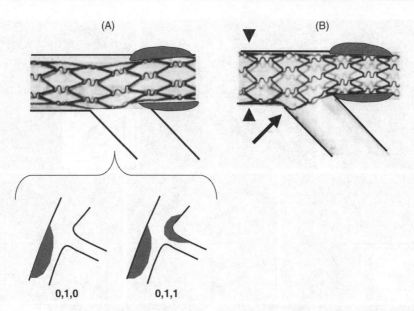

Figure 19.8 The role of final kissing balloon inflation in 0,1,0 and 0,1,1 bifurcations. (a) After main branch stent implantation in a 0,1,0 or 0,1,1 lesion, the proximal stent segment is not apposed to the vessel wall; (b) After final kissing balloon inflation the proximal stent segment is well apposed to the vessel wall (short arrows) with additional scaffolding of the side branch ostium (long arrow).

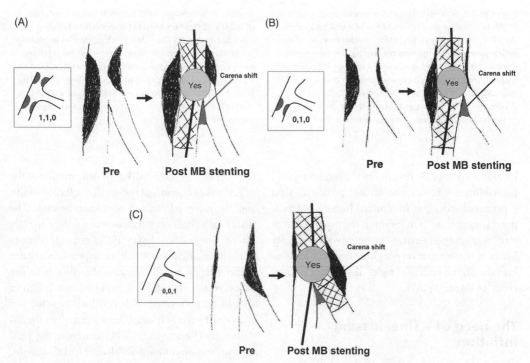

Figure 19.9 Utility of the zero length spherical, oversized, post-dilation balloon to discover a "proximal cross" in Medina 1,1,0 (a) in Medina 0,1,0; (b) and in Medina 0,0,1; (c) bifurcations.

Conclusions

Based on the results of six randomized controlled trials [2–7], a stepwise provisional SB stenting strategy with drug-eluting stents is consensually considered [8] a preferable technique to deliberate double stenting in bifurcation lesions suitable for both treatments. This strategy is applicable to over 90% non-selected coronary bifurcation lesions in the real world [35]. A new adjunctive tool (a spherical oversized balloon inflated at the carina after guide wire exchange and before the kissing balloon inflation) can be used to assist operators in identifying a wrong "proximal cross" versus a correct "distal cross" in coronary bifurcations with minimal or no disease at the ostium of the SB (1,1,0 or 0,1,0 as shown in Figure 19.9A and Figure 19.9B) or with disease in the SB ostium only (0,0,1 as shown in Figure 19.9C).

References

1 Tsuchida K, Colombo A, Lefevre T, *et al.* The clinical outcome of percutaneous treatment of bifurcation lesions in multivessel coronary artery disease with the sirolimus-eluting stent: insights from the Arterial Revascularization Therapies Study part II (ARTS II). Euro Heart J 2007;28(4):433–42.

2 Colombo A, Moses JW, Morice MC, *et al.* Randomized study to evaluate sirolimus-eluting stents implanted at coronary bifurcation lesions. Circulation 2004;109(10):1244–9.

3 Pan M, de Lezo JS, Medina A, *et al.* Rapamycin-eluting stents for the treatment of bifurcated coronary lesions: a randomized comparison of a simple versus complex strategy. Am Heart J 2004;148(5):857–64.

4 Steigen TK, Maeng M, Wiseth R, *et al.* Randomized study on simple versus complex stenting of coronary artery bifurcation lesions: the Nordic bifurcation study. Circulation 2006;114(18):1955–61.

5 Ferenc M, Gick M, Kienzle RP, *et al.* Randomized trial on routine vs. provisional T-stenting in the treatment of de novo coronary bifurcation lesions. Euro Heart J 2008;29(23):2859–67.

6 Colombo A, Bramucci E, Sacca S, *et al.* Randomized study of the crush technique versus provisional side-branch stenting in true coronary bifurcations: the CACTUS (Coronary Bifurcations: Application of the Crushing Technique Using Sirolimus-Eluting Stents) Study. Circulation 2009;119(1):71–8.

7 Hildick-Smith D. The British Bifurcation Coronary Study: old, new and evolving strategies (BBC ONE study).

Presented at Transcatheter Cardiovascular Therapeutics (TCT), Washington DC; 2008.

8 Legrand V, Thomas M, Zelisko M, *et al.* Percutaneous coronary intervention of bifurcation lesions: state-of-the-art. Insights from the second meeting of the European Bifurcation Club. EuroIntervention 2007;3(9):44–9.

9 Medina A, Suarez de Lezo J, Pan M. [A new classification of coronary bifurcation lesions]. Revista Espanola Cardiol 2006;59(2):183.

10 Thomas M, Hildick-Smith D, Louvard Y, *et al.* Percutaneous coronary intervention for bifurcation disease. A consensus view from the first meeting of the European Bifurcation Club. EuroIntervention 2006;2(6):149–53.

11 Kassab GS, Fung YC. The pattern of coronary arteriolar bifurcations and the uniform shear hypothesis. Ann Biomed Eng 1995;23(1):13–20.

12 Kimura BJ, Russo RJ, Bhargava V, McDaniel MB, Peterson KL, DeMaria AN. Atheroma morphology and distribution in proximal left anterior descending coronary artery: in vivo observations. J Am Coll Cardiol 1996;27(4):825–31.

13 Peacock J, Jones T, Tock C, Lutz R. An in vitro study on the effect of branch points on the stability of coronary artery flow. Med Eng Phys 1997;19(2):101–8.

14 Perktold K, Hofer M, Rappitsch G, Loew M, Kuban BD, Friedman MH. Validated computation of physiologic flow in a realistic coronary artery branch. J Biomech 1998;31(3):217–28.

15 Doriot P, Dorsaz P, Dorsaz L, Chatelain P. Accuracy of coronary flow measurements performed by means of Doppler wires. Ultrasound Med Biol 2000;26(2):221–8.

16 Weydahl ES, Moore JE. Dynamic curvature strongly affects wall shear rates in a coronary artery bifurcation model. J Biomech 2001;34(9):1189–96.

17 Jin S, Yang Y, Oshinski J, Tannenbaum A, Gruden J, Giddens D. Flow patterns and wall shear stress distributions at atherosclerotic-prone sites in a human left coronary artery–an exploration using combined methods of CT and computational fluid dynamics. Conf Proc IEEE Eng Med Biol Soc 2004;5:3789–91.

18 Fabregues S, Baijens K, Rieu R, Bergeron P. Hemodynamics of endovascular prostheses. J Biomech 1998;31(1):45–54.

19 Mallus MT, Kutryk MJ, Prati F, *et al.* Extent and distribution of atherosclerotic plaque in relation to major coronary side-branches: an intravascular ultrasound study in vivo. Giornale Italiano di Cardiologia 1998;28(9):961–9.

20 Wahle A, Lopez JJ, Olszewski ME, *et al.* Plaque development, vessel curvature, and wall shear stress in coronary arteries assessed by X-ray angiography and intravascular ultrasound. Med Image Anal 2006;10(4):615–31.

21 Papafaklis MI, Katsouras CS, Theodorakis PE, Bourantas CV, Fotiadis DI, Michalis LK. Coronary dilatation 10 weeks after paclitaxel-eluting stent implantation. No role of shear stress in lumen enlargement? Heart and Vessels 2007;22(4):268–73.

22 Banks J, Bressloff NW. Turbulence modeling in three-dimensional stenosed arterial bifurcations. J Biomech Eng 2007;129(1):40–50.

23 Montenegro MR, Eggen DA. Topography of atherosclerosis in the coronary arteries. Lab Invest; J Tech Meth Path 1968;18(5):586–93.

24 Caro CG, Fitz-Gerald JM, Schroter RC. Atheroma and arterial wall shear. Observation, correlation and proposal of a shear dependent mass transfer mechanism for atherogenesis. Proc R Soc Lond Series B 1971;177(46): 109–59.

25 Schwartz CJ, Mitchell Jr., Observations on localization of arterial plaques. Circ Res 1962;11:63–73.

26 Asakura T, Karino T. Flow patterns and spatial distribution of atherosclerotic lesions in human coronary arteries. Circ Res 1990;66(4):1045–66.

27 Oviedo C, Maehara A, Mintz G, et al. A critical intravascular ultrasound appraisal of the angiographic classification of bifurcation lesions: Where is the plaque really located? J Am Coll Cardiol 2008;51(Poster2902-16): B23–B98.

28 Lefevre T, Louvard Y, Morice MC, Loubeyre C, Piechaud JF, Dumas P. Stenting of bifurcation lesions: a rational approach. J Interv Cardiol 2001;14(6):573–85.

29 Burzotta F, Gwon HC, Hahn JY, et al. Modified T-stenting with intentional protrusion of the side-branch stent within the main vessel stent to ensure ostial coverage and facilitate final kissing balloon: the T-stenting and small protrusion technique (TAP-stenting). Report of bench testing and first clinical Italian-Korean two-centre experience. Catheter Cardiovasc Interv 2007;70(1): 75–82.

30 Koo BK, Kang HJ, Youn TJ, et al. Physiologic assessment of jailed side branch lesions using fractional flow reserve. J Am Coll Cardiol 2005;46(4):633–7.

31 Pan M, Suarez de Lezo J, Medina A, et al. A stepwise strategy for the stent treatment of bifurcated coronary lesions. Catheter Cardiovasc Interv 2002;55(1):50–7.

32 Ormiston JA, Webster MW, Ruygrok PN, Stewart JT, White HD, Scott DS. Stent deformation following simulated side-branch dilatation: a comparison of five stent designs. Catheter Cardiovasc Interv 1999;47(2): 258–64.

33 Brunel P, Lefevre T, Darremont O, Louvard Y. Provisional T-stenting and kissing balloon in the treatment of coronary bifurcation lesions: results of the French multicenter "TULIPE" study. Catheter Cardiovasc Interv 2006;68(1):67–73.

34 Ormiston JA, Webster MW, El Jack S, et al. Drug-eluting stents for coronary bifurcations: bench testing of provisional side-branch strategies. Catheter Cardiovasc Interv 2006;67(1):49–55.

35 Routledge HC, Morice MC, Lefèvre T, et al. 2-Year Outcome of Patients Treated for Bifurcation Coronary Disease With Provisional Side Branch T-Stenting Using Drug-Eluting Stents. J Am Coll Cardiol Intv 2008;1: 358–65.

CHAPTER 20

Axxess stent

Stefan Verheye, MD, PhD[1], *John E. Shulze,* BSEE, MBA[2] *and Brett Trauthen,* MS[3]

[1]Interventional Cardiology, Antwerp Cardiovascular Center, ZNA Middelheim, Antwerp, Belgium
[2]Biosensors International, Morges, Switzerland
[3]Devax Inc., Irvine, CA, USA

Overview of bifurcation lesions

Lesions located at bifurcations are frequently found on diagnostic coronary angiograms and occur in 10–20% percutaneous coronary interventions (PCI). A bifurcation lesion has been defined as lesion of a major epicardial coronary artery co-located with a branch vessel measuring at least 2.2 mm in diameter. In the metal stent era, a US study from the National Heart, Lung, and Blood Institute Dynamic Registry in patients undergoing PCI between 1997 and 1998, showed that 321 out of a total of 2,436 consecutive subjects (13.2%) had at least one bifurcation lesion treated [1]. Similar rates of intervention on bifurcation lesions (12.1%) were reported in a series of 3,082 patients in Europe [2]. In the DES era, the frequency of bifurcation lesion treatment appears to be increasing. A slide from the 2009 PCR (Figure 20.1) reflects the increasing prevalence of bifurcation lesions in post-market clinical studies as the time from DES market introduction in 2003 has lengthened. These studies suggest that as operators have become more comfortable with the efficacy of DES, more complex lesions are being included in routine PCI. As a result, the frequency of bifurcation lesions is in the 20% range.

As widely recognised, stenoses located at the bifurcation of the coronary artery are among the most technically challenging lesion subsets to treat by PCI. The main complexities in the management of bifurcation lesions include difficulty to access the side branch, occurrence of dissections, spasm, thrombus formation and/or plaque shifting. The latter represents the movement of atheromatous plaque towards the side branch that requires dilatation and/or stenting of the side branch ostium. Failure to restore the patency of the side branch is associated with a high incidence of procedure-related acute myocardial infarction (MI). Although the occlusion of small side branches may be well tolerated, occlusion or compromise of large side branches may have grave acute clinical events and higher restenosis rates. An analysis of 4,800 patients from the Cleveland Clinic Foundation showed that occlusion of side branches greater than 1 mm in diameter was associated with an incidence of MI of 14% [3].

Classification of bifurcation lesions

Bifurcation lesions are inherently complex and describing them is difficult. Many permutations are possible depending on the location of the plaque in the parent vessel (PV) and degree of involvement of the side branch (SB). Several classification systems have been proposed, but the simplest is the Medina system [4]. In the Medina schema, the basis of classification is the position of the SB relative to the lesion in the parent vessel and the involvement of the SB in the lesion. A "1" is assigned for presence of at least a 30% stenosis, and the PV is segmented into proximal and distal segments. For example, in Figure 20.2, bifurcation

Bifurcation Stenting, First Edition. Edited by Ron Waksman and John A. Ormiston.
© 2012 Blackwell Publishing Ltd. Published 2012 by Blackwell Publishing Ltd.

Bifurcation Lesions

- Remain a challenge to today's interventionalist.

Study	No. of patients	% Bifurcations
ARRIVE I & II	7,592	8%
e-CYPHER	15,157	9%
RESEARCH	508	16%
ARTS-II	607	22%
LEADERS	1,707	29%
SYNTAX	903	72%

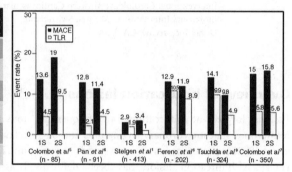

Figure 20.1 Prevalence of bifurcation lesions in post-market clinical studies.

types (1,1,0), (1,0,0) and (0,1,0) involve only the PV and are classified according to the lesion location relative to the SB. Bifurcation types (1,1,1), (1,0,1), and (0,0,1) all describe lesions where the SB is involved in the stenosis. The type (1,1,1) bifurcation is sometimes referred to as a "true" bifurcation because the stenosis involves both stegments of the PV and at least the ostium of the side branch. Approximately 60% of bifurcations fit the Type (1,1,1) classification.

Outcomes of patients treated with PCI using drug-eluting stents

Early interventional experience using balloon angioplasty (PTCA) for the treatment of bifurcation lesions using standard single wire and balloon technique were associated with higher rates of acute complications, restenosis and target vessel revascularization due to complications with the SB than in non bifurcation lesions. The optimal stent strategy for treating bifurcated lesions is unknown. Several dual vessel stenting techniques have been described, the so-called "T", "V", "Y", "culotte" and "crush" procedures. While stents provide an immediate angiographic result superior to that obtainable by PTCA alone, restenosis rates were high, especially in the side branch.

Given these complications, most studies of bifurcation stenting have found that optimal long-term results are obtained by stenting the main vessel and then performing balloon angioplasty of

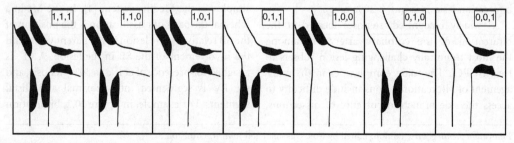

Figure 20.2 Medina classifications of bifurcation lesion types.

the SB. However, occlusion of the SB is a frequent complication of stenting the PV, possibly due to the multiple overlapping stents and repeated balloon inflations involved in T, V, Y, and other techniques. As a result, the SB is stented in approximately 50% of procedures even where PTCA alone was the intended procedure.

Drug-eluting stents (DES) have demonstrated dramatically reduced restenosis rates in patients with relatively simple lesions. The safety and efficacy of sirolimus-eluting stent (SES) was reported in a consecutive series of unselected patients with de-novo bifurcation lesions enrolled in the rapamycin-eluting stent evaluation at Rotterdam Cardiology Hospital (RESEARCH) registry. Of 563 consecutive patients treated solely with SES, 58 patients (10.3%) with 65 de-novo bifurcation lesions were treated with SES implantation in both the main and side branches. Of 65 lesions, 6-month angiographic follow-up was performed in 44 lesions. The binary restenosis rate was 22.7% (10/44 lesions). Angiographic restenosis occurred in four lesions within the main branch (one in the proximal segment, three in the in-stent segment), yielding a main branch restenosis rate of 9.1%. Angiographic restenosis occurred in six of the side branches, all within the in-stent segment, for a side branch restenosis rate of 13.6%. The restenosis rate in the side branch following T-stenting was 16.7% (5/30 lesions), whereas the restenosis rate following the other stent techniques (culotte stenting, kissing stents, or the "crush" technique) was 7.1% (1/14 lesions). At 6 months, the survival-free MACE rate was 89.7%. MACE included one case of death after bifurcation stent implantation of the left main stem in a patient presenting with acute myocardial infarction and cardiogenic shock pre-procedure and TLR in five patients (8.6%). There were no episodes of acute or subacute stent thrombosis, and no patient had a myocardial infarction [5].

A prospective randomized multicenter study evaluated the safety and efficacy of sirolimus-eluting stents (SES) for treatment of coronary bifurcation lesions [6]. A total of 85 patients with 86 bifurcation lesions were enrolled in the study and assigned to either double stenting (n = 43) or stent/PTCA (n = 43). There were high rates of cross-over from the stent/PTCA group to the stent/stent group (51.2%). Two patients crossed over from the stent/stent to the stent/PTCA group due to failed stent delivery to the side branch. When the results were evaluated according to the actual treatment implemented, lesion angiographic success defined as < 50% residual stenosis of both the main and side branches was achieved in 59 cases in the stent/stent group (93.6%) and 17 cases in the stent/PTCA group (77.3%) and procedural success in 58 (92.2%) and 17 (77.3%) cases, respectively. All cases without angiographic success were because of residual stenosis ≥ 50% in the side branch.

At 6-month angiographic follow-up (53 patients in the stent/stent group (84.1%) and 21 patients in the stent/PTCA group (95.4%)), the overall in-segment restenosis rate (of either the side branch or the main branch or both) was 25.7% among patients having index procedure angiographic success and 6-month angiographic follow-up. Fourteen of these cases were observed in the stent/stent group (28%) and three in the stent/PTCA group (18.7%, p = 0.53). At a mean follow-up of 6.4 months, there was one case of sudden death 4.5 months after the procedure, seven cases of TLR (8.2%), 15 cases of target vessel failure (TVF, [17.6%]), and three cases of stent thrombosis (3.5%), occurring 1, 3, and 32 days after the procedure. All three patients with thrombotic events and the patient with sudden death had stenting performed on both branches. Angina, class I–III by Canadian Cardiovascular Society Classification, was present in 17 patients in the stent/stent (27.4%) and three patients in the stent/PTCA (13.6%, p = 0.25) groups.

Another randomized study compared two strategies for the SES treatment of bifurcation lesions [7]: a simple approach (main vessel stenting and balloon dilation of the SB (n = 47)) versus complex reconstruction of the bifurcation (stenting both vessels (n = 44)) in a total of 91 patients. Primary success did not differ significantly between the two groups (94% vs 97%, respectively). Two patients from the stent/PTCA group developed a non-Q wave MI. One patient from the stent/stent group developed a subacute stent thrombosis on day 15 post procedure that resulted in MI and death from cardiogenic shock. At the mean follow up of 11 ± 3 months, additional MACE were observed in three patients: 1 patient from the stent/PTCA group and two patients from the stent/stent group had TLR. There were no significant differ-ences between groups regarding angiographic binary restenosis (7% vs 20%). Restenosis of the main vessel was observed in one patient from the stent/PTCA group (2%) and in four from the stent/stent group (10%). Restenosis of the side branch developed in two patients from the stent/ PTCA group (5%) and in six from the stent/stent group (15%).

The NORDIC trial compared a single PV siro-limus-eluting stent strategy (with kissing balloon angioplasty of the SB only if the flow was impaired, but not if there was a residual angiographically severe lesion) to a strategy of stenting both the PV and the SB with sirolimus-eluting stents (in this case different techniques were allowed) [8]. This trial showed good clinical results, with low 6-month TLR rates in both arms (1.9% in the PV stent arm and 1% in the PV + SB stent arm), not influenced by the angiographic follow-up, per-formed on purpose at 8 months. However, the overall MACE rates evaluated at 6 months (2.9% in the PV stent arm and 3.4% in the PV + SB stent arm) did not include the periprocedural MI, which were as high as 8% in the PV stent group and 18% in the PV + SB stent group. Moreover, post-proce-dural blood samples for myocardial enzymes were not available in the whole cohort, but only in around 68% of the patients, thus a risk of under-estimation of the event rate should also be consid-ered. Furthermore, the angiographic restenosis rate, evaluated at 8 months, remained elevated in both groups (22.5% in the PV stent group and 16% in the PV + SB stent group), and were mainly driven by the SB restenosis.

The most important findings with regard to the treatment of bifurcation lesions with DES were as follows: (1) the use of the SES in bifurcation lesions is associated with a restenosis rate of −10% in the main branch, a value close to the restenosis rate in the SIRIUS trial; (2) MACE rates at 6 months are in the range of 15–25%; (3) the TLR rate of 8–10% is seemingly diminished compared with historical controls; (4) elective side branch stenting seems to provide no advantages over the stenting of the main branch followed by ostial side branch balloon dilation, however, angioplasty at the ostium of the side branch frequently results in high residual stenosis, leading to implantation of an additional stent; (5) follow-up restenosis rates on the side branch are relatively high when an additional SES is implanted; and (6) the risk of stent thrombosis with the SES used in the side branch is of serious concern.

The Axxess bifurcation DES experience

The Axxess stent is made from a nickel-titanium alloy (nitinol) in the austenitic (super-elastic) phase. The stent elutes Biolimus A9® (Biosensors International, Ltd), a derivative of sirolimus, with similar anti-proliferative properties. Drug release is mediated by a bio-absorbable polylactic acid-based polymer (which is metabolized over time into carbon dioxide and water). This drug-polymer coating is applied to the abluminal surface of the stent. The nominal drug loading is 22 μg/mm of stent length for all sizes. The stent is kept in place on the delivery system by a covering sheath, which is gently retracted once the stent is in place at the level of the carina, allowing stent self-expansion and deployment (Figure 20.3). The stent has one radiopaque marker at the proximal edge and three markers at the distal edge to assist in accurate positioning and deployment at the target site. The Axxess stent's conical shape and self-expanding property allow it to cover the irregular anatomy of a bifurcation at the level of the carina. The stent is unique in that it spans both the PV and SB without obstructing access to either, and allows easy passage of additional stents in both branches. If needed, additional stents are implanted to complete lesion coverage. Because the branch vessel stents are implanted distal to the carina, flow to the side branch is unobstructed, and no strut deformation is induced by techniques such as post-implant kissing balloon dilation.

The Axxess stent has been evaluated in two studies enrolling over 400 patients. The first study, Axxess PLUS [9], was a prospective, single arm evaluation of the Axxess stent and procedure for treating de novo bifurcation lesions in native coronary vessels. At 13 centers located in Europe, New Zealand, and Brazil, 139 patients were enrolled in the study. Treated patients received the Axxess stent at the level of the carina. Depending on the lesion anatomy, additional stents were placed

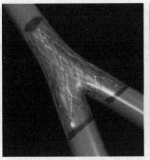
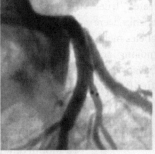
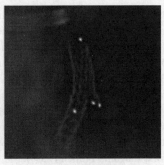

(A) Axxess stent   (B) Angiographic image   (C) Stent boost image

Figure 20.3 Axxess stent.

to complete treatment of the lesion. Choice of treatment in the side branch was left to the discretion of the operator. Approximately half (51.2%) of the patients received a stent to the side branch, 29.4% received PTCA, and 20.6% of the side branches were wired but not treated. While intended to be an all-drug-eluting stent trial, there were two patients who received metal stents. Six month clinical and angiographic follow-up was completed in July 2005.

The baseline clinical and angiographic characteristics suggest that this study included a complex set of lesions. Diabetes mellitus was present in 16.5% of patients, 38.8% had a history of smoking, 30.2% had undergone prior PCI, and 44% had disease in at least two of the primary epicardial vessels (LMCA, LAD, LCX, or RCA). Mean vessel reference diameter was 2.86 mm in the PV and 2.34 mm for the SB, and mean lesion length was 16.28 mm in the PV and 7.43 mm in the SB. The most common bifurcation treated was at the LAD and first diagonal branch (73%). A mean of 2.4 stents (length, 35.6 mm) were implanted per patient.

At six months, mean angiographic late loss in the Axxess stent was 0.09 mm, compared to 0.46 mm in the historical control, which consisted of 41 patients treated with bare metal Axxess stents in a previous study. Angiographic restenosis in all PV stents occurred in 7.1% of cases overall (and in only 5.6% of lesions excluding the two cases where bare metal stents were placed distal to the Axxess stent). Among the lesions in which stents were placed in the SB, the SB mean late loss was only 0.23 mm, with a corresponding restenosis rate of 9.2% (7.9% excluding the two cases where bare metal stents were placed in the SB). The SB restenosis rate was 25.0%

when treated by PTCA, and when the SB did not require interventional treatment, 12% of patients had a >50% SB diameter stenosis at 6-month follow-up. The cumulative MACE rate (as known by a follow-up rate of 136 subjects updated as long-term follow-up obtained data on additional subjects) was 11.0%, and target lesion revascularization (TLR) was required in 7.4% of patients. The cumulative stent thrombosis rate was 2.2%. There was no stent thrombosis within 30 days of the procedure and late stent thrombosis (>30 days) was observed in three cases (2.2%), two of which occurred in patients who had discontinued antiplatelet therapy (aspirin and/or clopidogrel).

At 12 months, the cumulative MACE rate (from enrollment through 12 months for 135 subjects with known status) was 14.1% and included a non-cardiac death. There were no cases of late stent thrombosis reported in the 6–12 month follow up interval. Additionally, the 3-year clinical outcomes continue to support the safety of the procedure. There were no additional patients with target lesion revascularization in the 1–3 year interval, however the rate appears to have increased from 9.6 to 10.7% (13/121) due to fewer patients completing the 3-year follow-up. The cumulative MACE to 3 years was 16.5% (20/121) and included two cardiac related deaths. There were no cases of late stent thrombosis reported in the 1–3 year follow-up interval.

A second study utilizing the Axxess stent, called DIVERGE [10], enrolled 302 subjects in Europe, Australia, and New Zealand between June 2006 and October 2007. Similar in design to the Axxess PLUS study, the subjects enrolled in the DIVERGE trial had complex bifurcation disease with 77.4% of the 302 populations exhibiting complicated "true" bifurcation lesions. Baseline characteristics were similar with 18.2% of subjects with diabetes mellitus present, 68.0% with a history of smoking, and 31.8% having undergone prior PCI. Mean vessel reference diameter was 2.90 mm in the PV and 2.29 mm for the SB. Mean lesion length was 14.62 mm in the PV and 6.91 mm in the SB. The most common bifurcation treated was at the LAD and first diagonal branch (73%).

The DIVERGE protocol called for placement of the Axxess stent at the level of the carina, followed by ad hoc additional stents in the PV and SB, depending on the lesion pattern. Based on an analysis of the angiographic data from the Axxess PLUS Trial, a strategy of stenting for an optimal angiographic outcome was recommended to the investigators. As a result, stents were used frequently, and the total number of stents implanted in this bifurcation set was higher than seen in the previous trial at 2.7 per patient, with a total stent length of 40 mm per patient.

Procedure success in the DIVERGE study was 96.7% and the primary endpoint of 9-month MACE was 7.7%. The study primary endpoint was met with treatment of bifurcations in the DIVERGE trial

demonstrating superiority in 9-month MACE as compared to the set historic bare-metal objective performance criteria of 20.5%. MACE at 12 months increased slightly from the 9 month level to 9.3%. The stent thrombosis rate in DIVERGE was 0.7% in the period 0–30 days, and 0.3% between 30 days and 12 months per the ARC definitions. In general, clinical outcomes for the DIVERGE study numerically improved compared to Axxess PLUS at the 12-month time point, although the differences were not statistically significant, as shown in Table 20.1.

At nine months, in correlation to the safety results, (binary) restenosis rate in the angiographic sub-population was 3.6% in the PV and 4.3% in the SB. On a per-patient basis, restenosis was seen in 6.4% of subjects seen for angiographic follow-up. This is substantially lower than the restenosis rates observed in the Axxess PLUS study, despite longer time to follow up. The differences were likely due to the increased frequency of side branch stenting in the DIVERGE study.

Summary

Despite the fact that there is no firm agreement on the standard treatment of bifurcation lesions,

Table 20.1 Comparative clinical endpoints at 1 year: Axxess PLUS and DIVERGE*

Variable description	DIVERGE	Axxess PLUS	Combined	P-value**
Death	0.7% (2)	1.5% (2)	0.9% (4)	0.5923
Cardiac	0.7% (2)	0.7% (1)	0.7% (3)	1.0000
Non-Cardiac	0.0% (0)	0.7% (1)	0.2% (1)	0.3125
MI	4.4% (13)	6.7% (9)	5.1% (22)	0.3475
Q-Wave	1.0% (3)	1.5% (2)	1.2% (5)	0.6499
Non Q-Wave	3.4% (10)	5.2% (7)	3.9% (17)	0.4246
TLR	5.7% (17)	9.6% (13)	6.9% (30)	0.1546
PCI	4.7% (14)	8.9% (12)	6.0% (26)	0.1244
CABG	1.0% (3)	0.7% (1)	0.9% (4)	1.0000
TVR	7.7% (23)	11.9% (16)	9.0% (39)	0.2042
PCI	6.7% (20)	11.1% (15)	8.1% (35)	0.1308
CABG	1.0% (3)	0.7% (1)	0.9% (4)	1.0000
MACE (Death/MI/TLR)	9.1% (27)	14.8% (20)	10.9% (47)	0.0948
Stent thrombosis				
ARC: Definite	1.0% (3)	1.5% (2)	1.2% (5)	0.6506
ARC: Probable	0.0% (0)	0.0% (0)	0.0% (0)	N/A
ARC: Possible	0.0% (0)	0.7% (1)	0.2% (1)	0.3132

*analyses done post-hoc
**P value calculated using Chi-square or Fisher's exact test where appropriate

there is some consensus that a strategy based on single stenting of the PV with provisional stenting of the SB is recommended; however, neither an advantage nor a disadvantage of stenting both branches has ever been shown.

The first-in-man Axxess PLUS trial, despite its non-randomized design, suggested improved angiographic outcomes in the SB if it was treated with a drug-eluting stent (with a restenosis rate of 7.9%) as compared with balloon angioplasty (with a restenosis rate of 25%). However, stenting of the SB in the Axxess PLUS trial occurred only in half of the cohort enrolled. In the DIVERGE trial, stents were used to obtain an optimal angiographic result in the bifurcation in the same way as would be done for a mid-vessel lesion. Using this approach, a single Ax stent was used in 12% of lesions, an additional stent was added in 21.5% of lesions, and a stent was added to both branches in 65% of lesions. The rationale behind this approach was to cover any diseased part of the bifurcation with both stent and drug and to obtain an angiographically "optimal" outcome at the end of the procedure. This strategy resulted in a TLR rate of 4.3%, a total bifurcation restenosis rate of 6.4%, and a SB restenosis rate of 4.3%.

One mechanistic explanation for these results could be the combination of the self-expanding properties of the study device with local drug delivery resulting in a large proximal PV lumen, coupled with lack of strut deformation, minimization of stent overlap, and undisturbed flow into the distal branch vessels.

Thus, it appears that dedicated stenting technology for bifurcation lesions in combination with site-specific drug delivery offers an excellent outcome in terms of clinical, angiographic and intravascular ultrasound endpoints. Based on these findings, there seems to be no penalty for stenting the side branch, but it remains to be seen in a randomized manner whether this strategy is superior to provisional stenting.

References

1 Al Suwaidi J, Yeh W, Cohen HA, Detre KM, Williams DO, Holmes DR, Jr., Immediate and one-year outcome in patients with coronary bifurcation lesions in the modern era (NHLBI dynamic registry). Am J Cardiol. 2001;87:1139–1144.

2 Lefevre T, Louvard Y, Morice MC, Dumas P, Loubeyre C, Benslimane A, Premchand RK, Guillard N, Piechaud JF. Stenting of bifurcation lesions: classification, treatments, and results. Catheter Cardiovasc Interv. 2000;49:274–283.

3 Arora RR, Raymond RE, Dimas AP, Bhadwar K, Simpfendorfer C. Side branch occlusion during coronary angioplasty: incidence, angiographic characteristics, and outcome. Cathet Cardiovasc Diagn 1989;18:210–12.

4 Medina A, Suarez de Lezo J, Pan M. A new classification of coronary bifurcation lesions. Rev Esp Cardiol 2006; 59(2):183.

5 Tanabe K, Hoye A, Lemos PA, Aoki J, Arampatzis CA, Saia F, Lee CH, Degertekin M, Hofma SH, Sianos G, McFadden E, Smits PC, van der Giessen WJ, de Feyter P, van Domburg RT, Serruys PW. Restenosis rates following bifurcation stenting with sirolimus-eluting stents for de novo narrowings. Am J Cardiol 2004;94:115–118.

6 Colombo A, Moses JW, Morice MC, Ludwig J, Holmes DR, Jr, Spanos V, Louvard Y, Desmedt B, Di Mario C, Leon MB. Randomized study to evaluate sirolimus-eluting stents implanted at coronary bifurcation lesions. Circulation 2004;109:1244–9.

7 Pan M, de Lezo JS, Medina A, Romero M, Segura J, Pavlovic D, Delgado A, Ojeda S, Melian F, Herrador J, Urena I, Burgos L. Rapamycin-eluting stents for the treatment of bifurcated coronary lesions: a randomized comparison of a simple versus complex strategy. Am Heart J 2004;148:857–64.

8 Steigen T, Thuesen L, et al. Randomized study on simple versus complex stenting of coronary artery bifurcation lesions; the Nordic bifurcation study. Circulation 2006;114:1955–61.

9 Grube E, Bullesfeld L, Verheye S, et al. Six month clinical and angiographic results for a dedicated drug eluting stent for the treatment of bifurcation narrowings. Am J Cardiol 2007;99:1691–7.

10 Verheye S, Agostoni P, et al. 9 Month clinical, angiographic, and intravascular ultrasound evaluation of the Axxess Biolimus A9 eluting self expanding stent in coronary artery lesions. J Am Coll Cardiol 2009;53:1031–9.

Index

Page numbers in *italic* denote figures, those in **bold** denote tables.

Bifurcation Stenting, First Edition. Edited by Ron Waksman and John A. Ormiston.
© 2012 Blackwell Publishing Ltd. Published 2012 by Blackwell Publishing Ltd.